A Clinical Guide to Rheumatoid Arthritis

A Clinical Guide to Rheumatoid Arthritis

Editor: Sindy Campling

AMERICAN
MEDICAL PUBLISHERS
www.americanmedicalpublishers.com

AMERICAN
MEDICAL PUBLISHERS
www.americanmedicalpublishers.com

Cataloging-in-Publication Data

A clinical guide to rheumatoid arthritis / edited by Sindy Campling.
p. cm.
Includes bibliographical references and index.
ISBN 979-8-88740-439-4
1. Rheumatoid arthritis. 2. Arthritis. 3. Rheumatism. 4. Autoimmune diseases. I. Campling, Sindy.
RC933 .C55 2023
616.722--dc23

American Medical Publishers,
41 Flatbush Avenue,
1st Floor, New York,
NY 11217, USA

ISBN 979-8-88740-439-4 (Hardback)

Contents

Preface

This book has been a concerted effort by a group of academicians, researchers and scientists, who have contributed their research works for the realization of the book. This book has materialized in the wake of emerging advancements and innovations in this field. Therefore, the need of the hour was to compile all the required researches and disseminate the knowledge to a broad spectrum of people comprising of students, researchers and specialists of the field.

Rheumatoid arthritis (RA) is a chronic autoimmune disease that affects the joints on both sides of the body. Some of its common symptoms are tenderness, pain and swelling in more than one joint, stiffness, weakness, fatigue and fever. There is no specific cause of rheumatoid arthritis, but factors like emotional or physical stress, smoking and infection may result in the immune system attacking the joints. The diagnosis includes physical exam based on symptoms and medical history. Blood tests like erythrocyte sedimentation rate (ESR) and C-reactive protein (CRP), along with imaging tests such as X-rays, ultrasounds and MRI scans are used to diagnose RA. Its treatment aims to prevent or improve joint function and damage. There are several medications like non-steroidal anti-inflammatory drugs (NSAIDs), COX-2 inhibitors, corticosteroids and disease-modifying antirheumatic drugs (DMARDs) that help to relieve the symptoms of RA. Treatment of severe RA includes surgeries, like synovectomy and total joint replacement to correct the deformity. This book is compiled in such a manner, that it will provide in-depth knowledge about rheumatoid arthritis. It will serve as a valuable source of reference for clinicians and medical students.

At the end of the preface, I would like to thank the authors for their brilliant chapters and the publisher for guiding us all-through the making of the book till its final stage. Also, I would like to thank my family for providing the support and encouragement throughout my academic career and research projects.

Editor

1

Bone Loss, Osteoporosis and Fractures in Patients with Rheumatoid Arthritis

Patrice Fardellone [1,*], Emad Salawati [2], Laure Le Monnier [1] and Vincent Goëb [1]

1 Department of Rheumatology, Picardie-Jules Verne University, University hospital of Amiens, 80054 Amiens, France; LeMonnier.Laure@chu-amiens.fr (L.L.M.); goeb.vincent@chu-amiens.fr (V.G.)
2 Assistant Professor, Faculty of Medicine, King Abdulaziz University, 21589 Jeddah, Saudi Arabia; esalawati@kau.edu.sa
* Correspondence: fardellone.patrice@chu-amiens.fr

Abstract: Rheumatoid arthritis (RA) is often characterized by bone loss and fragility fractures and is a frequent comorbidity. Compared with a matched population, RA patients with fractures have more common risk factors of osteoporosis and fragility fractures but also risk factors resulting from the disease itself such as duration, intensity of the inflammation and disability, and cachexia. The inflammatory reaction in the synovium results in the production of numerous cytokines (interleukin-1, interleukin-6, tumor necrosis factor) that activate osteoclasts and mediate cartilage and bone destruction of the joints, but also have a systemic effect leading to generalized bone loss. Regular bone mineral density (BMD) measurement, fracture risk assessment using tools such as the FRAX algorithm, and vertebral fracture assessment (VFA) should be performed for early detection of osteoporosis and accurate treatment in RA patients.

Keywords: rheumatoid arthritis; osteoporosis; fragility fractures; BMD; bone remodeling markers

1. Introduction

Rheumatoid arthritis is the most common immune disease of the skeleton. During the last three decades, many studies have shown that besides the joint inflammation and destruction, bone mass in patients with rheumatoid arthritis (RA) is lower than in the matched non-RA population [1–9] and the risk of osteoporosis is increased [8,10–19]. Similarly, the incidence of osteoporotic fractures is high [6,11,12,14–25] even when compared to the general population of the same age and sex [5,9,15,26–42]. Osteoporosis-related fragility fractures represent one of the most severe complications in RA patients [43]. They contribute to a significant decrease in the quality of life and can reduce life expectancy. In the United States, data from the National Data Bank for Rheumatic Diseases indicated that osteoporotic fractures are the third cause of mortality in RA patients [44]. The severe inflammatory reaction in the synovium results in the production of numerous cytokines (interleukin-1, interleukin-6, tumor necrosis factor) that mediate cartilage and bone destruction but also have a systemic effect leading to generalized bone loss. As in the general population, the highly sensitive C-reactive protein (CRP) level is a predictor of the risk of fracture that is underlying the role of systemic inflammation [45]. The mechanism of bone loss relies on increased bone resorption mediated by pro-inflammatory cytokines that activate osteoclasts, as well as by the frequent use of glucocorticoids or inactivity resulting from the disease. Some clues lowering the level of inflammation with potent drugs such as biologic agents can reduce the risk of osteoporosis and fractures. The literature provides interesting data on the prevalence of osteoporosis in RA patients, as well as the incidence of fragility fractures compared to a healthy population.

2. Epidemiology of Bone Loss and Fractures in Rheumatoid Patients

2.1. Low Bmd

According to the definition given by the WHO organization in 1994, based on a bone mineral density (BMD) T-score ≤ 2.5 SD measured by dual-energy X-ray absorptiometry (DEXA) in the spine and/or hip, it is possible to evaluate the prevalence of osteoporosis in the RA population. In this population, decreased mean BMD values of the spine and hips are known to be a very common feature and are more frequent than in a paired healthy control population (Table 1). A significant bone loss appears early in RA. After a two-year duration of the disease, the hip and spine BMD show an already significant loss in all locations, with a significantly greater BMD loss in the hands (BMD measured in metacarpals 2–4 by digital x-ray radiogrammetry) than a generalized BMD loss in the hip and spine [46]. In an established RA, observational and case-control studies estimate the prevalence of loss of BMD to be doubled in both male and female RA patients compared with healthy controls at both the lumbar spine and the hip (Tables 1 and 2). Results are expressed whether in T-score or Z-score. T-score is a young gender-matched population at peak bone mass, while the Z-score is derived from an age-matched reference population. Both T-scores and Z-scores are derived by comparison to the reference population on a standard deviation scale.

As shown in Table 1, among the classical risk factors of bone loss, glucocorticoids (GCs) commonly prescribed in RA patients are also well known for causing secondary osteoporosis with the long use of high dosage when comparing users with non-users [1,2,4]. Inversely, it seems that at low dosage, glucocorticoids exert a protective effect on the bone probably because the lowering of the inflammation is more beneficial than the deleterious effects of the drug [47].

2.2. Fragility Fractures

Epidemiological studies on the frequency of fractures in RA populations can be observational, case-controlled, conducted on databases, or prospective (Tables 3 and 4). Most epidemiological studies provide a fractures risk increased by 1.5- to 2-fold among patients with RA compared to the general population (Table 4).

Patients with RA are at a high risk of vertebral fractures. However, the prevalence of spine fractures varies enormously according to the population studied (age, women alone, or men and women), the way to assess fractures (radiographs or vertebral fracture assessment (VFA) for vertebral fractures), and the source of data (cohort, registry, randomized trial). This explains that the prevalence of vertebral fractures ranges from 8% to nearly 50% (Table 3).

On the other hand, the risk of fractures, despite the site, is always higher in RA patients than in the general population (Table 4). In a very large case-control study of 30,262 patients with RA using the British General Practice Research Database, the increased risk of fracture compared to the general population was most marked at the hip (RR: 2.0, 95% CI 1.8–2.3) and spine (RR: 2.4, 95% CI 2.0–2.8) [32]. The relationship between RA and the fracture was examined in the Women's Health Initiative prospective study (WHI). Compared to the non-arthritis group, the risk (HR (95% CI)) of sustaining any clinical fracture comprising self-reported spinal fractures in the RA group was 1.49 (1.26, 1.75) ($p < 0.001$). Moreover, the risk of sustaining a hip fracture significantly increased in the RA group (3.03 (2.03, 4.51)) ($p < 0.001$) [34].

Table 1. Bone mineral density (BMD) in rheumatoid arthritis (RA) patients: Observational studies.

Authors Country Year	Studied Population	Type of the Study	BMD		
			Sites		
			Total Hip	Femoral Neck	Lumbar Spine
Laan RFJM The Netherlands 1993 [10]	men and women (58.7%) mean age: women 57.5 95% CI 27 to 78 men 57 95% CI 30 to 80	longitudinal 97 RA	Z-score < −2 = 4.4% 95% CI 0.2 to 8.6		Z-score < −2 = 9.3% 95% CI 3.5 to 15.0
Sinigaglia L Italy 2000 [11]	women 20 to 70 years	observational 925 RA		36.2% T-score ≤ −2.5 SD	28.8% T-score ≤ −2.5 SD
Kvien TK Norway 2000 [12]	women mean age: 54.8 ± 11.6 years Oslo RA Register	observational 394 RA	14.7% T-score ≤ −2.5 SD 95% CI 11.1 to 18	14.7% 95% CI 11.1 to 18.3	16.8% 95% CI 13.1 to 20.5
Haugeberg G Norway 2000 [13]	women age: 20 to 70 years county RA register	observational 394 RA	all RA patients: 14.7% T-score ≤ −2.5 SD 95% CI 11.1 to 18.3 corticoid non-users: 5.8 T-score ≤ −2.5 SD 95% CI 1.9 to 9.7 corticoid users: 24.0 T-score ≤ −2.5 SD 95% CI 17.1 to 30.9	all RA patients: 14.7% T-score ≤ −2.5 SD 95% CI 11.1 to 18.3 corticoid non-users: 6.5 95% T-score ≤ −2.5 SD 95% CI 2.4 to 10.6 corticoid users: 24.7 T-score ≤ −2.5 SD 95% CI 17.7 to 31.7	all RA patients: 16.8% T-score ≤ −2.5 SD 95% CI 13.1 to 20.5 corticoid non-users: 8.6% T-score ≤ −2.5 SD 95% CI 3.9 to 13.3 corticoid users: 26.6% T-score ≤ −2.5 SD 95% CI 19.6 to 33.6
Lodder MC Norway, UK, The Netherlands 2003 [14]	women from OSTRA cohort mean age: 61.0 ± 5.8 years age: 50 to 70 years	observational 150 RA	8% T-score ≤ −2.5 SD	12% T-score ≤ −2.5 SD	10.7% T-score ≤ −2.5 SD
Ørstavik RE Norway 2003 [15]	women Oslo RA register mean age: 63.4 (51.4 to 73.6) years	observational 229 RA	16.6% T-score ≤ −2.5 SD	20.3% T-score ≤ −2.5 SD	21.8% T-score ≤ −2.5 SD
El Maghraoui Morocco 2010 [16]	women mean age: 49.4 ± 7.3 years age: 27 to 70 years	observational 172 RA	Any site: 44.2% T-score ≤ −2.5 SD		
Lee SG South Korea 2012 [8]	women age: 20 to 80 years	case-control 299 RA 246 non-RA controls	7.8% ** T-score ≤ −2.5 SD		18.2% T-score ≤ −2.5 SD $p = 0.067$

Table 1. *Cont.*

Brébant S France 2012 [17]	women mean age: 56.0 ± 13.5 years	observational 185 RA	21.2% T-score ≤ −2.5 SD	33.3% T-score ≤ −2.5 SD	24.2% T-score ≤ −2.5 SD
El Maghraoui Morocco 2015 [18]	men and women (82.6%) mean age: 54.1 ± 11.5 years age: 25 to 82 years	observational 178 RA	overall population: 29.2% T-score ≤ −2.5 SD		
Choi ST South Korea 2018 [19]	men and women (88.9%) mean age: 61.8 ± 11.5 years	retrospective cross-sectional study 479 RA	overall population: 91.3% T-score ≤ −2.5 SD men: 90% T-score ≤ −2 T.5 SD women: 91.3% T-score ≤ −2.5 SD		

Level of significance between RA and non-RA controls: ** $p < 0.02$; NS: Non-significant; OR: Odd ratio; RR: Relative risk; HR: Hazard ratio.

Table 2. BMD in RA patients: Case-control studies.

Authors Country Year (Ref)	Studied Population	Type of the Study *n* RA/ *n* Controls	BMD		
			Sites		
			Total Hip	**Femoral Neck**	**Lumbar Spine**
Garton MJ UK 1993 [1]	men age: 47 to 74 years	40 RA 20 non-RA controls	Trochanter RA corticoid users vs. non-RA: −15.9% ** RA non-users vs. non-RA: −10.1 *		RA corticoid users vs. non-RA: −12.0% ** RA non-users vs. non-RA: −11.2 **
Hall GM UK 1993 [2]	postmenopausal women	195 RA 597 non-RA controls	RA corticoid users vs. non-users: −7.4 *** 95% CI −1.2 to 13.6 RA corticoid non-users vs. non-RA: −6.9% * 95% CI 3.4 to 10.3 RA corticoid users vs. non-RA: −13.8% * 95% CI 8.6 to 19.0	RA corticoid users vs. RA non-users: −6.9 ** 95% CI −3.4 to −10.3	RA corticoid users vs. RA non-users: −6.5 * 95% CI 0 to 13.0 RA corticoid non-users vs. non-RA: NS RA corticoid users vs. non-RA: −7.5 * 95% CI 1.8 to 13.2

Table 2. *Cont.*

Gough AKS UK 1994 [3]	men and women (66.9%)	148 RA 50 non-RA controls	loss of BMD in 1-year at the trochanter all: −2.2 ± 0.5 *** male: −0.6 ± 0.6 *** female: −2.9 ± 0.6 ***	loss of BMD in 1-year all: −2.0 ± 0.4 male: −12 ± 0.7 female: −23 ± 0.6	loss of BMD in 1-year all: −1.0 ± 0.3 * male: −0.2 ± 0.5 * female: −13 ± 0.4 *
Lane NE USA 1995 [4]	non-black women ≥ 65 years SOF study	120 RA 7966 non-RA controls	RA corticoid non-users vs. non-RA: −7.3 * 95% CI −11.4 to −3.2 RA corticoid users vs. non-RA: −14.7 * 95% CI −23.4 to 5.9		RA corticoid non users vs. non-RA: −8.4 * 95% CI −13.4 to −3.4 RA corticoid users vs. non-RA: NS (too small number)
Martin JC UK 1997 [5]	caucasian postmenopausal women from EVOS	46 RA 29 non-RA controls		RA vs. non-RA: −15.4% **	RA vs. non-RA: −6.7%
Haugeberg G Norway 2000 [7]	men age: 20 to 70 years county RA register	case-control 94 RA men 1130 non-RA controls: European/United States reference population	age group 60–70 years: −6.9% *	age group 60–70 years: −5.2% *	NS
Ørstavik RE Norway 2004 [6]	women Oslo RA register mean age: 63.0 (50.7 to 73.6) years	249 RA	17.3% T-score ≤ −2.5 SD * OR = 5.8 95% CI 2.4 to 17.0	18.6% T-score ≤ −2.5 SD * OR = 4.1 95% CI 2.0 to 9.7	22.0% T-score ≤ −2.5 SD * OR = 2.0 95% CI 1.2 to 3.4
Lee SG South Korea 2012 [8]	women age: 20 to 80 years	299 RA 246 non-RA controls	7.8% ** T-score ≤ −2.5 SD		18.2% T-score ≤ −2.5 SD $p = 0.067$
Avouac J France 2012 [9]	women mean age: 61 ± 11 years	139 RA 227 non-RA controls	19% T-score ≤ −2.5 SD ***		21% T-score ≤ −2.5 SD ***

Level of significance between RA and non-RA controls: * $p < 0.05$; ** $p < 0.02$; *** $p < 0.001$; NS: Non-significant.

Table 3. Incidence, prevalence, and risk of fractures in RA patients: Observational studies.

Authors Country Year (Ref)	Studied Population	Type of Study *n* RA	Fractures Sites			
			Vertebral	Proximal Femur	Non-Vertebral	Any Site
Kvien TK Norway 2000 [12]	women age: 54.8 ± 11.6 years Oslo RA Register	observational 394 RA			21.2%	
Sinigaglia L Italy 2000 [11]	women 20 to 70 years	observational 925 RA	8.0%			
Lodder MC Norway UK, The Netherlands 2003 [14]	women from OSTRA cohort mean age: 61.0 ± 5.8 years age: 50 to 70 years	observational 150 RA	16%			
Ørstavik RE Norway 2002 [15]	women Oslo RA register mean age: 63.4 (51.4 to 73.6) years	observational 229 RA	48.9%			
Ørstavik RE Norway 2005 [6]	women Oslo RA register mean age: 53.0 ± 11.2 years	longitudinal 255 RA	15.0% (VFA) IR = 2.9/100 person-years			
El Maghraoui Morocco 2010 [16]	women mean age: 49.4 ± 7.3 years age: 27 to 70 years	observational 172 RA	36% (VFA)			
Vis M Norway, UK, The Netherlands 2011 [20]	women OSTRA cohort mean age: 61 years age: 20 to 70 years	Prospective 102 RA	33% IR = 3.7/100 person-year 95% CI 2.2 to 5.8		35% IR = 3.7/100 person-years 95% CI 2.2 to 5.8	
El Maghraoui Morocco 2015 [16]	men and women (82.8%) mean age: 54.1 ± 11.5 years	observational 178 RA	37% (VFA)			
Coulson KA USA 2009 [21]	women CORRONA registry	prospective 8419 RA	IR = 0.78/100 person-years	IR = 0.66/100 person-years	IR = 2.8/100 person-years	IR = 3.71/100 person-years
Brébant S France 2012 [17]	women 56.0 ± 13.5 years	observational 185 RA	17.8% (VFA)			31.3%

Table 3. *Cont.*

Dirven L The Netherlands 2012 [22]	BeSt study men and women (67%) mean age: 54 years	randomized trial 275 RA	15.0%			
El Maghraoui Morocco 2015 [18]	men and women (82.6%) mean age: 54.1 ± 11.5 years age: 25 to 82 years	observational 178 RA				
Rentero ML Spain 2015 [23]	Women age ≥ 18 years mean age: 59.6 ± 15.0 years	observational 480 RA	20.0% (VFA)		9.8%	
Choi YJ South Korea 2017 [24]	women age ≥ 50 years	observational 279 RA	12.5%			
Choi ST South Korea 2018 [19]	men and women (88.9%) age: 61.8 ± 11.5 years	retrospective cross-sectional study 479 RA	16.9%	0%	0%	
Phuan-udon R Thailand 2018 [25]	men and women (89%) Siriraj RA Cohort mean age: 61.6 ± 9.91 age: 40 to 90 years	232 RA				45.7%

Level of significance between RA and non-RA controls: ** $p < 0.02$; *** $p < 0.001$; NS: Non-significant; OR: Odd ratio; RR: Relative risk; HR: Hazard ratio; IR: Incidence rate; VFA: Vertebral fracture assessment.

Table 4. Incidence, prevalence, and risk of fractures in RA patients: Case-control studies.

Authors Country Year	Studied Population	Type of Study *n* RA/ *n* Controls	Fractures Sites			
			Vertebral	Proximal Femur	Non-Vertebral	Any Site
Hooyman JR USA 1984 [26]	women Rochester	population-based 388 RA	10.8%	7.5% RR = 1.51% * 95% CI 1.01 to 2.17	19.6%	30.4%
Verstraeten A Belgium 1986 [27]	postmenopausal women	case-control 104 RA 43 controls	7.7%	1.0%		
Spector UK 1993 [28]	postmenopausal women age 45 to 65 years RA: Five London hospitals controls: London practice register	case-control 149 RA 713 non-RA controls	12.1% OR = 2.1 95% CI 1.2 to 3.7			
Cooper C UK 1995 [29]	men and women (80%) age: 50 to 99 years	case-control 300 RA 600 non-RA controls		OR = 2.1 95% CI 1.0 to 4.7 $p = 0.06$ corticosteroids users: OR = 2.5 95% CI 1.1 to 5.5 *		
Peel NFA UK 1995 [30]	postmenopausal women mean age: 65 years (50 to 79) years	case-control 76 RA corticosteroids users 347 non-RA controls	27.6% OR = 6.2 95% CI 3.2 to 12.3			
Martin JC UK 1997 [5]	postmenopausal women from EVOS	case-control 46 RA 29 non-RA controls	corticosteroids users: 20% non-corticosteroids users: 23.8%			
Huusko TM Finland 2001 [31]	men and women (72%) mean age: Men 79 (62 to 92) women 77 (52 to 91)	case-control fractures Non-RA controls with hip fractures		OR = 3.26 95% CI 2.26 to 4.70		
Ørstavik RE Norway 2004 [6]	women Oslo RA register mean age: 63.0 (50.7 to 73.6) years	case-control 249 RA 249 non-RA controls	59.0%			

Table 4. *Cont.*

Van Staa TP UK 2006 [32]	General Practice Research Database men and women (71.1%) ≥ 40 years	case-control 30,262 RA 90,783 controls	RR = 2.4 95% CI 2.0 to 2.8	RR = 2.0 95% CI 1.8 to 2.3		RR = 1.5 95% CI 1.4 to 1.6
Kim SY USA 2010 [33]	men and women (73%) Health Core Integrated Research Database age ≥ 18 years median age: 55 years	case-control 92,827 RA 921,715 non-RA controls		men IR = 2.4/1000 person-years women IR = 3.8/1000 person-years HR = 1.44, 95% CI 1.24 to 1.67		1.4% IR = 9.6/1000 person-years HR = 1.26 95% CI 1.15 to 1.38 corticosteroids users: HR = 1.15 95% CI 1.03 to 1.27
Wright NC USA 2011 [34]	postmenopausal women 50 to 79 years WHI study	prospective 960 RA 83,295 non-RA controls	4.0% *** HR = 1.93 *** 95% CI 1.29 to 2.90	4.0%*** IR = 0.51/100 person-years HR = 3.03 2.03 to 4.51 ***		24.8% *** IR = 3.64/100 patient-years 95% CI 3.17 to 4.11 HR = 1.49 95% CI 1.26 to 1.75 ***
Ghazi M France 2012 [35]	women age 56.1 ± 14.2 years	case-control 101 RA 303 non-RA controls	21.8% (VFA) *** OR = 6.5 95% CI 3.1 to 13.9		28.71%	
Avouac J France 2012 [9]	Women mean age: 61 ± 11 years	case-control 139 RA 227 non-RA controls	19.0% ***		22.0% **	33.0% ***
Filho JCA Brazil 2013 [36]	men age 51.6 ± 9.3 years	case-control 50 RA 52 non-RA controls	36.0% *		4%	
Roussy JP Canada 2013 [37]	men and women Quebec healthcare databases age ≥ 50 years	case-control 27,076 RA non-RA controls		2.4%	5.6% IR = 11.0/1000 person-years 95% CI 10.4 to 11.5	
Brennan SL Australia 2014 [38]	women age ≥ 35 years database: Barwon Statistical Division	case-control 1008 RA 172,422 non-RA controls	31.7% ***	7.3% ***		1.9% IR = 114/10000 person-years RR = 1.43 95% CI 0.98–2.09 $p = 0.08$

Table 4. *Cont.*

Xue A-L USA, UK, Sweden, Norway, Finland, Australia, China 2017 [39]	men and women	meta-analysis (13 studies)	RR = 2.93 95% CI 2.25 to 3.83	RR = 2.41 95% CI 1.83 to 3.17	RR = 2.25 95% CI 1.76 to 2.87
Clynes MA UK 2019 [40]	men and women (70.1%) UK Biobank: Hospital Episode Statistics (HES)	case-control 5492 RA 497,051 non-RA controls			men: 5.1% OR = 1.46 95% CI 1.17 to 1.81 *** women: 5.5% OR = 1.71 95% CI 1.50 to 1.94 ***
Hong Taiwan 2019 [41]	men and women Nationwide database age ≥ 40 years	retrospective 30.507 RA	HR = 1.47 *** 95% CI 1.19 to 1.81		
Weiss RJ Sweden 2019 [42]	men and women (66%) Swedish National Hospital Discharge Register median age: 71 years	case-control 3379 RA 420,331 non-RA controls	OI = 2.7 * 95% CI 2.1 to 3.4	OI = 2.9 * 95% CI 2.7 to 3.1	OI = 2.9 * 95% CI 2.8 to 3.1

Level of significance between RA and non-RA controls: * $p < 0.05$; ** $p < 0.02$; *** $p < 0.001$; NS: Non- significant; OR: Odd ratio; RR: Relative risk; HR: Hazard ratio; IR: Incidence rate.

Cohort and registry studies allow calculating the incidence-rates of fractures mostly for peripheral fractures. A Canadian nested case-control study conducted using Quebec physician billing, pharmacy data from the "Régie de l'assurance maladie du Québec", and hospital discharge data found that the incidence rate of non-vertebral osteoporotic fractures is 11.0/1000 person-years in the population of RA patients aged 50 years and more [37]. In another large study conducted based on a USA health database on both men and women aged more than 18 years comparing 92,827 RA to 921,715 non-RA controls, the incidence rate of fracture at any of the four sites (wrist, humerus, hip, and pelvis) among RA patients was 9.6 per 1000 person-years and 1.5 times higher than that of non-RA patients (6.3 per 1000 person-years) [33].

In contrast with other peripheral sites, the incidence of wrist fracture decreased in RA as compared to the controls [6,32]. It could be due to different risk factors, especially for the mechanisms of fall. It was expected to find the same risk factors for a fracture in the RA population and the general population. Patients with incident vertebral deformities or peripheral fractures are significantly older [16,22], had lower BMD, higher disability and more often a previous fracture and a higher cumulative steroid [11,15,20], frequent falls [35], low body mass index (BMI), alcohol abuse, smoking [28], risk factors resulting from the disease itself such as the intensity of the inflammation and disability [29,36,40], duration of the disease [1,37], and cachexia [18].

Similar to the general population, patients with a morphometric, self-reported vertebral fracture or self-reported non-vertebral fracture have a higher statistically significant 10-year probability of sustaining a major osteoporotic fracture or hip fracture than patients without fractures [23].

According to Avouac et al. [9], BMD incompletely predicts patients who will suffer from an osteoporotic fracture, since only half of RA patients with fractures had BMD ≤ -2.5 SD. A higher proportion of RA patients have vertebral fractures, although their BMD is above the osteoporotic threshold. These data suggest that other parameters, especially the bone microarchitecture, have to be considered and underlines the need for other techniques and strategies to assess the risk of fracture in RA, such as the FRAXtool® or the trabecular bone score (TBS). The fracture risk assessment tool® developed by the World Health Organization (FRAXtool®) [48] computes the 10-year probability of a hip fracture or a major osteoporotic fracture. It integrates the risks associated with BMD at the femoral neck as well as clinical risk factors such as age, height, weight, sex, smoking status, alcohol drinking, use of glucocorticoids, and history of secondary osteoporosis. FRAXtool® is useful to set a threshold in order to screen candidates for pharmacological intervention and the proportion of RA patients with a greater risk of osteoporotic fractures detected with FRAXtool® is higher than with the WHO criteria [19]. When applied to 238 patients enrolled in the Canadian Early Arthritis Cohort (CATCH) study without using BMD measurements, FRAXtool® identified 5% to 13% of patients at a high risk for fracture [49]. Patients with a higher osteoporotic fracture risk determined by FRAXtool® are more likely to be female, especially postmenopausal women, with alcohol use, glucocorticoid use, proton pump inhibitor use, and had lower BMI (<25 kg/m^2) [19]. High fracture risk patients identified by the FRAXtool® was also statistically associated with disease duration, menopause duration, disease activity score (DAS28), and health assessment questionnaire (HAQ) [25].

The trabecular bone score (TBS) is also a useful, new tool to improve the prediction of fragility fracture. It is a parameter that can be automatically calculated during a BMD measurement. It assesses the quality of bone texture using the pixel gray-level variations in dual-energy X-ray absorptiometry images. A low TBS value suggests a low quality of bone texture. In the RA population, a low TBS is associated with a higher risk of having vertebral fractures even after adjusting for confounding factors such as age, DAS28, and BMD [17,24]. TBS can now be combined with the FRAXtool®. The TBS could be a supplementary tool for discriminating osteoporotic fractures risk in postmenopausal women with RA. It may have a nonlinear relationship with the cumulative dose of GCs, but not with the RA disease activity.

3. Physiopathology of Bone Loss in Rheumatoid Arthritis

As expected, classical risk factors for osteoporosis are still valuable to predict osteoporosis in patients with RA. In most of the studies, patients with spinal or femoral osteoporosis were more often female than male [3], were older [26], have a previous history of low trauma fracture, [12,17] had a lower BMI, a longer disease duration [10], a corticosteroid treatment [11], a high Larsen score [14], and a higher HAQ score [11,23,29]. There is an excess of bone loss among RA women compared to controls with post-menopausal status and HRT reduces bone resorption regardless of glucocorticoid therapy in post-menopausal RA patients [2]. There could also be an interaction between estrogen deficiency and RA-genetic risk alleles promoting enhanced Th17-cell autoreactivity, manifested by ACPA (+) RA that exacerbates the inflammatory conditions and enhances loss.

In addition to these classical risk factors, there is a crosstalk between bone cells and the immunity system and chronic inflammation that can perturb bone metabolism and promote an increase in bone loss. There is a consistent association between bone loss and the CRP reflecting disease activity [3,20,50].

The association between joint damage progression and both hand and generalized BMD loss in RA suggests common mechanisms, with hand BMD loss occurring earlier than generalized BMD loss in the disease course [51,52].

In the CATCH study, the disease activity score with 28 joint counts in the high-risk fracture group was significantly higher compared to the low-risk fracture group ($p = 0.048$) [49].

3.1. *Role of Cytokines*

Pro-inflammatory cytokines, particularly tumor necrosis factor (TNF) and interleukins IL-1, IL-6, and IL-17 play a key role in the pathogenesis of inflammation-induced bone loss. The TNF-α stimulates the receptor activator of nuclear factor kappa B ligand (RANKL), which is a membrane protein secreted by osteoblasts that binds to the RANK receptor on osteoclast precursors and induces osteoclast maturation and activation leading to bone resorption and inhibits osteoblast function thus bone formation [53]. In addition, osteoprotegerin (OPG) acts as a decoy receptor, the RANKL/OPG being of major importance to assess the balance between bone formation and resorption. OPG expression is increased in anti-TNF treated patients while RANKL is not decreased even if its level can predict the therapeutic response to anti-TNF therapy.

In mice, despite TNF-mediated inflammatory arthritis, systemic bone is fully protected by the absence of interleukin-1 (IL-1), which suggests that IL-1 is an essential mediator of inflammatory osteopenia [54]. Thus, both TNF-α and IL1 play a key role in the pathogenesis of inflammation-induced bone loss in RA patients.

The Wnt/B catenin pathway is a crucial regulatory pathway for bone formation inhibiting osteoblastic differentiation and activity. Dickkopf-1 (Dkk-1) and sclerostin (SCL) are blockers of the Wnt-signaling pathway and play an important role in RA. TNF-α increases Dkk-1 which down regulates the Wnt pathway, blocking osteoblast differentiation and inducing expression of SCL leading to the apoptosis of osteocytes.

3.2. *Bone Remodeling Markers in Ra*

Histomorphometric analysis from trans-iliac bone biopsies show that the low bone mass was not only due to an increased bone resorption but also due to reduced bone formation [55]. These mechanisms of bone loss have been assessed in many studies [56] by measuring bone remodeling markers: Osteocalcin, bone alkaline phosphatase (BAP), carboxy-terminal collagen cross links (CTX), carboxy-terminal propeptides of type 1 collagen (ICTP), and deoxypyridinoline. These bone remodeling markers are surrogates to evaluate bone formation, resorption, and further risk of fractures. I-CTX, which is derived from a matrix metalloprotease activity (MMPs), reflects joint erosions while I-CTX, produced by cathepsin K, gives evidence of general osteoporosis.

In the COBRA study, high levels of measured I-CTX and II-CTX were strong and independent predictors of articular damages [57].

4. Effects on Bone of Treatments for Rheumatoid Arthritis

The DMARDs reduce the inflammation and by the way are associated with a reduced bone loss in RA patients [40]. In some studies, BMD is decreased in RA according to corticosteroid usage, especially at the lumbar spine in both females and males with RA, and in those who are current users of steroids [1,9,11] with an increased risk of fracture [21]. The effect of corticosteroid may vary according to skeletal sites [4].

4.1. Corticosteroids

Other authors were not able to show a detrimental effect of corticosteroids on bone in RA patients [32,58] and some showed even a protective effect probably mediated by a better control of inflammation [35], which is known to be associated with a decrease in structural damage and bone loss [59,60].

In the Canadian Early Arthritis Cohort (CATCH), there was a significant correlation between increased fracture risk groups measured by the FRAXtool® and oral glucocorticoid use ($p = 0.012$) and baseline erosions ($p = 0.040$) [49].

The use of corticosteroids may be an indicator of more severe disease and a poorer functional status if the degree of systemic inflammation and the severity of RA correlated with the risk of fracture. Their detrimental effect on the fracture might have been confounded if the drug was selectively given to patients with a higher degree of systemic inflammation and RA severity [33].

In contrast, several studies recently reported a potentially beneficial effect of low-dose, short-term systemic glucocorticoids on BMD in RA suggesting that the deleterious effect of prednisolone on bone may be counteracted by its anti-inflammatory effect [47,60,61].

Other drugs, used specifically or not for RA, have been suspected to be detrimental for bone such as opioids, selective serotonin reuptake inhibitors (SSRIs), and anticonvulsants. All were associated with an increased risk of fracture in patients with RA [37,62].

4.2. Biological Agents

In RA patients, BMD is inversely correlated to serum levels of TNF-α and an optimal control of inflammation has been shown to reduce bone loss in this inflammatory disease.

Some observational or randomized study designs have reported that inflammatory generalized bone loss is suppressed by biological DMARDs targeting pro-inflammatory mediators such as the TNF-α (adalimumab, certolizumab, etanercept, golimumab, and infliximab), CD80/CD86 (abatacept), IL-6 (tocilizumab), CD20 (rituximab), and IL-1 (anakinra) both at the hip and lumbar spine. Nevertheless, this global protective effect was associated with a continuing bone loss in the BMD of the hands, which could reflect a suboptimal suppression of local inflammation [63–65]. This effect on BMD is accompanied by a significant increase in osteocalcin serum levels and a significant decrease in markers for bone resorption [66].

5. Conclusions

Bone loss in RA patients is well documented and is a frequent comorbidity. Fractures resulting from osteoporosis ranked high among comorbidities in contributing to mortality, future hospitalizations, and increased disability. Regular bone mineral density (BMD) measurements and fracture risk assessments using tools such as the FRAX algorithm should be performed for an early detection of osteoporosis in RA patients. Furthermore, the VFA technology on DXA devices should be used in these patients at the time of BMD measurement. We presume that with a lesser use of corticosteroids due to a better control of the inflammation and the potential protective effect of biologic agents that the prevalence of osteoporosis will slightly decrease. However, the risk of fractures remains high in this population highlighting the need for monitoring osteoporosis among RA patients and justifying its prevention and treatment.

Author Contributions: Writing—original draft, writing—review and editing, P.F.; co-writing—original draft, supervision, writing—review and editing, E.S.; writing—review and editing, L.L.M.; supervision, writing—review and editing, V.G. All authors have read and agreed to the published version of the manuscript.

References

1. Garton:, M.J.; Reid, D.M. Bone Mineral Density of the Hip and of the Anteroposterior and Lateral Dimensions of the Spine in Men with Rheumatoid Arthritis: Effects of Low-Dose Corticosteroids. *Arthritis Rheum.* **1993**, *36*, 222–228. [CrossRef] [PubMed]
2. Hall, G.M.; Spector, T.D.; Jane Griffin, A.; SM Jawad, A.; Hall, M.L.; Doyle, D.V. The Effect of Rheumatoid Arthritis and Steroid Therapy on Bone Density in Postmenopausal Women. *Arthritis Rheum.* **1993**, *36*, 1510–1516. [CrossRef] [PubMed]
3. Gough, A. Generalised Bone Loss in Patients with Early Rheumatoid Arthritis. *The Lancet* **1994**, *344*, 23–27. [CrossRef]
4. Lane, N.E.; Pressman, A.R.; Star, V.L.; Cummings, S.R.; Nevitt, M.C. Rheumatoid Arthritis and Bone Mineral Density in Elderly Women. The Study of Osteoporotic Fractures Research Group. *J. Bone Miner. Res. Off. J. Am. Soc. Bone Miner. Res.* **1995**, *10*, 257–263. [CrossRef]
5. Martin, J.C.; Munro, R.; Campbell, M.K.; Reid, D.M. Effects of Disease and Corticosteroids on Appendicular Bone Mass in Postmenopausal Women with Rheumatoid Arthritis: Comparison with Axial Measurements. *Br. J. Rheumatol.* **1997**, *36*, 43–49. [CrossRef]
6. Ørstavik, R.E.; Haugeberg, G.; Mowinckel, P.; Høiseth, A.; Uhlig, T.; Falch, J.A.; Halse, J.I.; McCloskey, E.; Kvien, T.K. Vertebral Deformities in Rheumatoid Arthritis: A Comparison with Population-Based Controls. *Arch. Intern. Med.* **2004**, *164*, 420–425. [CrossRef]
7. Haugeberg, G.; Uhlig, T.; Falch, J.A.; Halse, J.I.; Kvien, T.K. Reduced Bone Mineral Density in Male Rheumatoid Arthritis Patients: Frequencies and Associations with Demographic and Disease Variables in Ninety-Four Patients in the Oslo County Rheumatoid Arthritis Register. *Arthritis Rheum.* **2000**, *43*, 2776–2784. [CrossRef]
8. Lee, S.-G.; Park, Y.-E.; Park, S.-H.; Kim, T.-K.; Choi, H.-J.; Lee, S.-J.; Kim, S.-I.; Lee, S.-H.; Kim, G.-T.; Lee, J.-W.; et al. Increased Frequency of Osteoporosis and BMD below the Expected Range for Age among South Korean Women with Rheumatoid Arthritis. *Int. J. Rheum. Dis.* **2012**, *15*, 289–296. [CrossRef]
9. Avouac, J.; Koumakis, E.; Toth, E.; Meunier, M.; Maury, E.; Kahan, A.; Cormier, C.; Allanore, Y. Increased Risk of Osteoporosis and Fracture in Women with Systemic Sclerosis: A Comparative Study with Rheumatoid Arthritis. *Arthritis Care Res.* **2012**, *64*, 1871–1878. [CrossRef]
10. Laan, R.F.; Buijs, W.C.; Verbeek, A.L.; Draad, M.P.; Corstens, F.H.; van de Putte, L.B.; van Riel, P.L. Bone Mineral Density in Patients with Recent Onset Rheumatoid Arthritis: Influence of Disease Activity and Functional Capacity. *Ann. Rheum. Dis.* **1993**, *52*, 21–26. [CrossRef]
11. Sinigaglia, L.; Nervetti, A.; Mela, Q.; Bianchi, G.; Del Puente, A.; Di Munno, O.; Frediani, B.; Cantatore, F.; Pellerito, R.; Bartolone, S.; et al. A Multicenter Cross Sectional Study on Bone Mineral Density in Rheumatoid Arthritis. Italian Study Group on Bone Mass in Rheumatoid Arthritis. *J. Rheumatol.* **2000**, *27*, 2582–2589. [PubMed]
12. Kvien, T.K.; Haugeberg, G.; Uhlig, T.; Falch, J.A.; Halse, J.I.; Lems, W.F.; Dijkmans, B.A.; Woolf, A.D. Data Driven Attempt to Create a Clinical Algorithm for Identification of Women with Rheumatoid Arthritis at High Risk of Osteoporosis. *Ann. Rheum. Dis.* **2000**, *59*, 805–811. [CrossRef] [PubMed]
13. Haugeberg, G.; Uhlig, T.; Falch, J.A.; Halse, J.I.; Kvien, T.K. Bone Mineral Density and Frequency of Osteoporosis in Female Patients with Rheumatoid Arthritis: Results from 394 Patients in the Oslo County Rheumatoid Arthritis Register. *Arthritis Rheum.* **2000**, *43*, 522–530. [CrossRef]

14. Lodder, M.C.; Haugeberg, G.; Lems, W.F.; Uhlig, T.; Orstavik, R.E.; Kostense, P.J.; Dijkmans, B.A.C.; Kvien, T.K.; Woolf, A.D.; Oslo-Truro-Amsterdam (OSTRA) Collaborative Study. Radiographic Damage Associated with Low Bone Mineral Density and Vertebral Deformities in Rheumatoid Arthritis: The Oslo-Truro-Amsterdam (OSTRA) Collaborative Study. *Arthritis Rheum.* **2003**, *49*, 209–215. [CrossRef] [PubMed]
15. Ørstavik, R.E.; Haugeberg, G.; Uhlig, T.; Falch, J.A.; Halse, J.I.; Høiseth, A.; Lilleås, F.; Kvien, T.K. Vertebral Deformities in 229 Female Patients with Rheumatoid Arthritis: Associations with Clinical Variables and Bone Mineral Density. *Arthritis Rheum.* **2003**, *49*, 355–360. [CrossRef] [PubMed]
16. El Maghraoui, A.; Rezqi, A.; Mounach, A.; Achemlal, L.; Bezza, A.; Ghozlani, I. Prevalence and Risk Factors of Vertebral Fractures in Women with Rheumatoid Arthritis Using Vertebral Fracture Assessment. *Rheumatol. Oxf. Engl.* **2010**, *49*, 1303–1310. [CrossRef]
17. Bréban, S.; Briot, K.; Kolta, S.; Paternotte, S.; Ghazi, M.; Fechtenbaum, J.; Roux, C. Identification of Rheumatoid Arthritis Patients With Vertebral Fractures Using Bone Mineral Density and Trabecular Bone Score. *J. Clin. Densitom.* **2012**, *15*, 260–266. [CrossRef]
18. El Maghraoui, A.; Sadni, S.; Rezqi, A.; Bezza, A.; Achemlal, L.; Mounach, A. Does Rheumatoid Cachexia Predispose Patients with Rheumatoid Arthritis to Osteoporosis and Vertebral Fractures? *J. Rheumatol.* **2015**, *42*, 1556–1562. [CrossRef]
19. Choi, S.; Kwon, S.-R.; Jung, J.-Y.; Kim, H.-A.; Kim, S.-S.; Kim, S.; Kim, J.-M.; Park, J.-H.; Suh, C.-H. Prevalence and Fracture Risk of Osteoporosis in Patients with Rheumatoid Arthritis: A Multicenter Comparative Study of the FRAX and WHO Criteria. *J. Clin. Med.* **2018**, *7*, 507. [CrossRef]
20. Vis, M.; Haavardsholm, E.A.; Bøyesen, P.; Haugeberg, G.; Uhlig, T.; Hoff, M.; Woolf, A.; Dijkmans, B.; Lems, W.; Kvien, T.K. High Incidence of Vertebral and Non-Vertebral Fractures in the OSTRA Cohort Study: A 5-Year Follow-up Study in Postmenopausal Women with Rheumatoid Arthritis. *Osteoporos. Int. J. Establ. Result Coop. Eur. Found. Osteoporos. Natl. Osteoporos. Found. USA* **2011**, *22*, 2413–2419. [CrossRef]
21. Coulson, K.A.; Reed, G.; Gilliam, B.E.; Kremer, J.M.; Pepmueller, P.H. Factors Influencing Fracture Risk, T Score, and Management of Osteoporosis in Patients with Rheumatoid Arthritis in the Consortium of Rheumatology Researchers of North America (CORRONA) Registry. *J. Clin. Rheumatol. Pract. Rep. Rheum. Musculoskelet. Dis.* **2009**, *15*, 155–160. [CrossRef] [PubMed]
22. Dirven, L.; van den Broek, M.; van Groenendael, J.H.L.M.; de Beus, W.M.; Kerstens, P.J.S.M.; Huizinga, T.W.J.; Allaart, C.F.; Lems, W.F. Prevalence of Vertebral Fractures in a Disease Activity Steered Cohort of Patients with Early Active Rheumatoid Arthritis. *BMC Musculoskelet. Disord.* **2012**, *13*, 125. [CrossRef] [PubMed]
23. Rentero, M.L.; Amigo, E.; Chozas, N.; Fernández Prada, M.; Silva-Fernández, L.; Abad Hernandez, M.A.; Rodriguez Barrera, J.M.; del Pino-Montes, J.; GHDP Study Group. Prevalence of Fractures in Women with Rheumatoid Arthritis and/or Systemic Lupus Erythematosus on Chronic Glucocorticoid Therapy. *BMC Musculoskelet. Disord.* **2015**, *16*, 300. [CrossRef] [PubMed]
24. Choi, Y.J.; Chung, Y.-S.; Suh, C.-H.; Jung, J.-Y.; Kim, H.-A. Trabecular Bone Score as a Supplementary Tool for the Discrimination of Osteoporotic Fractures in Postmenopausal Women with Rheumatoid Arthritis. *Medicine* **2017**, *96*, e8661. [CrossRef]
25. Phuan-Udom, R.; Lektrakul, N.; Katchamart, W. The Association between 10-Year Fracture Risk by FRAX and Osteoporotic Fractures with Disease Activity in Patients with Rheumatoid Arthritis. *Clin. Rheumatol.* **2018**, *37*, 2603–2610. [CrossRef]
26. Hooyman, J.R.; Melton, L.J.; Nelson, A.M.; O'Fallon, W.M.; Riggs, B.L. Fractures after Rheumatoid Arthritis. A Population-Based Study. *Arthritis Rheum.* **1984**, *27*, 1353–1361. [CrossRef]
27. Verstraeten, A.; Dequeker, J. Vertebral and Peripheral Bone Mineral Content and Fracture Incidence in Postmenopausal Patients with Rheumatoid Arthritis: Effect of Low Dose Corticosteroids. *Ann. Rheum. Dis.* **1986**, *45*, 852–857. [CrossRef]
28. Spector, T.D.; Hall, G.M.; McCloskey, E.V.; Kanis, J.A. Risk of Vertebral Fracture in Women with Rheumatoid Arthritis. *BMJ* **1993**, *306*, 558. [CrossRef]
29. Cooper, C.; Coupland, C.; Mitchell, M. Rheumatoid Arthritis, Corticosteroid Therapy and Hip Fracture. *Ann. Rheum. Dis.* **1995**, *54*, 49–52. [CrossRef]

30. Peel, N.F.; Moore, D.J.; Barrington, N.A.; Bax, D.E.; Eastell, R. Risk of Vertebral Fracture and Relationship to Bone Mineral Density in Steroid Treated Rheumatoid Arthritis. *Ann. Rheum. Dis.* **1995**, *54*, 801–806. [CrossRef]
31. Huusko, T.M.; Korpela, M.; Karppi, P.; Avikainen, V.; Kautiainen, H.; Sulkava, R. Threefold Increased Risk of Hip Fractures with Rheumatoid Arthritis in Central Finland. *Ann. Rheum. Dis.* **2001**, *60*, 521–522. [CrossRef] [PubMed]
32. van Staa, T.P.; Geusens, P.; Bijlsma, J.W.J.; Leufkens, H.G.M.; Cooper, C. Clinical Assessment of the Long-Term Risk of Fracture in Patients with Rheumatoid Arthritis. *Arthritis Rheum.* **2006**, *54*, 3104–3112. [CrossRef] [PubMed]
33. Kim, S.Y.; Schneeweiss, S.; Liu, J.; Daniel, G.W.; Chang, C.-L.; Garneau, K.; Solomon, D.H. Risk of Osteoporotic Fracture in a Large Population-Based Cohort of Patients with Rheumatoid Arthritis. *Arthritis Res. Ther.* **2010**, *12*, R154. [CrossRef] [PubMed]
34. Wright, N.C.; Lisse, J.R.; Walitt, B.T.; Eaton, C.B.; Chen, Z.; Women's Health Initiative Investigators. Arthritis Increases the Risk for Fractures–Results from the Women's Health Initiative. *J. Rheumatol.* **2011**, *38*, 1680–1688. [CrossRef]
35. Ghazi, M.; Kolta, S.; Briot, K.; Fechtenbaum, J.; Paternotte, S.; Roux, C. Prevalence of Vertebral Fractures in Patients with Rheumatoid Arthritis: Revisiting the Role of Glucocorticoids. *Osteoporos. Int. J. Establ. Result Coop. Eur. Found. Osteoporos. Natl. Osteoporos. Found. USA* **2012**, *23*, 581–587. [CrossRef] [PubMed]
36. Filho, J.C.A.; Pinheiro, M.M.; de Moura Castro, C.H.; Szejnfeld, V.L. Prevalence and Risk Factors Associated with Low-Impact Fractures in Men with Rheumatoid Arthritis. *Clin. Rheumatol.* **2014**, *33*, 1389–1395. [CrossRef]
37. Roussy, J.-P.; Bessette, L.; Bernatsky, S.; Rahme, E.; Lachaine, J. Biologic Disease-Modifying Anti-Rheumatic Drugs and the Risk of Non-Vertebral Osteoporotic Fractures in Patients with Rheumatoid Arthritis Aged 50 Years and Over. *Osteoporos. Int. J. Establ. Result Coop. Eur. Found. Osteoporos. Natl. Osteoporos. Found. USA* **2013**, *24*, 2483–2492. [CrossRef]
38. Brennan, S.L.; Toomey, L.; Kotowicz, M.A.; Henry, M.J.; Griffiths, H.; Pasco, J.A. Rheumatoid Arthritis and Incident Fracture in Women: A Case-Control Study. *BMC Musculoskelet. Disord.* **2014**, *15*, 13. [CrossRef]
39. Xue, A.-L.; Wu, S.-Y.; Jiang, L.; Feng, A.-M.; Guo, H.-F.; Zhao, P. Bone Fracture Risk in Patients with Rheumatoid Arthritis: A Meta-Analysis. *Medicine* **2017**, *96*, e6983. [CrossRef]
40. Clynes, M.A.; Jameson, K.; Prieto-Alhambra, D.; Harvey, N.C.; Cooper, C.; Dennison, E.M. Impact of Rheumatoid Arthritis and Its Management on Falls, Fracture and Bone Mineral Density in UK Biobank. *Front. Endocrinol.* **2019**, *10*, 817. [CrossRef]
41. Hong, W.-J.; Chen, W.; Yeo, K.-J.; Huang, P.-H.; Chen, D.-Y.; Lan, J.-L. Increased Risk of Osteoporotic Vertebral Fracture in Rheumatoid Arthritis Patients with New-Onset Cardiovascular Diseases: A Retrospective Nationwide Cohort Study in Taiwan. *Osteoporos. Int. J. Establ. Result Coop. Eur. Found. Osteoporos. Natl. Osteoporos. Found. USA* **2019**, *30*, 1617–1625. [CrossRef] [PubMed]
42. Weiss, R.J.; Wick, M.C.; Ackermann, P.W.; Montgomery, S.M. Increased Fracture Risk in Patients with Rheumatic Disorders and Other Inflammatory Diseases—A Case-Control Study with 53,108 Patients with Fracture. *J. Rheumatol.* **2010**, *37*, 2247–2250. [CrossRef] [PubMed]
43. Bultink, I.E.M.; Vis, M.; van der Horst-Bruinsma, I.E.; Lems, W.F. Inflammatory Rheumatic Disorders and Bone. *Curr. Rheumatol. Rep.* **2012**, *14*, 224–230. [CrossRef] [PubMed]
44. Michaud, K.; Wolfe, F. Comorbidities in Rheumatoid Arthritis. *Best Pract. Res. Clin. Rheumatol.* **2007**, *21*, 885–906. [CrossRef]
45. Schett, G.; Kiechl, S.; Weger, S.; Pederiva, A.; Mayr, A.; Petrangeli, M.; Oberhollenzer, F.; Lorenzini, R.; Redlich, K.; Axmann, R.; et al. High-Sensitivity C-Reactive Protein and Risk of Nontraumatic Fractures in the Bruneck Study. *Arch. Intern. Med.* **2006**, *166*, 2495–2501. [CrossRef]
46. Güler-Yüksel, M.; Allaart, C.F.; Goekoop-Ruiterman, Y.P.M.; de Vries-Bouwstra, J.K.; van Groenendael, J.H.L.M.; Mallée, C.; de Bois, M.H.W.; Breedveld, F.C.; Dijkmans, B.A.C.; Lems, W.F. Changes in Hand and Generalised Bone Mineral Density in Patients with Recent-Onset Rheumatoid Arthritis. *Ann. Rheum. Dis.* **2009**, *68*, 330–336. [CrossRef]

47. Engvall, I.-L.; Svensson, B.; Tengstrand, B.; Brismar, K.; Hafström, I.; Better Anti-Rheumatic FarmacO Therapy Study Group. Impact of Low-Dose Prednisolone on Bone Synthesis and Resorption in Early Rheumatoid Arthritis: Experiences from a Two-Year Randomized Study. *Arthritis Res. Ther.* **2008**, *10*, R128. [CrossRef]
48. Kanis, J.A.; McCloskey, E.V.; Johansson, H.; Oden, A.; Ström, O.; Borgström, F. Development and Use of FRAX in Osteoporosis. *Osteoporos. Int. J. Establ. Result Coop. Eur. Found. Osteoporos. Natl. Osteoporos. Found. USA* **2010**, *21* (Suppl. 2), 407–413. [CrossRef]
49. Cheng, C.K.; McDonald-Blumer, H.; Boire, G.; Pope, J.E.; Haraoui, B.; Hitchon, C.A.; Thorne, C.; Sun, Y.; Bykerk, V.P. Care Gap in Patients with Early Inflammatory Arthritis with a High Fracture Risk Identified Using FRAX(®). *J. Rheumatol.* **2010**, *37*, 2221–2225. [CrossRef]
50. Cauley, J.A.; Danielson, M.E.; Boudreau, R.M.; Forrest, K.Y.Z.; Zmuda, J.M.; Pahor, M.; Tylavsky, F.A.; Cummings, S.R.; Harris, T.B.; Newman, A.B. Inflammatory Markers and Incident Fracture Risk in Older Men and Women: The Health Aging and Body Composition Study. *J. Bone Miner. Res.* **2007**, *22*, 1088–1095. [CrossRef]
51. Takayanagi, H. Osteoimmunology and the Effects of the Immune System on Bone. *Nat. Rev. Rheumatol.* **2009**, *5*, 667–676. [CrossRef] [PubMed]
52. Kleyer, A.; Finzel, S.; Rech, J.; Manger, B.; Krieter, M.; Faustini, F.; Araujo, E.; Hueber, A.J.; Harre, U.; Engelke, K.; et al. Bone Loss before the Clinical Onset of Rheumatoid Arthritis in Subjects with Anticitrullinated Protein Antibodies. *Ann. Rheum. Dis.* **2014**, *73*, 854–860. [CrossRef] [PubMed]
53. Redlich, K.; Smolen, J.S. Inflammatory Bone Loss: Pathogenesis and Therapeutic Intervention. *Nat. Rev. Drug Discov.* **2012**, *11*, 234–250. [CrossRef]
54. Polzer, K.; Joosten, L.; Gasser, J.; Distler, J.H.; Ruiz, G.; Baum, W.; Redlich, K.; Bobacz, K.; Smolen, J.S.; van den Berg, W.; et al. Interleukin-1 Is Essential for Systemic Inflammatory Bone Loss. *Ann. Rheum. Dis.* **2010**, *69*, 284–290. [CrossRef] [PubMed]
55. Compston, J.E.; Vedi, S.; Croucher, P.I.; Garrahan, N.J.; O'Sullivan, M.M. Bone Turnover in Non-Steroid Treated Rheumatoid Arthritis. *Ann. Rheum. Dis.* **1994**, *53*, 163–166. [CrossRef] [PubMed]
56. Fardellone, P.; Séjourné, A.; Paccou, J.; Goëb, V. Bone Remodelling Markers in Rheumatoid Arthritis. *Mediators Inflamm.* **2014**, *2014*, 484280. [CrossRef] [PubMed]
57. van Tuyl, L.H.D.; Voskuyl, A.E.; Boers, M.; Geusens, P.; Landewé, R.B.M.; Dijkmans, B.A.C.; Lems, W.F. Baseline RANKL:OPG Ratio and Markers of Bone and Cartilage Degradation Predict Annual Radiological Progression over 11 Years in Rheumatoid Arthritis. *Ann. Rheum. Dis.* **2010**, *69*, 1623–1628. [CrossRef]
58. Kröger, H.; Honkanen, R.; Saarikoski, S.; Alhava, E. Decreased Axial Bone Mineral Density in Perimenopausal Women with Rheumatoid Arthritis–a Population Based Study. *Ann. Rheum. Dis.* **1994**, *53*, 18–23. [CrossRef] [PubMed]
59. Roux, C. Osteoporosis in Inflammatory Joint Diseases. *Osteoporos. Int. J. Establ. Result Coop. Eur. Found. Osteoporos. Natl. Osteoporos. Found. USA* **2011**, *22*, 421–433. [CrossRef] [PubMed]
60. Korczowska, I.; Olewicz-Gawlik, A.; Trefler, J.; Hrycaj, P.; Krzysztof Łacki, J. Does Low-Dose and Short-Term Glucocorticoids Treatment Increase the Risk of Osteoporosis in Rheumatoid Arthritis Female Patients? *Clin. Rheumatol.* **2008**, *27*, 565–572. [CrossRef]
61. Haugeberg, G.; Strand, A.; Kvien, T.K.; Kirwan, J.R. Reduced Loss of Hand Bone Density with Prednisolone in Early Rheumatoid Arthritis: Results from a Randomized Placebo-Controlled Trial. *Arch. Intern. Med.* **2005**, *165*, 1293–1297. [CrossRef]
62. Ozen, G.; Pedro, S.; Wolfe, F.; Michaud, K. Medications Associated with Fracture Risk in Patients with Rheumatoid Arthritis. *Ann. Rheum. Dis.* **2019**, *78*, 1041–1047. [CrossRef] [PubMed]
63. Vis, M.; Havaardsholm, E.A.; Haugeberg, G.; Uhlig, T.; Voskuyl, A.E.; van de Stadt, R.J.; Dijkmans, B.A.C.; Woolf, A.D.; Kvien, T.K.; Lems, W.F. Evaluation of Bone Mineral Density, Bone Metabolism, Osteoprotegerin and Receptor Activator of the NFkappaB Ligand Serum Levels during Treatment with Infliximab in Patients with Rheumatoid Arthritis. *Ann. Rheum. Dis.* **2006**, *65*, 1495–1499. [CrossRef] [PubMed]
64. Wijbrandts, C.A.; Klaasen, R.; Dijkgraaf, M.G.W.; Gerlag, D.M.; van Eck-Smit, B.L.F.; Tak, P.P. Bone Mineral Density in Rheumatoid Arthritis Patients 1 Year after Adalimumab Therapy: Arrest of Bone Loss. *Ann. Rheum. Dis.* **2009**, *68*, 373–376. [CrossRef]

65. Eekman, D.A.; Vis, M.; Bultink, I.E.M.; Kuik, D.J.; Voskuyl, A.E.; Dijkmans, B.A.C.; Lems, W.F. Stable Bone Mineral Density in Lumbar Spine and Hip in Contrast to Bone Loss in the Hands during Long-Term Treatment with Infliximab in Patients with Rheumatoid Arthritis. *Ann. Rheum. Dis.* **2011**, *70*, 389–390. [CrossRef] [PubMed]
66. Lange, U.; Teichmann, J.; Müller-Ladner, U.; Strunk, J. Increase in Bone Mineral Density of Patients with Rheumatoid Arthritis Treated with Anti-TNF-Alpha Antibody: A Prospective Open-Label Pilot Study. *Rheumatol. Oxf. Engl.* **2005**, *44*, 1546–1548. [CrossRef]

2

Therapeutic Maintenance of Baricitinib and Tofacitinib in Real Life

Valentine Deprez [1,*], Laure Le Monnier [1], Jean-Marc Sobhy-Danial [1], Franck Grados [1], Isabelle Henry-Desailly [1], Sarah Salomon-Goëb [1], Thibault Rabin [1], Sanja Ristic [1], Mathurin Fumery [2], Patrice Fardellone [1] and Vincent Goëb [1]

1 Department of Rheumatology, Amiens University Hospital, 80000 Amiens, France; LeMonnier.Laure@chu-amiens.fr (L.L.M.); SobhyDanial.Jean-Marc@chu-amiens.fr (J.-M.S.-D.); Grados.Franck@chu-amiens.fr (F.G.); DesaillyHenry.Isabelle@chu-amiens.fr (I.H.-D.); Salomon.Sarah@chu-amiens.fr (S.S.-G.); Rabin.Thibault@chu-amiens.fr (T.R.); Ristic.Sanja@chu-amiens.fr (S.R.); fardellone.patrice@chu-amiens.fr (P.F.); goeb.vincent@chu-amiens.fr (V.G.)

2 Department of Gastroenterology, Amiens University Hospital, 80000 Amiens, France; fumery.mathurin@chu-amiens.fr

* Correspondence: deprez.valentine@chu-amiens.fr

Abstract: Background: Janus kinase inhibitors (JAKis) represent a new alternative to treat rheumatoid arthritis (RA). The objective of this study was to evaluate the effectiveness, tolerance profile, and maintenance of these treatments (tofacitinib and baricitinib) in real life. Methods: All patients in the rheumatology department of Amiens University Hospital treated by JAKis for RA were included from 1 October 2017 to 20 May 2020. Clinical and biological data were provided retrospectively in this observational and single-center study. We aimed to study the JAKi maintenance rate at 12 months and their clinical and biological safety profiles. Results: Fifty-five patients were included. Drug maintenance at 12 months was 67.6%. Factors associated with poorer maintenance were a higher Charlson comorbidity index (HR 1.311 (1.089–1.579); $p = 0.0042$), a higher age (HR 1.055 (1.015–1.096); $p = 0.0067$), and corticosteroids therapy at initiation (HR 2.722 (1.006–7.365); $p = 0.0487$). The clinical and biological safety profile was generally good. Conclusions: Our study found that a higher Charlson index, age, and corticosteroids appeared to be associated with the earlier discontinuation of treatment. JAKis had a response and tolerance profile in real life at least equivalent to that of biological disease-modifying antirheumatic drugs (bDMARDs).

Keywords: rheumatoid arthritis; JAK inhibitors; baricitinib; tofacitinib; therapeutic maintenance

1. Introduction

Rheumatoid arthritis (RA) is the most common chronic inflammatory rheumatic disease [1]. It can cause structural damages, reduce quality of life, and lead to permanent disability. The therapeutic management of RA is therefore essential in rheumatology research and has undergone profound changes over the past few decades. Biological agents have rapidly multiplied, and a new therapeutic class has recently emerged: Janus kinase inhibitors (JAKis).

Janus kinases (JAKs) are essential enzymes in the signaling pathways of many surface cytokine receptors, including those in the inflammatory physiology. JAKis reduce inflammation by modulating the intracellular activity of JAKs and disrupting the signaling of multiple pro-inflammatory cytokines. In France in 2017, two molecules became available in current practice: baricitinib and tofacitinib; these can be prescribed as second-line therapy after conventional synthetic disease-modifying antirheumatic drug (csDMARD) failure [2–5].

Some information about the efficacy and safety profile of these molecules in current practice are now available, but there is still a lack of data about therapeutic maintenance [6–8]. The European League against Rheumatism (EULAR) recommendations in 2019 also raised some concerns about the safety and effectiveness profile of using JAKis after an interleukin 6 (IL6) failure or after another JAKi failure [4].

The main objective of this study was to study JAKi persistence at 12 months as a reflection of the effectiveness and safety profile in real life. The secondary objectives were to identify the factors associated with discontinuation of JAKi therapy, the potential biological issues, the effectiveness profile, and the collection of adverse effects.

2. Materials and Methods

2.1. Patient Selection

This observational, single-center, and retrospective study included all patients having benefited from the introduction of a JAKi for RA in the Rheumatology department of Amiens University Hospital from 1 October 2017 to 20 May 2020. The choice of treatment was left to the discretion of prescribing physicians according to the recommendations of the French Rheumatology Society [9].

All patients were informed about the study's objectives and agreed to the anonymous use of the collected data. The study was conducted in accordance with the Declaration of Helsinki. The protocol was approved by the Ethics Committee of Department of Clinical Research and Innovation (DRCI) of the Amiens-Picardie University Hospital, and a conformity declaration to a reference methodology to the National Commission for Computing and Civil Liberties (CNIL) was made (Project identification code: PI2020_843_0024).

Inclusion criteria for the patients were:

- RA according to the 2010 ACR/EULAR criteria [10].
- Age 18 years or older.
- Initiation of JAKi therapy.
- No objection to the use of their data.

Non-inclusion criteria were a refusal to participate and patients under legal protection measures.

2.2. Data Recorded

Data were collected as part of routine clinical practice, and electronic medical records were obtained. For each patient, the following variables were recorded from the medical file:

- Baseline characteristics (age, sex, body mass index, history of pulmonary, digestive and urogenital infections, neoplastic history, Charlson comorbidity index [11], and smoking).
- Disease characteristics (duration of RA, positivity of rheumatoid factor (RF) and anticitrullinated protein antibodies (ACPA), presence of extra-articular manifestation, presence of erosion, prior treatments, and concomitant treatments).
- Clinical data at baseline, 3 months, 6 months, and 12 months (number of nocturnal awakenings, duration of morning rusting, pain Visual Analog Scale (VAS), patient global health VAS, disease activity score in 28 joints using erythrocyte sedimentation rate (DAS-28 ESR), disease activity score in 28 joints using C-reactive protein (DAS-28 CRP), number of swollen joints (NSJ), number of tender joints (NTJ), and secondary effects (infections, neoplasia or cardiovascular events)).
- Biological data at baseline, 3 months, 6 months, and 12 months (complete blood count (CBC), sedimentation rate (ESR), C-reactive protein (CRP), liver function, creatinine, modification of diet in renal disease (MDRD) clearance, and lipid profile including total cholesterol, triglycerides, low density lipoprotein cholesterol (LDLc), and high density lipoprotein cholesterol (HDLc)).

2.3. Statistical Analysis

Quantitative variables are expressed as median and quartiles, and categorical variables are expressed as number and percentage. Missing data were not replaced. Drug maintenance was analyzed by the Kaplan–Meier method. The association between treatment discontinuation and baseline characteristics was assessed using a univariate Cox model and presented in terms of a hazard ratio (HR) with 95% confidence interval (CI). $p < 0.05$ was considered statistically significant. All statistical analyses were performed using SAS software version 9.4 (SAS Institute Inc, Cary, NC, USA).

3. Results

3.1. Patient Selection and Characteristics

Among 56 patients who met the inclusion criteria, only 55 were included because one patient refused to participate. Seven patients received 5 mg of tofacitinib twice daily, and 48 patients received 4 or 2 mg of baricitinib daily. We observed that six patients (12.5%) received a daily half-dose of 2 mg due to either an age over 75 years or a moderate renal failure, according to the recommendations. Only two out of six patients were able to benefit from the maximum dose of baricitinib due to a good clinical and biological safety profile. Four patients remained on 2 mg of baricitinib daily because of persistent renal failure but with controlled rheumatism at this posology for two patients. The characteristics at baseline of the 55 patients are shown in Table 1. Due to this small sample of patients receiving tofacitinib and the similarity of their characteristics, this study analyzed both molecules together. We could notice that four patients received baricitinib and then tofacitinib with same effectiveness and safety profile (primary inefficacy of two molecules for one patient, secondary inefficacy for another patient, and digestive adverse effects for a third patient). Only one patient with the treatment failure of baricitinib was still on tofacitinib at the time of data collection, i.e., at one year and two months after its introduction. These four patients were analyzed once in the baricitinib group.

Table 1. Baseline characteristics of the study population.

	Whole Population (n = 55)
Female sex, n (%)	45 (81.8%)
Age (years), *med [Q1–Q3]*	58.0 [46.0–67.0]
Body mass index (kg/m^2), *med [Q1–Q3]*	25.9 [22.9–30.5] *
Disease duration (years), *med [Q1–Q3]*	11.0 [4.0–18.0]
Personal medical history	
Infection, n (%)	18/49 (36.7%)
Neoplasia, n (%)	4 (7.3%)
Smoking, n (%)	12/49 (24.5%)
Charlson comorbidity index, *med [Q1–Q3]*	2.0 [0.0–3.0]
DAS-28 ESR, *med [Q1–Q3]*	4.2 [3.5–4.9]
DAS-28 CRP, *med [Q1–Q3]*	4.2 [3.3–4.8]
Extra-articular manifestations, n (%)	8/53 (15.1%)
Treatment	
Methotrexate at initiation, n (%)	30 (54.5%)
Methotrexate dose (mg/week), *med (min–max)*	20.0 (7.5–25.0)
Corticosteroids at initiation	23 (41.8%)
Corticosteroids dose (mg/day), *med (min–max)*	7 (2–20)
RF positive, n (%)	44 (80.0%)
ACPA positive, n (%)	43 (78.2%)
Erosion presence, n (%)	34 (61.8%)

N: number; *med*: median value; *Q1*: first quartile; *Q3*: third quartile; RF: rheumatoid factor; ACPA: anticitrullinated protein antibodies; DAS-28 ESR: disease activity score in 28 joints using erythrocyte sedimentation rate; DAS-28 CRP: disease activity score in 28 joints using C-reactive protein; * missing data for 21 patients.

3.2. *JAKi Maintenance*

The following-up median was 11.2 months (3.3–12.0). As shown in Table 2 and Figure 1, the rate of drug maintenance at 12 months was 67.6% (52.47–78.85).

Table 2. Therapeutic maintenance of Janus kinase inhibitors.

	Total	Baricitinib	Tofacitinib
Stop/Censure	16/39	13/35	3/4
		Kaplan–Meier (CI 95%)	
3 months	86.89% [74.43–93.53]	84.9% [70.88–92.51]	100.0% [100.0–100.0]
6 months	74.45% [59.99–84.33]	75.1% [59.41–85.43]	71.43% [25.82–91.98]
9 months	69.93% [55.0–80.74]	69.74% [53.4–81.29]	71.43% [25.82–91.98]
12 months	67.6% [52.47–78.85]	69.74% [53.4–81.29]	53.57% [13.2–82.5]

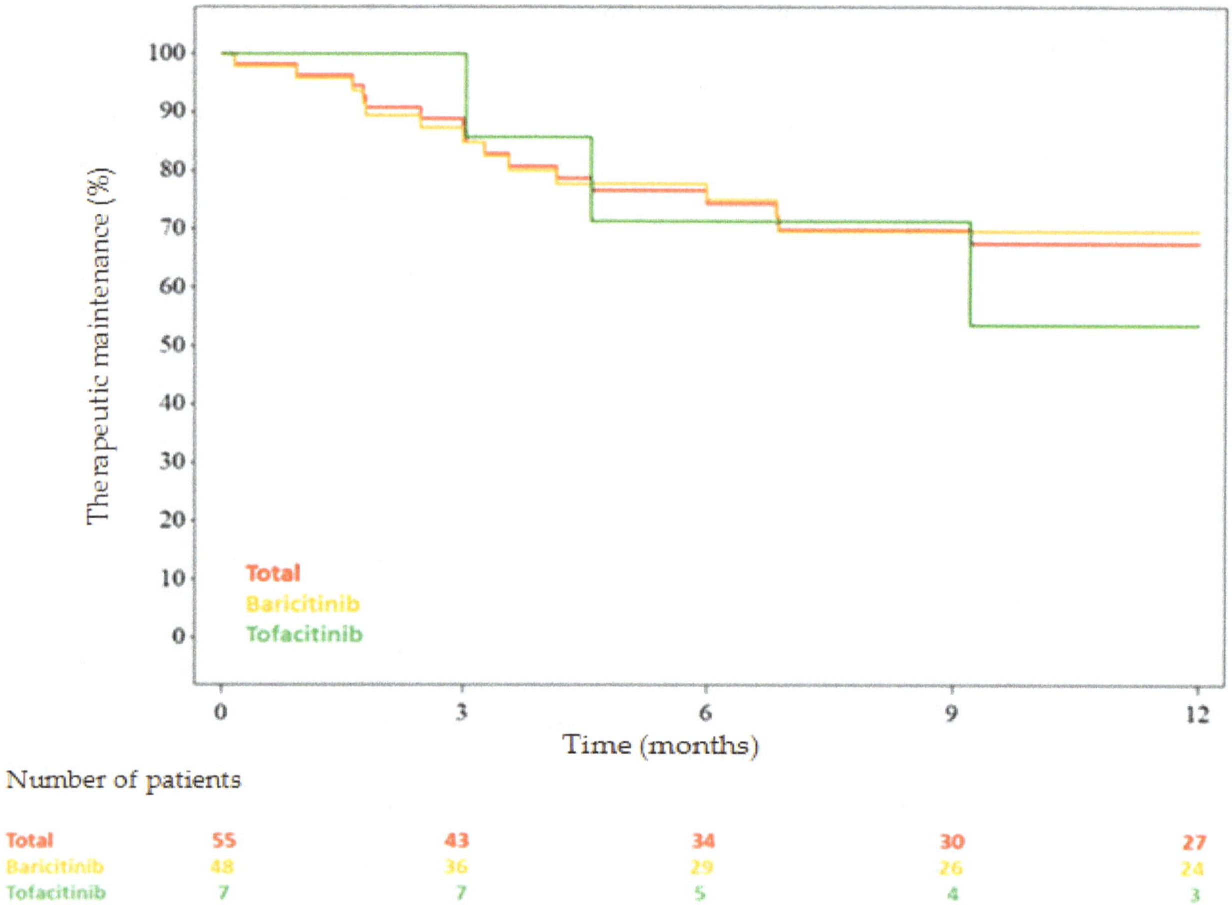

Figure 1. Janus kinase inhibitor maintenance in time.

3.3. *Factors Associated with Discontinuation of JAKis and Adverse Effects*

Our univariate analysis revealed three factors statistically associated with JAKi discontinuation: the Charlson comorbidity index (HR 1.358 (1.126–1.638); $p = 0.0014$), age (HR 1.055 (1.015–1.096); $p = 0.0067$), and corticosteroids at initiation (HR 2.722 (1.006–7.365); $p = 0.0487$) (Table 3). No other demographic, clinical, or paraclinical characteristics were found to be associated with drug discontinuation.

Table 3. Factors associated with therapy discontinuation.

Parameters	HR	Lower 95% CI	Upper 95% CI	*p*-Value
Age (for 1 year)	1.055	1.015	1.096	0.0067
Female vs. male sex	1.851	0.420	8.164	0.4159
Disease duration (for 1 year)	1.021	0.964	1.083	0.4763
Personal medical history				
Infections	1.264	0.438	3.645	0.6647
Neoplasia	0.806	0.106	6.108	0.8349
Smoking	0.390	0.089	1.717	0.2132
Charlson comorbidity index (for 1 point)	1.358	1.126	1.638	0.0014
DAS28-ESR at initiation (for 1 point)	1.324	0.882	1.987	0.1753
DAS28-CRP (at initiation (for 1 point)	1.091	0.709	1.680	0.6925
Prior treatment				
No prior biological treatment	0.705	0.160	3.102	0.6438
1 tumor necrosis factor inhibitor versus none	0.573	0.143	2.296	0.4316
2 or more tumor necrosis factor inhibitors versus none	1.151	0.346	3.830	0.8190
Interleukin 6 inhibitor	1.167	0.434	3.137	0.7598
Rituximab	1.498	0.520	4.315	0.4541
Abatacept	0.955	0.358	2.551	0.9273
Corticosteroids at initiation	2.722	1.006	7.365	
Methotrexate at initiation	0.547	0.203	1.474	0.2330
RF and/or ACPA positive	1.318	0.299	5.809	0.7151
Erosion presence	1.116	0.405	3.072	0.8317

RF: rheumatoid factor; ACPA: anticitrullinated protein antibodies; DAS-28 ESR: disease activity score in 28 joints using erythrocyte sedimentation rate; DAS-28 CRP: disease activity score in 28 joints using C-reactive protein.

No significant statistical link was found between therapeutic maintenance and prior treatment by IL6 inhibitors ($p = 0.7598$) either with treatment by methotrexate at initiation ($p = 0.2330$) or the absence of prior biological disease-modifying antirheumatic drugs (bDMARDs) ($p = 0.6438$).

The reasons for JAKi discontinuation within 12 months were: primary inefficacy in seven patients (43.8%), digestive intolerance in six (37.5%), infectious adverse effects in three (18.8%), secondary inefficacy in one (6.3%), cardiovascular events in one (6.3%), and biological abnormalities in one (6.3%).

The cardiovascular events listed in our study during the 12 months follow-up were: unbalanced arterial hypertension and a myocardial infarction.

The infectious adverse effects listed in our study were: exacerbations of chronic obstructive pulmonary disease, pneumonia, recurrent upper airway infections, recurrent urinary tract infections, and recurrent herpes labialis. No herpetic zoster was recorded.

The laboratory abnormality that led to the discontinuation of treatment was the worsening of chronic renal failure (change from stage 3 to stage 4 of chronic kidney disease).

No patient presented with neoplasia during follow-up.

3.4. Biological Data

The safety of JAKis was evaluated using biological data and the difference between the initiation of treatment and three and six months (Table 4). This study showed a slight decrease in hemoglobin (mean of −0.5 g/dL at six months), but we observed that the anemia present at the initiation of treatment in five patients (9.1%) was corrected for all at six months. We also found an elevation of platelets (mean of 41,032/mm^3 at six months) and a diminution of polynuclear neutrophils (mean of −383.4/mm^3 at six months) but no difference in liver function, renal function, or lipid profile.

3.5. Effectiveness Profile

The proportion of moderate and good responders, according to the EULAR response criteria, was on the DAS-28 ESR and CRP, respectively, 44.4% and 48.1% at 3 months, 71% and 68.8% at 6 months, and 78.9% and 76.2% at 12 months (Figures 2 and 3) [12]. The clinical parameter evolution is summarized in Figure 4. There is a clinical report of improvement in a patient's rheumatoid nodules in terms of the size and functional discomfort in the upper limbs. Regarding corticosteroid withdrawal, 23 patients (41.8% of the population) had corticosteroid therapy associated with JAKis at baseline, 20 patients were analyzed at six months, and eight of them (40%) were weaned off corticosteroids. However, the 12 patients still with corticosteroids had a decreased dosage for eight of them, with an average of 4.8 mg (median of 5 mg with a range of 1–10 mg) against a baseline mean of 8.3 mg (median of 7 mg with a range of 2–20 mg). No difference in methotrexate posology was observed in this study after JAKi initiation.

Table 4. Biological evolution between baseline, 3 months, and 6 months.

	Difference between Baseline and 3 Months	Difference between Baseline and 6 Months
Hemoglobin (g/dL), *med [Q1–Q3]*	−0.4 [−1.0–0.1] **	−0.8 [−1.1–0.1] *
Platelets (/mm^3), *med [Q1–Q3]*	56,000 [6000–82,000] *	38,500 [−12,000–76,000]
Leukocytes (/mm^3), *med [Q1–Q3]*	−300.0 [−1800–500] *	−105.0 [−1410–420]
Polynuclear neutrophils (/mm^3), *med [Q1–Q3]*	−488.5 [−1229.5–516.5] *	85.5 [−1040–655]
Eosinophilic cells (/mm^3), *med [Q1–Q3]*	−40.5 [−91–145] *	−24.0 [−91–−1.0]
Lymphocytes (/mm^3), *med [Q1–Q3]*	41.0 [−400–792] *	−181.5 [−501–430]
ESR, *med [Q1–Q3]*	0.0 [−4.0–4.0] *	−0.5 [−5.0–3.0]
CRP, *med [Q1–Q3]*	−1.1 [−5.9–0.0] *	−3.1 [−7.2–0.0]
Aspartate transaminase (UI/L), *med [Q1–Q3]*	3.0 [−3.0–7.0] **	4.0 [−2.0–6.0]
Alanine transaminase (UI/L), *med [Q1–Q3]*	1.0 [−31.0–24.0] **	0.0 [−6.0–7.0]
Creatinine (μmol/L), *med [Q1–Q3]*	2.6 [−2.5–7.0] **	0.0 [−4.5–7.9]
Creatinine clearance (mL/min), *med [Q1–Q3]*	−2.3 [−7.8–7.3] **	0.0 [−11.0–7.7]
Total cholesterol (g/L), *med [Q1–Q3]*	0.1 [−0.2–0.2] †	0.1 [−0.1–0.2] †
Triglycerides (g/L), *med [Q1–Q3]*	0.0 [−0.6–0.2] †	−0.3 [−0.6–0.2] †
LDL cholesterol (g/L), *med [Q1–Q3]*	0.0 [−0.2–0.2] †	0.0 [−0.1–0.1] †
HDL cholesterol (g/L), *med [Q1–Q3]*	0.0 [−0.4–0.4] †	0.0 [0.0–0.1] †

med: median value; *Q1*: first quartile; *Q3*: third quartile; ESR: erythrocyte sedimentation rate; CRP: C-reactive protein; LDL: low-density lipoprotein; HDL: high-density lipoprotein; * missing data for 7 patients; ** missing data for 10 patients; † missing data for 25 patients.

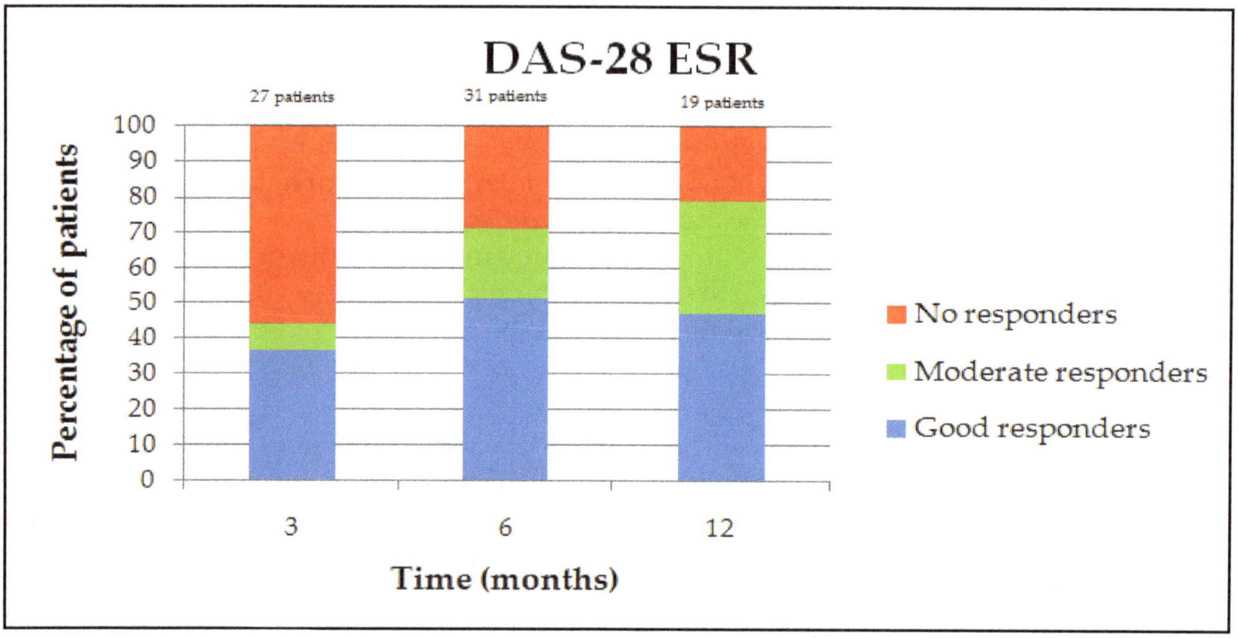

Figure 2. European League against Rheumatism (EULAR) response variation on DAS-28 ESR.

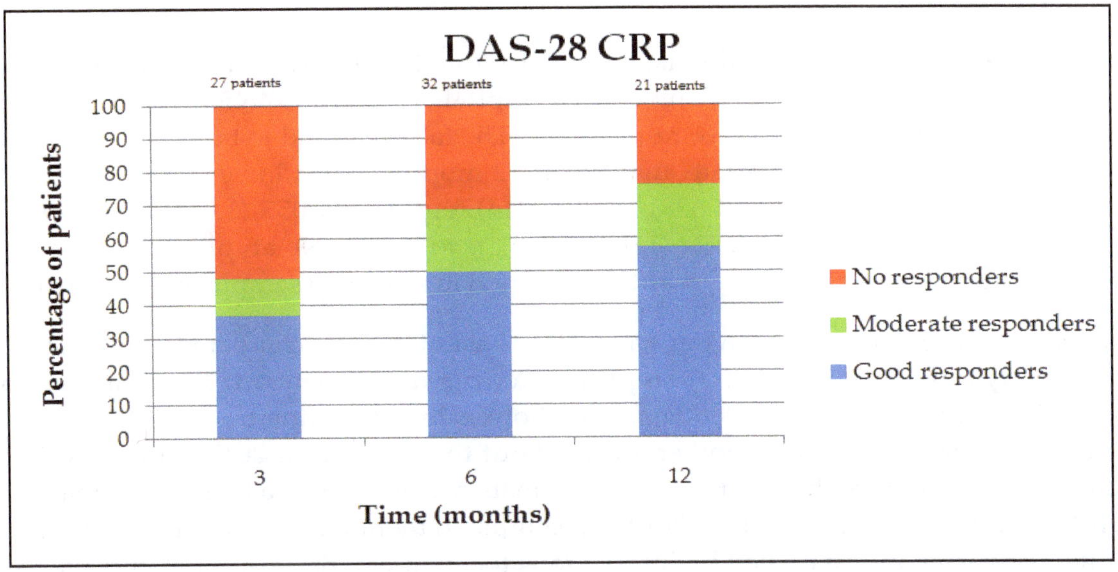

Figure 3. EULAR response variation on DAS-28 CRP.

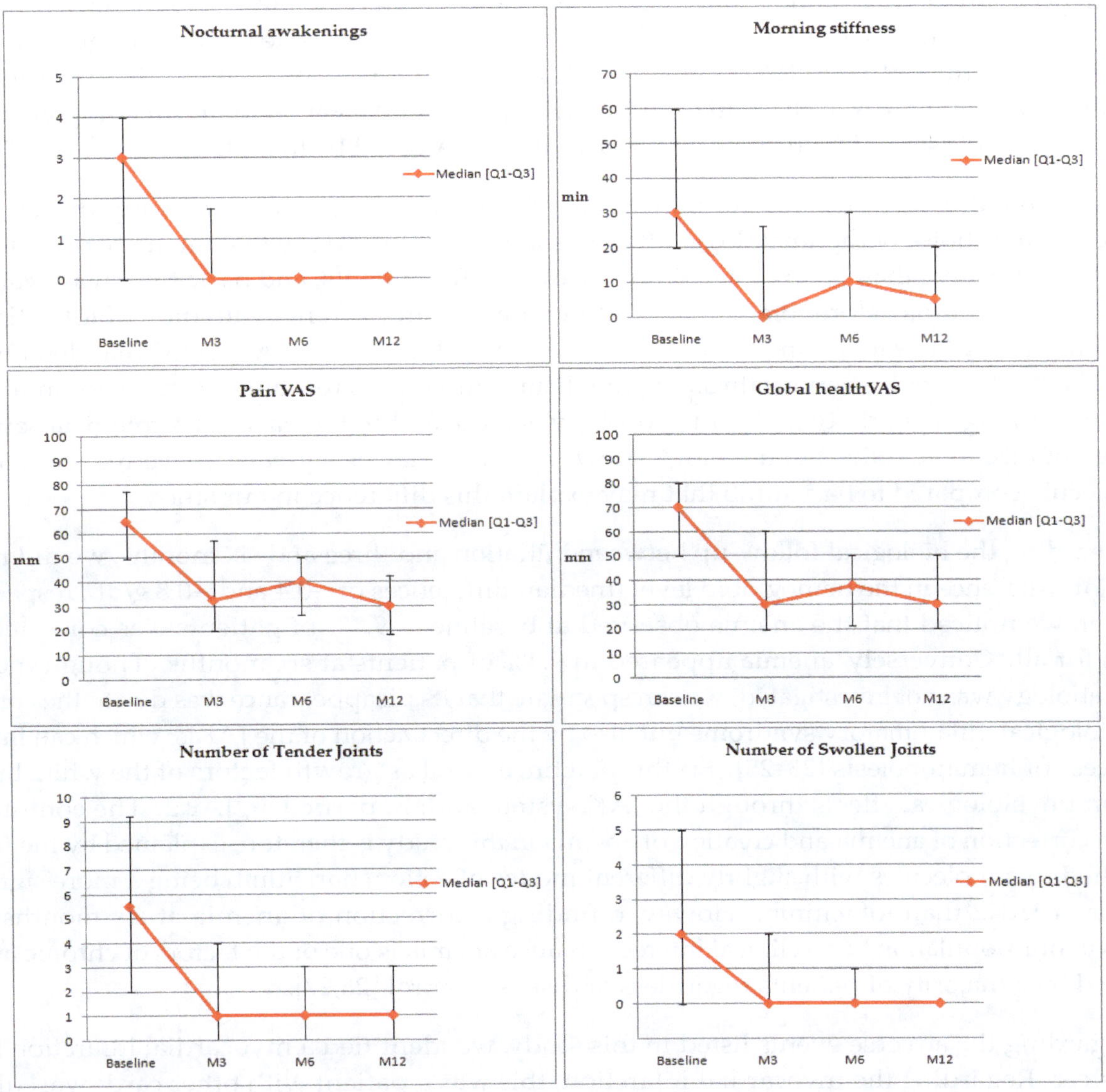

Figure 4. Clinical parameter variation. VAS: Visual Analog Scale.

4. Discussion

Our study evaluated JAKi maintenance in 55 patients with RA in routine practice in the Rheumatology department of Amiens University Hospital. We found 74.45% and 67.6% of patients continuing treatment at 6 and 12 months, respectively. The factors found to be significantly associated with drug discontinuation in univariate analysis at 12 months was a lower Charlson comorbidity index at initiation (HR 1.358 (1.126–1.638); $p = 0.0014$), age (HR 1.055 (1.015–1.096); $p = 0.0067$), and corticosteroids at initiation (HR 2.722 (1.006–7.365); $p = 0.0487$). No atypia was found in adverse events recorded, but the presence of a myocardial infarction in this small sample needs to be highlighted.

Drug maintenance at 12 months in our patients was slightly lower compared to published studies, except for a study published in May 2020 reporting a drug maintenance at 12 months of abatacept of 68% [13]. A study published in 2006 about methotrexate, a first-line treatment for RA, found a therapeutic maintenance of 76%. Another study about tocilizumab in 2017 showed a therapeutic maintenance of 82.9%, and another study about infliximab in 2008 showed a therapeutic maintenance of 78% [14–16]. We can also quote a study of 2019 that compared therapeutic maintenance for tocilizumab at 12 months between patients treated by intravenous tocilizumab (80%) and patients who switched for subcutaneous tocilizumab (77.7%) [17].

Our population was similar concerning baseline characteristics in comparison with patients in the RA-BEAM study about baricitinib, but our population was older with a longer duration of RA compared to the ORAL-STRATEGY study about tofacitinib [18,19]. Patients in our study had a generally lower active RA at the initiation of JAKis [18–21]. We can explain this difference by the real-life type of this study in which no severe activity of RA could be tolerated.

We included a small number of patients treated by tofacitinib, but our study design had no influence on the choice of rheumatologist. It seems fairly intuitive to say that taking baricitinib once a day is more attractive than taking tofacitinib twice a day for patients, and baricitinib was available in France several months before tofacitinib. Additionally, a European re-evaluation of tofacitinib was carried out in May 2019 following the interim analyses of clinical study A3921133 that demonstrated an increased risk of severe venous thromboembolism compared to tumor necrosis factor inhibitors at a dosage of 10 mg twice daily [22]. This posology is indicated in the gastroenterological setting for treatment of ulcerative colitis but not of RA. However, there may be a greater concern about the use of this molecule compared to baricitinib that may explain this difference in our study.

Regarding the biological follow-up between initiation and three and six months, we did not find any major difference in the hemoglobin level (median differences of −0.4 and −0.8 g/dL, respectively). However, we noticed that the anemia observed at baseline in 9.1% of patients was corrected at six months for all. Conversely, anemia appeared in 9.4% of patients at six months. Though the initial anemia etiology was not investigated, we can speculate that its disappearance was due to the correction of the biological inflammatory syndrome but also by the direct action of the JAKis, which can influence the process of hematopoiesis [23–25]. Erythropoietin, as well as growth factors of the white line, acts to obtain physiological effects through the JAK system and, in particular, JAK2. The contradiction between correction of anemia and creation of anemia in this study is therefore explained by the fact that we studied two molecules with slightly different modes of action, baricitinib being a more significant inhibitor of JAK2 than tofacitinib. However, finding a correction of anemia at six months for all patients in our population has a clinical interest because anemia is one of the factors of chronic asthenia expressed by a majority of patients regardless of disease control [26,27].

Regarding the adverse events listed in this study, we identified a myocardial infarction and an antral ulcer. Regarding the myocardial infarction, this was a patient with other cardiovascular risk factors, and all studies have been reassuring about the cardiovascular risk of JAKis. This isolated case does not challenge the available large-scale data [7,8]. Likewise, there was a case of antral ulcers in a patient with concomitant use of non-steroidal anti-inflammatory drugs. This type of adverse event is known and described in the literature under JAKis [28]. The main hypothesis regarding the physiology of digestive perforations is that the inhibition of the JAK–STAT system is partly responsible for the inhibition of IL6 signaling, and digestive perforations are a known and frequent risk with IL6 inhibitors.

Our study found a higher Charlson comorbidity index as a statistically significant factor associated with lower therapeutic maintenance (HR 1.358 (1.126–1.638); $p = 0.0014$). Age, that is part of the Charlson index, and treatment by corticosteroids at baseline were also factors that were statistically associated with lower therapeutic maintenance in our univariate analysis. We could therefore suggest that, according to our study, a higher patient's Charlson index at the start of treatment is associated with a greater probability of stopping treatment. In other words, the introduction of JAKis in patients with numerous co-morbidities should be discussed. This original sighting has never been described, to our knowledge, in JAKi treatments. Likewise, another Japanese study from 2014 showed a poorer response to biological DMARDs with a higher Charlson index in terms of DAS-28 evolution and quality of life [29]. Conversely, a German study from 2014 found no association between the Charlson index and therapeutic maintenance with adalimumab, etanercept, and infliximab [30]. Our study did not find any statistical difference of therapeutic maintenance for patients with a history of IL6 inhibitor therapy, for patients treated by JAKis with methotrexate, or for patients without prior bDMARDs.

Our study had several limitations. The retrospective characteristic induced a large variation in the duration of treatment, and many patients were censured. The small size of our single-center cohort did not allow us to perform multivariate analysis. Therefore, the association between characteristics at baseline and therapy discontinuation must be interpreted with caution and should be confirmed in multicenter studies of larger scales and longer follow-ups.

5. Conclusions

In view of our study, JAKis had a response and tolerance profile in real life at least equivalent to that of biological disease-modifying antirheumatic drugs. To optimize their prescription, it is suggested to take the patient's age, his Charlson comorbidity index, and any received corticosteroids therapy into account.

Our study did not find any difference in therapeutic maintenance whether JAKis were administered first-line after the failure of methotrexate, after a history of IL6 inhibitor treatment, or in combination with methotrexate, but these data must be confirmed by other teams on a larger scale.

Author Contributions: Conceptualization, V.G. and V.D.; methodology, V.G. and V.D.; validation and inclusion, all authors; formal analysis, S.R. and V.D.; writing—original draft preparation, V.D.; writing—review and editing, all authors. All authors have read and agreed to the published version of the manuscript.

References

1. Smolen, J.S.; Aletaha, D.; McInnes, I.B. Rheumatoid arthritis. *Lancet* **2016**, *388*, 2023–2038. [CrossRef]
2. Malemud, C.J. The role of the JAK/STAT signal pathway in rheumatoid arthritis. *Ther. Adv. Musculoskelet Dis.* **2018**, *10*, 117–127. [CrossRef]
3. Dowty, M.E.; Lin, T.H.; Jesson, M.I.; Hegen, M.; Martin, D.A.; Katkade, V.; Menon, S.; Telliez, J. Janus kinase inhibitors for the treatment of rheumatoid arthritis demonstrate similar profiles of in vitro cytokine receptor inhibition. *Pharmacol. Res. Perspect.* **2019**, *7*. [CrossRef] [PubMed]

4. Smolen, J.S.; Landewé, R.B.M.; Bijlsma, J.W.J.; Burmester, G.R.; Dougados, M.; Kerschbaumer, A.; McInnes, I.B.; Sepriano, A.; van Vollenhoven, R.F.; de Wit, M.; et al. EULAR recommendations for the management of rheumatoid arthritis with synthetic and biological disease-modifying antirheumatic drugs: 2019 update. *Ann. Rheum. Dis.* **2020**. [CrossRef] [PubMed]
5. Walker, J.G.; Ahern, M.J.; Coleman, M.; Weedon, H.; Papangelis, V.; Beroukas, D.; Roberts-Thomson, P.J.; Smith, M.D. Changes in synovial tissue Jak-STAT expression in rheumatoid arthritis in response to successful DMARD treatment. *Ann. Rheum. Dis.* **2006**, *65*, 1558–1564. [CrossRef] [PubMed]
6. Verden, A.; Dimbil, M.; Kyle, R.; Overstreet, B.; Hoffman, K.B. Analysis of Spontaneous Postmarket Case Reports Submitted to the FDA Regarding Thromboembolic Adverse Events and JAK Inhibitors. *Drug Saf.* **2018**, *41*, 357–361. [CrossRef]
7. Taylor, P.C.; Weinblatt, M.E.; Burmester, G.R.; Rooney, T.P.; Witt, S.; Walls, C.D.; Issa, M.; Salinas, C.A.; Saifan, C.; Zhang, X.; et al. Cardiovascular Safety during Treatment with Baricitinib in Rheumatoid Arthritis. *Arthritis Rheumatol.* **2019**, *71*, 1042–1055. [CrossRef]
8. Cohen, S.B.; Tanaka, Y.; Mariette, X.; Curtis, J.R.; Lee, E.B.; Nash, P.; Winthrop, K.L.; Charles-Schoeman, C.; Thirunavukkarasu, K.; DeMasi, R.; et al. Long-term safety of tofacitinib for the treatment of rheumatoid arthritis up to 8.5 years: Integrated analysis of data from the global clinical trials. *Ann. Rheum. Dis.* **2017**, *76*, 1253–1262. [CrossRef]
9. Daien, C.; Hua, C.; Gaujoux-Viala, C.; Cantagrel, A.; Dubremetz, M.; Dougados, M.; Fautrel, B.; Mariette, X.; Nayral, N.; Richez, C.; et al. Update of French society for rheumatology recommendations for managing rheumatoid arthritis. *Jt. Bone Spine* **2019**, *86*, 135–150. [CrossRef]
10. Aletaha, D.; Neogi, T.; Silman, A.J.; Funovits, J.; Felson, D.T.; Bingham, C.O.; Birnbaum, N.S.; Burmester, G.R.; Bykerk, V.P.; Cohen, M.D.; et al. 2010 rheumatoid arthritis classification criteria: An American College of Rheumatology/European League Against Rheumatism collaborative initiative. *Ann. Rheum. Dis.* **2010**, *69*, 1580–1588. [CrossRef]
11. Charlson, M.E.; Pompei, P.; Ales, K.L.; MacKenzie, C.R. A new method of classifying prognostic comorbidity in longitudinal studies: Development and validation. *J. Chronic. Dis.* **1987**, *40*, 373–383. [CrossRef]
12. Prevoo, M.L.; van't Hof, M.A.; Kuper, H.H.; van Leeuwen, M.A.; van de Putte, L.B.; van Riel, P.L. Modified disease activity scores that include twenty-eight-joint counts. Development and validation in a prospective longitudinal study of patients with rheumatoid arthritis. *Arthritis Rheum.* **1995**, *38*, 44–48. [CrossRef] [PubMed]
13. Salmon, J.-H.; Letarouilly, J.-G.; Goëb, V.; Kanagaratnam, L.; Coquerelle, P.; Guyot, M.-H.; Houvenagel, E.; Lecuyer, N.; Marguerie, L.; Morel, G.; et al. Actual Persistence of Abatacept in Rheumatoid Arthritis: Results of the French-Ric Network. *J. Clin. Med.* **2020**, *9*, 1528. [CrossRef] [PubMed]
14. Tahiri, L.; Allali, F.; Jroundi, I.; Abouqal, R.; Hajjaj-Hassouni, N. Therapeutic maintenance level of methotrexate in rheumatoid arthritis. *Sante* **2006**, *16*, 167–172. [CrossRef] [PubMed]
15. Chopin, C.; Pauvele, L.; Jaulerry, S.; Brochot, P.; Eschard, J.-P.; Salmon, J.-H. Effectiveness, therapeutic maintenance and reasons for stopping tocilizumab (TCZ): A retrospective and monocentric study in 88 patients followed for rheumatoid arthritis (RA) at the Reims university hospital. *Therapie* **2018**, *73*, 231–236. [CrossRef]
16. Figueiredo, I.T.; Morel, J.; Sany, J.; Combe, B. Maintenance and tolerability of infliximab in a cohort of 152 patients with rheumatoid arthritis. *Clin. Exp. Rheumatol.* **2008**, *26*, 18–23. [PubMed]
17. Darloy, J.; Segaud, N.; Salmon, J.-H.; Eschard, J.-P.; Goëb, V.; Deprez, X.; Guyot, M.-H.; Houvenagel, E.; Lecuyer, N.; Marguerie, L.; et al. Tocilizumab Effectiveness after Switching from Intravenous to Subcutaneous Route in Patients with Rheumatoid Arthritis: The RoSwitch Study. *Rheumatol. Ther.* **2019**, *6*, 61–75. [CrossRef] [PubMed]
18. Taylor, P.C.; Keystone, E.C.; van der Heijde, D.; Weinblatt, M.E.; Del Carmen Morales, L.; Reyes Gonzaga, J.; Yakushin, S.; Ishii, T.; Emoto, K.; Beattie, S.; et al. Baricitinib versus Placebo or Adalimumab in Rheumatoid Arthritis. *N. Engl. J. Med.* **2017**, *376*, 652–662. [CrossRef]
19. Fleischmann, R.; Mysler, E.; Hall, S.; Kivitz, A.J.; Moots, R.J.; Luo, Z.; DeMasi, R.; Soma, K.; Zhang, R.; Takiya, L.; et al. Efficacy and safety of tofacitinib monotherapy, tofacitinib with methotrexate, and adalimumab with methotrexate in patients with rheumatoid arthritis (ORAL Strategy): A phase 3b/4, double-blind, head-to-head, randomised controlled trial. *Lancet* **2017**, *390*, 457–468. [CrossRef]

20. Genovese, M.C.; Kremer, J.; Zamani, O.; Ludivico, C.; Krogulec, M.; Xie, L.; Beattie, S.D.; Koch, A.E.; Cardillo, T.E.; Rooney, T.P.; et al. Baricitinib in Patients with Refractory Rheumatoid Arthritis. *N. Engl. J. Med.* **2016**, *374*, 1243–1252. [CrossRef]
21. Keystone, E.C.; Taylor, P.C.; Drescher, E.; Schlichting, D.E.; Beattie, S.D.; Berclaz, P.-Y.; Lee, C.H.; Fidelus-Gort, R.K.; Luchi, M.E.; Rooney, T.P.; et al. Safety and efficacy of baricitinib at 24 weeks in patients with rheumatoid arthritis who have had an inadequate response to methotrexate. *Ann. Rheum. Dis.* **2015**, *74*, 333–340. [CrossRef] [PubMed]
22. XELJANZ (tofacitinib): Restriction d'Utilisation en cas de Risque élevé d'Embolie Pulmonaire. Available online: https://www.vidal.fr/actualites/23360/xeljanz_tofacitinib_restriction_d_utilisation_en_cas_de_risque_eleve_d_embolie_pulmonaire/ (accessed on 5 August 2020).
23. Paul, S.K.; Montvida, O.; Best, J.H.; Gale, S.; Pethoe-Schramm, A.; Sarsour, K. Effectiveness of biologic and non-biologic antirheumatic drugs on anaemia markers in 153,788 patients with rheumatoid arthritis: New evidence from real-world data. *Semin. Arthritis Rheum.* **2018**, *47*, 478–484. [CrossRef] [PubMed]
24. Choy, E.H. Clinical significance of Janus Kinase inhibitor selectivity. *Rheumatology* **2019**, *58*, 953–962. [CrossRef] [PubMed]
25. Smolen, J.S.; Genovese, M.C.; Takeuchi, T.; Hyslop, D.L.; Macias, W.L.; Rooney, T.; Chen, L.; Dickson, C.L.; Riddle Camp, J.; Cardillo, T.E.; et al. Safety Profile of Baricitinib in Patients with Active Rheumatoid Arthritis with over 2 Years Median Time in Treatment. *J. Rheumatol.* **2019**, *46*, 7–18. [CrossRef]
26. Taylor, P.C.; Moore, A.; Vasilescu, R.; Alvir, J.; Tarallo, M. A structured literature review of the burden of illness and unmet needs in patients with rheumatoid arthritis: A current perspective. *Rheumatol. Int.* **2016**, *36*, 685–695. [CrossRef]
27. Hewlett, S.; Cockshott, Z.; Byron, M.; Kitchen, K.; Tipler, S.; Pope, D.; Hehir, M. Patients' perceptions of fatigue in rheumatoid arthritis: Overwhelming, uncontrollable, ignored. *Arthritis Rheum.* **2005**, *53*, 697–702. [CrossRef]
28. Xie, F.; Yun, H.; Bernatsky, S.; Curtis, J.R. Brief Report: Risk of Gastrointestinal Perforation among Rheumatoid Arthritis Patients Receiving Tofacitinib, Tocilizumab, or Other Biologic Treatments. *Arthritis Rheumatol.* **2016**, *68*, 2612–2617. [CrossRef]
29. Nakajima, A.; Inoue, E.; Shimizu, Y.; Kobayashi, A.; Shidara, K.; Sugimoto, N.; Seto, Y.; Tanaka, E.; Taniguchi, A.; Momohara, S.; et al. Presence of comorbidity affects both treatment strategies and outcomes in disease activity, physical function, and quality of life in patients with rheumatoid arthritis. *Clin. Rheumatol.* **2015**, *34*, 441–449. [CrossRef] [PubMed]
30. Neubauer, S.; Cifaldi, M.; Mittendorf, T.; Ganguli, A.; Wolff, M.; Zeidler, J. Biologic TNF inhibiting agents for treatment of rheumatoid arthritis: Persistence and dosing patterns in Germany. *Health Econ. Rev.* **2014**, *4*, 32. [CrossRef] [PubMed]

3

Predictors of Flares in Patients with Rheumatoid Arthritis Who Exhibit Low Disease Activity

Yoon-Jeong Oh and Ki Won Moon *

Division of Rheumatology, Department of Internal Medicine, Kangwon National University School of Medicine, Chuncheon 24289, Korea; yjgark640@gmail.com
* Correspondence: kiwonmoon@kangwon.ac.kr;

Abstract: Using nationwide cohort data, this study evaluated predictors of flares in patients with rheumatoid arthritis (RA) who exhibit low disease activity (LDA) and the effects of flares on clinical outcomes. The Korean Observational Study Network for Arthritis (KORONA) registry is a nationwide Korean RA-specific cohort registry that collects data annually from 5.077 patients, with RA in 23 centers across South Korea. This study used data from 1.717 patients with RA who exhibited LDA [28–joint disease activity score (DAS28) < 3.2] at enrollment. Flares were defined as an increase in DAS28, compared with the previous value of > 1.2 or > 0.6, if the concurrent DAS28 was ≥ 3.2. Cox regression analysis was used to identify baseline predictors of flares. Of the 1.717 patients with RA, 566 (33.0%) experienced flares during the 2-year study period. An analysis of baseline characteristics of flare and non-flare groups revealed that more women and non-smokers were present in the flare group than in the non-flare group; the flare group also had higher scores on physician's and patient's pain and fatigue visual analogue scales (VAS) and the health assessment questionnaire (HAQ). In a multivariate analysis, physician's VAS score, hemoglobin level, and HAQ score were significant predictors of flares. A high physician's VAS score, low hemoglobin, and high HAQ score at baseline were significant predictors of flares in patients with RA who exhibited LDA.

Keywords: rheumatoid arthritis; flare; prediction

---

1. Introduction

The treatment of rheumatoid arthritis (RA) should target remission or low disease activity (LDA) in every patient [1]. If remission or LDA is reached, this state should be maintained. However, some patients with RA who exhibit LDA experience flares in their disease; up to 30% of patients with RA experience flares [2]. RA flares are typically defined as enhanced joint pain, joint swelling, and elevated levels of acute phase reactants. There is evidence that flares contribute to the worsening of subjective symptoms, joint damage, and other long-term outcomes [3]. In contrast, some patients remain in remission or exhibit LDA. The ability to predict flares when patients reach remission or LDA could facilitate decisions regarding treatment maintenance or reduction. There have been many studies about prediction for remission, but few studies about prediction for flare in RA. Bechman et al. evaluated predictors for flare in 97 RA patients who tapered tumor necrosis inhibitors after they reached sustained LDA [4]. They found baseline DAS28 and mental health status were predictors for flare. The results of another study of 93 RA patients with remission showed that ultrasound might be a useful tool for flare prediction [5]. In a recent study of 152 RA patients with LDA, health assessment questionnaire (HAQ) was a significant predictor for flare [6]. However, they were relatively small-sized and short-term observation studies. It is necessary to evaluate predicting factors for flare with large scale cohort database for long term period. Therefore, using nationwide cohort data, this study investigated predictors of flares in patients with RA who exhibited established LDA and the effects of flares on clinical outcomes in those patients.

2. Materials and Methods

2.1. *Study Subjects*

The Korean Observational Study Network for Arthritis (KORONA) is a nationwide Korean RA-specific cohort based on a prospective protocol and standard, with defined data collection instruments and annual patient follow-up. The KORONA cohort was established in July 2009 and enrolled patients with RA from July 2009 to December 2012. Patients aged 18 years or older who met the 1987 American College of Rheumatology criteria for diagnosis of RA were recruited by rheumatologists in 23 centers. KORONA is the largest nation-wide multicenter cohort; the demographic distribution of patients by age and sex in this cohort is comparable to that of all patients with RA in Korea. Demographic data, clinical features, laboratory data, radiologic findings, health-related outcomes, treatment modality, resource utilization, and health behaviors were collected from enrolled patients. A total of 5.077 patients were enrolled at baseline and participated in annual follow-ups. The KORONA protocol was approved by the Institutional Review Board (IRB) of all participating hospitals, and all participants were provided informed consent prior to enrollment in the study. This study was approved by the IRB of Kangwon National University Hospital.

2.2. *Clinical Assessment*

Data were collected regarding demographic and socioeconomic factors (i.e., sex, age, body mass index (BMI), smoking, marital status, regular exercise, and monthly income), as well as clinical factors (i.e., disease duration, familial history, side effects, poor adherence, malignancy, operation history, fracture history, and number of combined disorders). Disease activity and functional disability were measured using a physician's visual analogue scale (VAS), patient's pain VAS, global health VAS, fatigue VAS, 28-joint count disease activity score (DAS28)-ESR, EuroQol-5D (EQ-5D), and HAQ. Laboratory data were collected regarding rheumatoid factor, anti-citrullinated protein antibody (ACPA), hemoglobin, erythrocyte sedimentation rate (ESR), and C-reactive protein (CRP); medication data were collected regarding methotrexate, disease-modifying anti-rheumatic drugs, nonsteroidal anti-inflammatory drugs, steroids, and biologics.

2.3. *Definitions of LDA and RA Flares*

We enrolled patients with RA who exhibited LDA and had a baseline DAS28-ESR of <3.2. Flares were defined using validated criteria as a DAS28 increase of >1.2, compared with the previous value, or a DAS28 increase of >0.6 with concurrent DAS28 of ≥3.2 [7]. We investigated flares in patients with RA who exhibited LDA for total 2 years. After 1 year, we separated patients with and without flares into flare and non-flare groups according to a reported definition; patients without flares at 1 year were divided into flare and non-flare groups after 2 years. We allocated patients who had not experienced a flare for 2 years into the non-flare group and patients who had experienced at least one flare into the flare group (Figure 1). We compared their clinical outcomes after 2 years, including changes in physician's VAS score, patient's pain VAS score, global health VAS score, fatigue VAS score, DAS28-ESR, EQ-5D score, and HAQ score.

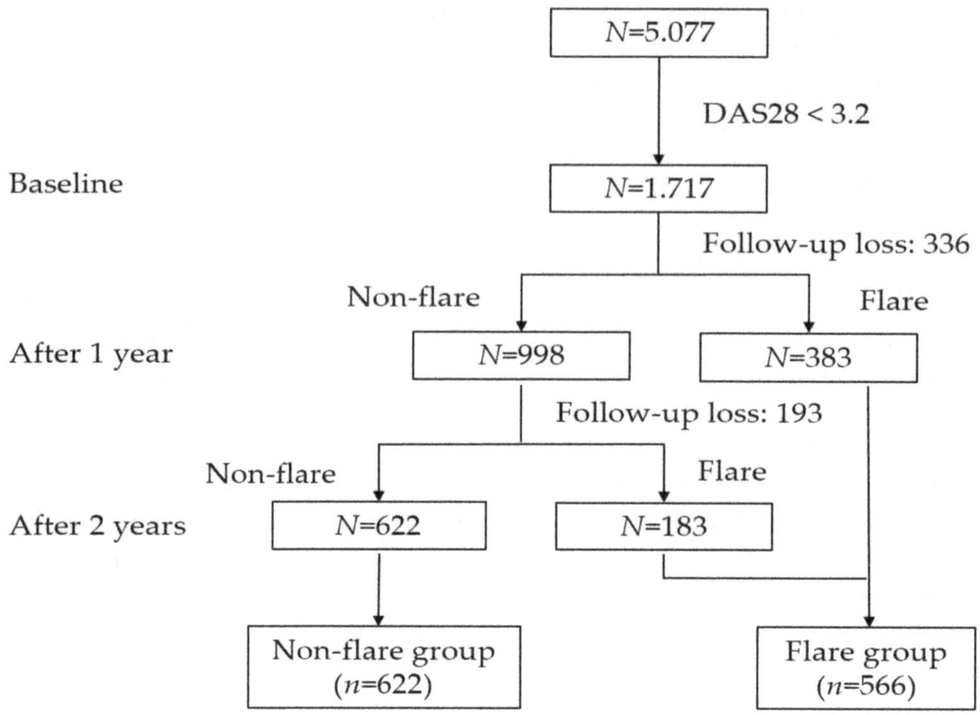

Figure 1. Flow chart of enrolled patients with rheumatoid arthritis during the 2-year study period.

2.4. Statistical Analysis

Descriptive analysis was used to summarize the baseline characteristics of both groups. The chi-squared test and Student's *t*-test were used to compare categorical and continuous variables, respectively. The multiple imputation method was used to input missing continuous values. To identify significant predictors of flares, univariate and multivariate Cox regression analyses were performed. These results were expressed as hazard ratios with 95% confidence intervals. Student's *t*-test was used to compare changes in clinical outcomes between groups at 2 years. Results with p-values < 0.05 were considered statistically significant. All analyses were performed using IBM SPSS ver. 24.0 (IBM Corp., Armonk, NY, USA).

3. Results

From the 5.077 patients with RA, we selected 1.717 patients who had DAS28-ESR < 3.2 at baseline. After 1 year, 336 patients were lost to follow-up, 338 patients had a flare, and 998 patients remained in a non-flare state. After the 2-year follow-up, 193 patients were lost to follow-up, 183 patients had a flare, and 622 patients remained in a non-flare state. Consequently, 622 patients were allocated to the non-flare group and 566 patients were allocated to the flare group (Figure 1).

Table 1 shows the baseline characteristics of both groups. The proportions of women and non-smokers were higher in the flare group, while the proportion of past smokers was higher in the non-flare group. The physician's VAS, patient's pain VAS, and fatigue VAS scores were higher in the flare group. The EQ-5D score was higher in the non-flare group, while the HAQ score was higher in the flare group. The proportion of ACPA-positive patients and levels of hemoglobin were both higher in the non-flare group. The flare group tended to have a longer disease duration and greater incidence of side effects, although these differences were not statistically significant. We divided flare group into first year and second year flare group to find out differences in patients flaring after first or second year (Supplementary Table S1). Most of baseline characteristics were not significantly different, except the frequency of poor adherents and NSAID users. The frequency of poor adherents was higher in second year flare group, and that of NSAID users was higher in first year flare group.

Table 1. Baseline characteristics of non-flare and flare groups.

	Non-Flare Group (n = 622)	Flare Group (n = 566)	p-Value
Female sex (%)	474 (76.2)	461 (81.4)	0.028 *
Age	52.55 ± 11.86	52.43 ± 12.11	0.862
BMI (kg/m^2)	22.68 ± 3.06	22.64 ± 3.38	0.817
Socioeconomic data			
Smoking status (%)			
Non-smoker	470 (75.6)	469 (82.9)	
Past smoker	87 (14.0)	45 (8.0)	0.002 **
Current smoker	65 (10.5)	52 (9.2)	
Married (%)	507 (81.5)	462 (81.6)	1.000
Regular exercise (%)	314 (50.5)	273 (48.2)	0.450
Monthly income (USD, %)			
<2.000	377 (60.6)	359 (63.4)	
2.000–4.999	212 (34.1)	188 (33.2)	0.221
≥5.000	33 (5.3)	19 (3.4)	
Clinical data			
Disease duration (years)	5.94 ± 6.02	6.56 ± 6.25	0.082
Familial history (%)	86 (13.8)	73 (12.9)	0.670
Side effects (%)	179 (28.8)	192 (33.9)	0.060
Poor adherent (%)	25 (4.0)	30 (5.3)	0.334
Malignancy (%)	50 (8.0)	50 (8.8)	0.676
Operation history (%)	73 (11.7)	83 (14.7)	0.144
Fracture history (%)	96 (15.4)	89 (15.7)	0.936
Number of combined disorders	0.88 ± 1.09	0.88 ± 1.03	0.953
Physician's VAS score (mm)	15.07 ± 12.90	18.73 ± 13.18	0.000 **
Pain VAS score (mm)	19.75 ± 20.63	22.28 ± 21.44	0.038 *
Global health VAS score (mm)	23.87 ± 20.55	24.80 ± 19.91	0.431
Fatigue VAS score (mm)	31.29 ± 26.25	35.14 ± 27.26	0.014 *
DAS28-ESR	2.32 ± 0.64	2.37 ± 0.63	0.299
EQ-5D score	0.82 ± 0.17	0.78 ± 0.17	0.001 **
HAQ score	0.27 ± 0.36	0.38 ± 0.45	0.000 **
Laboratory data			
RF (%)	310 (49.8)	279 (49.3)	0.862
ACPA (%)	447 (71.9)	372 (65.7)	0.024 *
Hemoglobin (g/dL)	13.02 ± 1.36	12.83 ± 1.26	0.015 *
ESR (mm/h)	14.26 ± 12.83	15.29 ± 12.28	0.157
CRP (mg/dL)	0.29 ± 1.01	0.31 ± 0.63	0.723
Medication data			
Methotrexate (%)	543 (87.3)	492 (86.9)	0.863
Number of DMARDs	1.76 ± 0.65	1.78 ± 0.65	0.625
NSAIDs (%)	483 (77.7)	431 (76.1)	0.581
Steroids (%)	426 (68.5)	382 (67.5)	0.756
Biologics (%)	37 (5.9)	28 (4.9)	0.523

ACPA, anti-citrullinated protein antibody; BMI, body mass index; CRP, C-reactive protein; DAS28, 28-joint count disease activity score; DMARD, disease modifying anti-rheumatic drug; ESR, erythrocyte sedimentation rate; EQ-5D, EuroQol-5D; HAQ, health assessment questionnaire; NSAID, non-steroidal anti-inflammatory drug; RF, rheumatoid factor; VAS, visual analogue scale; * $p < 0.05$; ** $p < 0.01$.

Table 2 shows the results of Cox proportional hazards analyses. A univariate analysis revealed that female sex, past smoker status, physician's VAS score, pain VAS score, fatigue VAS score, hemoglobin level, EQ-5D score, and HAQ score at baseline were significant predictors of flares. These variables were then entered into multivariate analysis. Flares were associated with enhancements of physician's VAS and HAQ scores, as well as with the reduction of hemoglobin level. We reanalyzed the data from 687 RA patients who exhibit remission (DAS28 < 2.6) at baseline level, with univariate and multivariate Cox regression models for flare prediction (Supplementary Table S2). The results were similar with those of data from RA patient with LDA. Physician's VAS, hemoglobin, and HAQ were still significant predictors for flare.

Table 2. Cox proportional hazards model of flares in patients with RA who exhibit low disease activity.

Variables	Univariate Analysis		Multivariate Analysis	
	HR (95% CI)	*p*-Value	HR (95% CI)	*p*-Value
Female sex	1.29 (1.04–1.59)	0.019 *	0.85 (0.60–1.21)	0.367
Smoking status				
Non-smoker	1 (reference)			
Past smoker	0.68 (0.50–0.93)	0.014 *	0.69 (0.46–1.03)	0.068
Current smoker	0.76 (0.57–1.01)	0.059	0.84 (0.57–1.22)	0.355
ACPA	0.86 (0.72–1.03)	0.095	0.92 (0.77–1.09)	0.324
Physician's VAS score	1.02 (1.01–1.02)	0.000 **	1.01 (1.01–1.02)	0.000 **
Pain VAS score	1.01 (1.00–1.01)	0.012 *	0.99 (0.99–1.00)	0.506
Fatigue VAS score	1.01 (1.00–1.01)	0.012 *	1.01 (0.99–1.01)	0.146
Hemoglobin	0.90 (0.84–0.95)	0.001 **	0.93 (0.87–0.99)	0.047 *
EQ–5D score	0.46 (0.29–0.73)	0.001 **	0.90 (0.49–1.65)	0.732
HAQ score	1.55 (1.30–1.86)	0.000 **	1.41 (1.12–1.78)	0.003 **

Acpa, anti-citrullinated protein antibody; CI, confidence interval, EQ-5D, EuroQol-5D; HAQ, health assessment questionnaire; HR, hazard ratio; VAS, visual analogue scale; * $p < 0.05$; ** $p < 0.01$.

Table 3 shows the changes in clinical outcomes at 2 years in the non-flare and flare groups. The changes in physician's VAS score, patient's pain VAS score, global health VAS score, fatigue VAS score, DAS28, EQ-5D score, and HAQ score differed significantly between the two groups.

Table 3. Changes from baseline levels for 2-year clinical outcomes in non-flare and flare groups.

Clinical Outcome	Non-Flare Group	Flare Group	*p*-Value
Physician's VAS score change	−4.40 ± 14.11	−1.18 ± 16.85	0.000 **
Pain VAS score change	0.83 ± 23.01	12.78 ± 28.77	0.000 **
Global health VAS score change	1.52 ± 22.72	15.20 ± 27.61	0.000 **
Fatigue VAS score change	−0.25 ± 31.35	7.81 ± 31.35	0.000 **
DAS28 change	−0.14 ± 0.71	1.07 ± 1.02	0.000 **
EQ-5D score change	0.01 ± 0.19	−0.05 ± 0.22	0.000 **
HAQ score change	0.00 ± 0.38	0.12 ± 0.49	0.000 **

DAS28, 28-joint count disease activity score; EQ-5D, EuroQol-5D; HAQ, health assessment questionnaire; VAS, visual analogue scale; ** $p < 0.01$.

4. Discussion

This study investigated the predictors of flare in patients with RA who exhibited LDA for 2 years using data from a large cohort. Of 1.717 patients with RA, 566 (33.0%) experienced a flare at least once during the 2-year study period. The prevalence of flare differs according to the follow-up interval, observation period, and flare definition. Flares can be defined based on subjective symptom worsening, a questionnaire, or a disease activity score, such as the DAS28. By investigating flares using a questionnaire every 6 months, Bykerk et al. reported that 95% of patients experienced at least one flare, with a frequency of 54~74% per evaluation during a 3-year study period [2]. However, in another study where flare was defined based on the DAS28, 46 (30%) of 152 patients experienced a flare within the 1-year study period [6]. Flares seem to be more frequent when defined based on subjective symptoms, rather than objective disease activity. The Outcome Measures in Rheumatology (OMERACT) initiative classified the RA flare criteria based on changes in the DAS28 [7]; therefore, we applied the flare criteria suggested by OMERACT. Recently, the OMERACT initiative recognized the limitations of the DAS28 in defining flare events and suggested a consensus-based core domain set to identify flares in patients with RA [8].

The baseline characteristics flare and non-flare groups were significantly different in regard to sex, smoking, subjective symptom, functional status, and laboratory results. However, when compared to the baseline characteristics of first year and second year flare groups, the only differences were adherence and NSAID use. The percentage of NSAID users were higher in first year flare group, which would have artificially lowered the baseline DAS28, leading to flare in earlier time. Our results indicated that baseline physician's VAS score, hemoglobin, and HAQ score predicted flares in patients with RA who exhibited LDA. Notably, the physician's VAS score predicted flares in patients with RA, whereas the patient's VAS score did not. Some studies have reported a discrepancy between patient's VAS and physician's VAS scores. Furu et al. reported that the inflammatory burden (e.g., swollen joint count, tender joint count, and CRP) mainly contributed to the physician's VAS score, whereas non-inflammatory variables (e.g., pain and functional disability) influenced the patient's VAS score [9]. The physician's VAS score could predict flares, whereas the patient's VAS score could not, because flares were defined based on DAS28-ESR in our study. The hemoglobin level is known to be negatively correlated with disease activity [10]. A low hemoglobin level has also been shown to predict radiographic progression in patients with RA. Möller et al. reported that a lower hemoglobin level was associated with greater radiographic damage, even in patients with LDA [11]. Furthermore, there have been reports that HAQ score is an independent predictor of flares in patients with RA. Bechman et al. investigated predictors of flares in 152 patients with RA who exhibited LDA; they found that a higher baseline HAQ score was a modest predictor of flares [6]. Another Korean study investigated potential predictors of sustained remission in 290 patients with RA from one center; the findings suggested that only the baseline HAQ score was independently associated with sustained remission (according to the DAS28-CRP) for 2 years [12]. Moreover, the HAQ score has been associated with mortality in patients with RA. Michaud et al. evaluated whether functional disability could predict mortality in 10.319 patients with RA from the USA; they found that HAQ and short-form 36 questionnaire scores were strongly associated with mortality risk in patients with RA [13]. Many other variables are known to predict flares in patients with RA. A study in the UK revealed that female sex, higher tender joint count, higher HAQ score, obesity, hypertension, and depression were independent predictors of flares [14]. Power Doppler activity has also been reported to predict flares. Saleem et al. showed that elevated baseline ultrasound power Doppler activity and functional disability were independently associated with the risk of flares [5]. Overall, the HAQ score appears to be an important predictor of flares, clinical outcomes, and radiographic progression.

We demonstrated that flares affected the clinical outcome in patients with RA who exhibited LDA for a relatively long duration. There were significant differences in clinical outcomes over 2 years between the non-flare and flare groups; these outcomes included changes in the physician's VAS score, patient's pain VAS score, global health VAS score, fatigue VAS score, EAS28, EQ-5D score, and HAQ score. Thus, flares contribute to worsening subjective symptoms, disease activity, quality of life, and functional capability; these results are consistent with the findings of other studies. One study evaluated the long-term effect of flares in 508 patients with RA (using data from The BeSt Study) over a period of 10 years. Greater numbers of flares were associated with greater disease activity, pain, morning stiffness, functional deterioration, and radiographic progression [3]. Another study observed 268 patients with RA who exhibited LDA for 2 years; the incidences of radiographic progression and functional impairment were higher in patients with flares than in patients without flares [15]. These results suggested that flares negatively affect clinical outcomes in patients with LDA, as well as patients with high disease activity.

There were some limitations in this study. First, we did not reflect a change in medication as a predictor of flares. However, our purpose was to identify significant predictors of flares at baseline. Second, we did not evaluate radiographic progression because the KORONA registry does not provide a quantitative measure of radiographic damage. Third, we could not monitor short-term flares, because a 1-year follow-up interval was used. However, we presume that our data provide an important perspective regarding the treatment of patients with RA who exhibit LDA. When patients with RA reach remission or LDA, many physicians consider reducing their medication in accordance with the management guidelines for RA [1]. However, it is necessary to individualize the treatment plans of patients who are expected to have flares, because flares are associated with symptom worsening, functional disability, and radiographic progression. Physicians should exercise caution when reducing the dose of medication if patients have a high physician's VAS score, low hemoglobin level, and high HAQ score in conjunction with LDA.

Author Contributions: Conceptualization, Y.-J.O. and K.W.M.; Data curation, Y.-J.O.; Formal analysis, Y.-J.O.; Methodology, Y.-J.O. and K.W.M.; Writing—original draft, Y.-J.O.; Writing—review and editing, K.W.M. All authors have read and agreed to the published version of the manuscript.

Acknowledgments: The authors acknowledge the invaluable contributions of all investigators in the Korean Observational Study Network for Arthritis (KORONA).

References

1. Smolen, J.S.; Landewe, R.B.M.; Bijlsma, J.W.J.; Burmester, G.R.; Dougados, M.; Kerschbaumer, A.; McInnes, I.B.; Sepriano, A.; van Vollenhoven, R.F.; de Wit, M.; et al. EULAR recommendations for the management of rheumatoid arthritis with synthetic and biological disease-modifying antirheumatic drugs: 2019 update. *Ann. Rheum. Dis.* **2020**, *79*, 685–699. [CrossRef] [PubMed]
2. Bykerk, V.P.; Shadick, N.; Frits, M.; Bingham, C.O., 3rd; Jeffery, I.; Iannaccone, C.; Weinblatt, M.; Solomon, D.H. Flares in rheumatoid arthritis: Frequency and management. A report from the BRASS registry. *J. Rheumatol.* **2014**, *41*, 227–234. [CrossRef] [PubMed]
3. Markusse, I.M.; Dirven, L.; Gerards, A.H.; van Groenendael, J.H.; Ronday, H.K.; Kerstens, P.J.; Lems, W.F.; Huizinga, T.W.; Allaart, C.F. Disease flares in rheumatoid arthritis are associated with joint damage progression and disability: 10-year results from the BeSt study. *Arthritis Res. Ther.* **2015**, *17*, 232. [CrossRef] [PubMed]
4. Bechman, K.; Sin, F.E.; Ibrahim, F.; Norton, S.; Matcham, F.; Scott, D.L.; Cope, A.; Galloway, J. Mental health, fatigue and function are associated with increased risk of disease flare following TNF inhibitor tapering in patients with rheumatoid arthritis: An exploratory analysis of data from the Optimizing TNF Tapering in RA (OPTTIRA) trial. *RMD Open* **2018**, *4*, e000676. [CrossRef] [PubMed]
5. Saleem, B.; Brown, A.K.; Quinn, M.; Karim, Z.; Hensor, E.M.; Conaghan, P.; Peterfy, C.; Wakefield, R.J.; Emery, P. Can flare be predicted in DMARD treated RA patients in remission, and is it important? A cohort study. *Ann. Rheum. Dis.* **2012**, *71*, 1316–1321. [CrossRef] [PubMed]
6. Bechman, K.; Tweehuysen, L.; Garrood, T.; Scott, D.L.; Cope, A.P.; Galloway, J.B.; Ma, M.H.Y. Flares in Rheumatoid Arthritis Patients with Low Disease Activity: Predictability and Association with Worse Clinical Outcomes. *J. Rheumatol.* **2018**, *45*, 1515–1521. [CrossRef] [PubMed]
7. van der Maas, A.; Lie, E.; Christensen, R.; Choy, E.; de Man, Y.A.; van Riel, P.; Woodworth, T.; den Broeder, A.A. Construct and criterion validity of several proposed DAS28-based rheumatoid arthritis flare criteria: An OMERACT cohort validation study. *Ann. Rheum. Dis.* **2013**, *72*, 1800–1805. [CrossRef] [PubMed]
8. Bartlett, S.J.; Barbic, S.P.; Bykerk, V.P.; Choy, E.H.; Alten, R.; Christensen, R.; den Broeder, A.; Fautrel, B.; Furst, D.E.; Guillemin, F.; et al. Content and Construct Validity, Reliability, and Responsiveness of the Rheumatoid Arthritis Flare Questionnaire: OMERACT 2016 Workshop Report. *J. Rheumatol.* **2017**, *44*, 1536–1543. [CrossRef]
9. Furu, M.; Hashimoto, M.; Ito, H.; Fujii, T.; Terao, C.; Yamakawa, N.; Yoshitomi, H.; Ogino, H.; Ishikawa, M.; Matsuda, S.; et al. Discordance and accordance between patient's and physician's assessments in rheumatoid arthritis. *Scand. J. Rheumatol.* **2014**, *43*, 291–295. [CrossRef] [PubMed]
10. Goyal, L.; Shah, P.J.; Yadav, R.N.; Saigal, R.; Agarwal, A.; Banerjee, S. Anaemia in Newly Diagnosed Patients of Rheumatoid Arthritis and its Correlation with Disease Activity. *J. Assoc. Physicians India* **2018**, *66*, 26–29. [PubMed]
11. Moller, B.; Everts-Graber, J.; Florentinus, S.; Li, Y.; Kupper, H.; Finckh, A. Low Hemoglobin and Radiographic Damage Progression in Early Rheumatoid Arthritis: Secondary Analysis From a Phase III Trial. *Arthritis Care Res.* **2018**, *70*, 861–868. [CrossRef] [PubMed]

12. Lee, K.E.; Choi, S.E.; Xu, H.; Kang, J.H.; Park, D.J.; Lee, S.S. HAQ score is an independent predictor of sustained remission in patients with rheumatoid arthritis. *Rheumatol. Int.* **2017**, *37*, 2027–2034. [CrossRef] [PubMed]
13. Michaud, K.; Vera-Llonch, M.; Oster, G. Mortality risk by functional status and health-related quality of life in patients with rheumatoid arthritis. *J. Rheumatol.* **2012**, *39*, 54–59. [CrossRef] [PubMed]
14. Cook, M.J.; Diffin, J.; Scire, C.A.; Lunt, M.; MacGregor, A.J.; Symmons, D.P.; Verstappen, S.M. Predictors and outcomes of sustained, intermittent or never achieving remission in patients with recent onset inflammatory polyarthritis: Results from the Norfolk Arthritis Register. *Rheumatology* **2016**, *55*, 1601–1609. [CrossRef] [PubMed]
15. Smolen, J.S.; Pedersen, R.; Jones, H.; Mahgoub, E.; Marshall, L. Impact of flare on radiographic progression after etanercept continuation, tapering or withdrawal in patients with rheumatoid arthritis. *Rheumatology* **2020**, *59*, 153–164. [CrossRef] [PubMed]

4

Sleep Quality in Patients with Rheumatoid Arthritis and Associations with Pain, Disability, Disease Duration and Activity

Igor Grabovac [1], Sandra Haider [1,*], Carolin Berner [2], Thomas Lamprecht [3], Karl-Heinrich Fenzl [3], Ludwig Erlacher [2,3], Michael Quittan [4,5] and Thomas E. Dorner [1]

1 Department of Social and Preventive Medicine, Centre for Public Health, Medical University of Vienna, Kinderspitalgasse 15, 1090 Vienna, Austria; igor.grabovac@meduniwien.ac.at (I.G.); thomas.dorner@meduniwien.ac.at (T.E.D.)

2 Department of Rheumatology and Osteology, Kaiser Franz Josef Hospital, Sozialmedizinisches Zentrum Süd, Kundratstrasse 3, 1100 Vienna, Austria; carolin.berner@gmx.net (C.B.); ludwig.erlacher@wienkav.at (L.E.)

3 Karl Landsteiner Institute for Autoimmune Diseases and Rheumatology, Kundratstrasse 3, 1100 Vienna, Austria; t.lamprecht@sportunion.at (T.L.); karlhfenzl@gmail.com (K.-H.F.)

4 Karl Landsteiner Institute for Remobilisation and Functional Health, Kundratstrasse 3, 1100 Vienna, Austria; michael.quittan@wienkav.at

5 Department of Physical Medicine and Rehabilitation, Kaiser-Franz-Josef-Hospital, Sozialmedizinisches Zentrum Süd, Kundratstrasse 3, 1100 Vienna, Austria

* Correspondence: sandra.a.haider@meduniwien.ac.at

Abstract: We aimed to assess the subjective sleep quality in patients with rheumatoid arthritis (RA) and its correlation with disease activity, pain, inflammatory parameters, and functional disability. In a cross-sectional study, patients with confirmed RA diagnosis responded to a questionnaire (consisting of socio-demographic data, the Health Assessment Questionnaire Disability Index, and the Medical Outcome Study Sleep Scale). Disease activity was assessed with the Clinical Disease Activity Index, and pain levels using the visual analogue scale. In addition, inflammatory markers (C-reactive protein, interleukin-6, and tumor necrosis factor alpha) were analyzed. Ninety-five patients were analyzed, predominantly female, with an average age of 50.59 (9.61) years. Fifty-seven percent reported non-optimal sleep duration, where functional disability (92.7% vs. 69.8%; $p = 0.006$) and higher median pain levels (3.75 (2.3–6.0) vs. 2.5 (2.0–3.5); $p = 0.003$) were also more prevalent. No differences in sociodemographic variables, disease duration or activity, inflammatory parameters, or use of biological and corticosteroid therapy were observed. The multivariate regression analysis showed that more intense pain was associated with a lower likelihood of optimal sleep (odds ratio (OR) = 0.68, 95% confidence interval (CI) 0.47–0.98, $p = 0.038$). Patients with RA report a high prevalence of non-optimal sleep, which is linked to pain level. Clinicians need to be aware of this issue and the potential effects on health and functional status.

Keywords: rheumatoid arthritis; sleep; sleep disorders; pain

---

1. Introduction

Rheumatoid arthritis (RA) is a chronic autoimmune disease characterized by changes in the synovium followed by joint swelling, pain, cartilage and bone destruction, and subsequent systemic inflammation [1]. The exact etiology is still unknown; however, 50% of the risk is attributable to genetics [2]. The incidence of RA has proven difficult to determine due to the wide variety of symptoms with which patients seek medical help and the associated delay in seeking medical help. However, the prevalence of RA has been reported at around 1% globally, with some countries showing reduced prevalence [3]. Overall, the disease is more prevalent in women and has been found to increase in prevalence with age, with the highest rates found in women older than 65 years [2]. Patients with RA have a higher mortality and morbidity burden, reduced quality of life, and higher disability [4].

As in other pain conditions, issues of sleep disturbance are of major concern in RA patients, who often report problems with poor sleep quality, issues with falling asleep, as well as feeling unrested and fatigued after sleep [5–8]. These subjective findings have been supported by polysomnographic studies where, compared to healthy controls, patients with RA showed lower overall sleep efficiency and more awakenings [9]. Sleep problems in people with chronic illness are associated with a variety of problems, including lower quality of life, psychological issues, cognitive decline, as well as higher morbidity and mortality [10]. In addition, patients with RA have reported that issues with sleep are of high personal importance [6].

A commonly reported symptom of RA is fatigue, which is described as an overwhelming feeling and different from normal tiredness, and is a multifactorial phenomenon associated with sleep issues, pain, depression, and functional limitations [11–13]. RA patients that experience fatigue, pain, and depression also have higher levels of physical disability. Several studies have indicated that pain and depression, as well as sleep quality through its relationship with pain and fatigue, are associated with functional disability [7].

Studies have shown that most sleep issues experienced in patients with RA stem from pain. In particular, difficulties with falling asleep and feeling tired after sleep have been found to be associated with lower pain threshold, pain severity, depression, and inflammation in patients with RA [14–17]. Pain has also been found to predict sleep disturbance over time, even without sleep issues affecting pain. Both pain and sleep issues were found to be associated with depression after a 2-year follow-up [18]. Interestingly, poor clinical management and increased disease activity of RA were found to be associated with lower daytime sleepiness (but also, as expected, with sleep problems), which may be explained by pain-related alertness [19]. However, the exact mechanisms of disease activity and sleep issues are not known. Sleep problems may also be of concern for clinicians working with RA patients, as reduced sleepiness was found in studies of patients taking certain biopharmaceutical therapies [17,20]. For instance, studies on abatacept have shown a positive influence on some aspects of sleep quality [21].

Sleep quality and its associations with disease activity parameters has not yet been researched in Austria. This paper presents the results of a larger cross-sectional study in patients with from RA. The complete study protocol was previously published [22]. The aim of the present study was to determine the prevalence of problems with sleep and its association with disease activity, pain levels, inflammatory parameters, and functional disability in patients with RA.

2. Materials and Methods

2.1. Participants

One hundred participants visiting the rheumatology outpatient clinic of the Kaiser Franz Josef Hospital in Vienna during their regularly scheduled visits were recruited for the purposes of this study [22]. Inclusion criteria were: age between 18 and 65 years; and fulfilled the RA diagnostic criteria according to the 2010 European League Against Rheumatism (EULAR) classification at the time of inclusion [23]. Additionally, patients with severe comorbidities (fibromyalgia, cancer, severe cardiovascular illness) as well as those that could affect handgrip strength measurements, and patients who refused or were not able to sign the informed consent were excluded from the study. The study took place from November 2015 to August 2016.

2.2. Methods

In this monocentric cross-sectional study, patients were approached during their regularly scheduled visits to a rheumatology outpatient clinic, and if they fitted the inclusion criteria, were asked to participate in the study. After informed consent was given, the participants were asked to fill out a questionnaire, after which measurements were taken.

2.3. *Questionnaire*

The questionnaire was made up of four parts and had 49 items in total—multiple choice and open-end questions—and took around 10 min to finish. The questionnaire was designed for self-reporting, with measurements of disease activity undertaken by a member of the study team. The questionnaire was provided in several languages, including German, English, and Turkish, and one with a combination of both Serbian and Croatian.

2.3.1. Socio-Demographic Data

This part consisted of multiple choice and open-end questions and was made up of 13 items covering socio-demographic characteristics of the sample (age, sex, marital status, education level, and current occupation). Additional questions on disease duration, as well as current therapy and comorbidities, were also asked.

2.3.2. Functional Disability

The Health Assessment Questionnaire Disability Index (HAQ-DI) was used to assess the patients' self-reported functional disability. This validated instrument consists of 20 questions divided into eight categories of functioning: dressing, rising, eating, walking, hygiene, reach, grip, and usual activities. The overall functional disability index is given as a final score, with values between 0 (no functional disability) and 3 (severe functional disability) [24].

2.3.3. Sleep Quality

Quality of sleep was assessed using the Medical Outcome Study Sleep Scale (MOS-SS). This questionnaire is recommended for use in RA patients and is made up of 12 items regarding the patient's sleep over the last 4 weeks. MOS-SS is a self-report questionnaire that scores six different sleep dimensions as scales and two additional indices: sleep disturbance (four items), daytime somnolence (three items), snoring (one item), awakening short of breath or with a headache (1 item), sleep adequacy (two items), and quantity of sleep (one item, which is not scored, but is an average number of hours spent asleep over the past 4 weeks). Optimal sleep is an added dichotomized variable derived from the quantity of sleep, where sleep is considered optimal if the reported duration is between 7 and 8 h, otherwise it is non-optimal. All items in the MOS-SS, expect for quantity of sleep, are given a numerical score, and the result is the sum of the individual scores, with the minimum value being 0 and the maximum 100. Higher scores indicate more of the named dimension, i.e., more sleep problems. The two indices—sleep problem indices I and II—are derived from several items, with sleep problem index I being derived from six items and sleep problem index II from nine items of the MOS-SS. As with the other items, higher values indicate more sleep problems [25]. Patients were also asked about their use of sleeping pills or pain medication.

2.4. *Measurements*

2.4.1. Disease Activity

Overall disease activity was measured by the Clinical Disease Activity Index (CDAI), which is a widely used and validated instrument. The CDAI score is derived as a sum of the subscales (Swollen 28-Joint Count, Tender 28-Joint Count, Patient Global Disease Activity, and Evaluator's Global disease Activity). Scores ≤ 2.8 are considered as remission, >2.8 and ≤ 10 as low disease activity, >10 and ≤ 22

as moderate, and >22 as high disease activity [26]. For the purposes of our study, we grouped the participants into two categories: remission and low disease activity in one group, and moderate and high disease activity as the other group.

2.4.2. Pain Intensity

Pain was assessed using the visual analogue scale (VAS), ranging from 0 to 10, whereby a higher number indicates a higher pain intensity [27].

2.4.3. Inflammatory Parameters

The inflammatory parameters of C-reactive protein (CRP; mg/dL), interleukin-6 (IL-6; pg/mL), and tumor necrosis factor alpha (TNF-alpha; ng/mL) were obtained through analysis of the patients' blood samples at the Department of Laboratory Medicine of Kaiser Franz Josef Hospital, where the research was conducted on the same day.

2.5. Statistical Analysis

Kolmogorov-Smirnov tests, Shapiro-Wilk tests, and histogram analysis were employed to determine the data distribution. Descriptive statistics were recorded for each variable, with the quantitative variables shown as mean values and standard deviation, and in the case of a non-normal distribution, as median and 25–75 percentile values. Differences between groups were calculated with T-tests or Mann-Whitney U-tests, depending on the data distribution. Chi-square tests were used for the differences between categorical variables. Spearman's rank order correlation was used for the possible correlations between the dimensions of sleep quality, as derived from the MOS-SS, and the other scores (age, disease duration, pain, CDAI score and HAQ-DI score). A multivariate logistical regression analysis was performed in order to assess the characteristics that were associated with the MOS-SS-derived dichotomized variable of optimal sleep (reported sleep between 7 and 8 h was deemed "optimal", while reported sleep under 7 h and more than 8 h was deemed "non-optimal"). Variables which showed significant correlations in the univariate correlation analysis were included in the multivariate logistic regression model. All *p*-values under 0.05 were considered statistically significant. The analysis was performed using SPSS for Windows version 24.0 software (IBM, Armonk, NY, USA).

2.6. Ethics Approval

The study complied with Good Clinical Practice standards and the Helsinki Declaration. The study was approved by the Ethical Committee of the City of Vienna (number: EK 15-173-0915).

3. Results

A total of 140 patients that fulfilled the inclusion criteria were approached and asked to participate. However, 14 (10%) were not interested to take part, 6 (4.3%) declined due to time constraints, 4 (2.9%) didn't speak any of the languages the surveys were available in and 22 (15.7%) did not complete the necessary measurements, which left 95 (67.9%) patients available for analysis. Approximately two-thirds of the study population were female, with an age range from 22 to 65 years. The mean duration of the disease in our population was around 9 years, with 80% receiving therapy with disease-modifying anti-rheumatic drugs (DMRAD). According to the HAQ-DI score, 21.4% of the participants had a level of functional disability, and the median pain score was 3.0 (2.0–5.0) out of 10. Differences according to optimal sleep duration were found in pain intensity, level of functional disability, and use of non-steroidal anti-inflammatory drugs (NSAID) and disease-modifying drugs. Additional information about the study participants is provided in Table 1.

Table 1. Sociodemographic and disease-related variables stratified by optimal sleep duration.

Variable	Total (n = 95)	Non-Optimal Sleep Duration (n = 54)	Optimal Sleep Duration (n = 41)	p
Age; mean (SD)	50.59 (9.61)	49.98 (9.14)	51.39 (10.25)	0.482
Sex				
Male	32.6%	33.3%	31.7%	0.867
Female	67.4%	66.7%	68.3%	
Relationship status				
In a relationship	73.7%	77.8%	68.3%	0.298
Not in a relationship	26.3%	22.2%	31.7%	
Education level				
Primary level	15.8%	13.0%	19.5%	0.434
Secondary level	72.6%	77.8%	65.9%	
Tertiary level	11.6%	9.3%	14.6%	
Employment status				
Employed	61.1%	63.0%	58.5%	0.661
Unemployed	38.9%	37.0%	41.5%	
Disease duration in months; median (Q_{25}–Q_{75})	72.0 (36.0–141.0)	78.0 (36.0–144.0)	60.0 (28.50–138.0)	0.452
Pain intensity; median (Q_{25}–Q_{75})	3.0 (2.0–5.0)	3.75 (2.3–6.0)	2.5 (2.0–3.5)	0.003
Functional disability				
No disability	79.8%	69.8%	92.7%	0.006
Disability	20.2%	30.2%	7.3%	
Disease activity				
Remission	29.5%	29.6%	30.8%	0.726
Low	33.7%	31.5%	38.5%	
Moderate	26.3%	27.8%	25.6%	
High	8.4%	11.1%	5.1%	
Inflammatory parameters				
CRP (mg/dL); median (Q_{25}–Q_{75})	3.20 (1.10–6.70)	3.05 (1.07–7.05)	2.70 (1.00–5.55)	0.594
TNF-α (g/mL); median (Q_{25}–Q_{75})	1.60 (0.56–2.35)	1.65 (0.54–2.89)	1.60 (0.64–2.32)	0.884
IL-6 (pg/mL); median (Q_{25}–Q_{75})	3.89 (1.98–7.91)	4.47 (2.04–9.67)	3.44 (1.72–6.18)	0.179
Therapy				
Disease-modifying drugs	81.1%	72.2%	92.7%	0.012
Biologicals	43.2%	50.0%	34.1%	0.122
Corticosteroid	16.8%	18.5%	14.6%	0.616
Non-steroidal anti-inflammatory	14.7	7.4%	24.4%	0.021
Other medication	55.8%	55.6%	56.1%	0.958

SD = standard deviation. Differences between groups were calculated with the T-test, Mann-Whitney U test dependent on data distribution. Chi-square test was used for differences between categorical variables.

Overall, our patients reported non-optimal sleep duration in 56.8% of cases, with a mean duration of sleep over the past 4 weeks of 6.5 (1.3) h. The median score of sleep problem index I was 30.0, with the score of sleep problem index II being slightly higher at 32.2 points. The highest reported median value of the six items was in sleep adequacy, which indicates that our patients, in general, feel well rested and have enough sleep during the night. Furthermore, most of the participants did not take pain medication or sleeping pills. Other results regarding the MOS-SS score and the other sleep quality variables are presented in Table 2. In terms of disease activity, patients with moderate and high disease activity reported fewer hours asleep in comparison to patients with low disease activity or in remission (6.7 (1.2) vs. 6.0 (1.2); p = 0.009).

Table 2. Sleep characteristics of the study participants.

Sleep-Related Variables	$n = 95$
Sleep disturbance median (Q_{25}–Q_{75})	32.5 (15.0–51.2)
Snoring; median (Q_{25}–Q_{75})	40.0 (20.0–60.0)
Shortness of breath or headache; median (Q_{25}–Q_{75})	20.0 (0.0–30.0)
Sleep adequacy; median (Q_{25}–Q_{75})	60.0 (30.0–80.0)
Somnolence; median (Q_{25}–Q_{75})	26.6 (13.3–46.6)
Sleep problem index I; median (Q_{25}–Q_{75})	30.0 (16.6–46.6)
Sleep problem index II; median (Q_{25}–Q_{75})	32.2 (18.3–47.8)
Optimal sleep	
Yes	43.2%
No	56.8%
Pain medication for sleep	
Daily	8.2%
Up to 3 times a week	7.2%
More than 3 times a week	5.2%
Up to 3 times a month	12.4%
Never	67.0%
Sleeping pills	
Daily	9.3%
Up to 3 times a week	2.1%
More than 3 times a week	1.0%
Up to 3 times a month	4.1%
Never	83.5%
Hours asleep; mean (SD)	6.5 (1.3)

SD = standard deviation.

The relationship between the sleep domains of the MOS-SS and age, disease duration in months, pain intensity, disease activity, and functional disability scores was investigated, as seen in Table 3. Pain intensity was the only variable that was correlated with all the MOS-SS domains, with the highest coefficient being a medium positive correlation with sleep problem index II ($r = 0.406$; $p < 0.001$). Overall, the strongest relationship was found between functional disability and sleep problem index II ($r = 0.516$; $p < 0.001$). Disease activity had significant small to medium positive correlations with sleep disturbance, snoring, shortness of breath or snoring, and sleep problem indices I and II, while a significant negative correlation was observed between sleep duration and the sleep adequacy domains of the MOS-SS, as seen in Table 3.

Table 3. Spearman's rank order correlation of variables that correlate with the sleep domains.

Variable	Hours Asleep	Sleep Disturbance	Snoring	Awakening Short of Breath or with Headache	Sleep Adequacy	Sleep Somnolence	Sleep Problem Index I	Sleep Problem Index II
Age	0.077	−0.007	0.204 *	−0.012	0.043	−0.027	−0.050	−0.040
Disease duration	−0.177	0.201 *	−0.037	0.134	−0.066	0.184	0.173	0.149
Pain intensity (VAS)	−0.350 **	0.379 **	0.228 *	0.279 **	−0.297 **	0.305 **	0.374 **	0.406 **
CDAI Score	−0.304 **	0.324 **	0.210 *	0.249 *	−0.275 **	0.148	0.293 **	0.322 **
HAQ-DI Score	0.247 *	0.459 **	0.090	0.298 **	−0.436 **	0.390 **	0.495 **	0.516 **

* $p < 0.005$; ** $p < 0.001$; VAS: visual analogue scale, CDAI: Clinical Disease Activity Index, HAQ-DI: Health Assessment Questionnaire Disability Index.

According to the multivariate logistical regression analysis, pain intensity was the only variable that was significantly associated with optimal sleep duration, where more severe pain was associated with a reduced likelihood of optimal sleep, as seen in Table 4.

Table 4. Logistic regression model of variables associated with optimal sleep duration.

Variable	OR	95% CI	*p*
Age	1.03	0.99–1.09	0.162
Pain VAS scale	0.68	0.47–0.98	0.038
HAQ-DI score	0.53	0.19–1.45	0.215
CDAI score	1.02	0.95–1.11	0.544
Disease duration	1.00	0.99–1.01	0.756

OR: odds ratio, 95% CI: 95% confidence interval, VAS: visual analogue scale, CDAI: Clinical Disease Activity Index, HAQ-DI: Health Assessment Questionnaire Disability Index.

4. Discussion

Our study showed that, in an investigated sample of patients with RA, problems with sleep are common, with 56.8% of the participants reporting non-optimal sleep duration. Interestingly, the MOSS-SS sleep adequacy scale showed high results, meaning that our participants were, overall, satisfied with their sleep quality. Studies have shown that up to 70% of patients with RA suffer from problems with sleep, ranging from difficulty falling asleep to difficulty maintaining sleep or suffering from daytime sleepiness [6,28]. Several studies found that higher disease activity is associated with sleep problems [9,29,30]. A study by Wolfe et al. [8] showed that sleep disturbance could be attributed to RA in up to 42% of cases, linking sleep disturbance to pain, mood, and disease activity. Similarly, a Korean study found decreasing subjective sleep quality as the disease activity was increasing [30]. Conversely, studies have also found that reducing the active inflammatory disease and the arthritic process have a positive effect on sleep quality [31]. However, a connection between disease activity and sleep quality has not been universally reported in studies. For example, Hirsch et al. [5] reported overall disturbed sleep in patients with RA, but found no association with inflammatory disease activity. These results have often been questioned as the study population was very small (only 19 patients), which may be the reason for the lack of association. Our study, although five times larger in terms of the sample size, also found no difference in sleep quality in patients with different disease activity, as shown in Table 1. In terms of the relationship between the CDAI scores and the sleep domains of the MOS-SS, seen in Table 3, only low to moderate correlations were found. The only significant difference in sleep characteristics between patients with different disease activity was found in sleep duration, where patients in the moderate/high disease activity group reported shorter sleep duration.

The mechanism of how disease activity influences sleep quality is not completely clear; however, most studies have suggested the connection with joint stiffness and pain. In a study by Wolfe and Michaud [8], pain was shown to be one of the most common underlying reasons leading to problems with sleep, with a recent study of Austrian patients with chronic pain also reporting notable sleep disturbance [32]. Chronic pain and associated sleep issues are a risk for developing depressive symptoms in patients with RA, which in turn may have an additional influence as depression has been reported as being a predictive factor for poor quality of sleep [15,19]. In our study population, pain levels were generally low; however, there was a significant difference based on reported optimal sleep duration, as seen in Table 1, where lower pain levels were found in those patients who reported optimal sleep duration. The multivariate logistic regression model showed pain intensity to be a predictor for non-optimal sleep in our population, as shown in Table 4. Furthermore, pain was found to be correlated with all the domains of sleep quality in the MOS-SS, having a negative relationship with hours spent sleeping and the sleep adequacy domain. More pain intensity is positively correlated with sleep disturbance, snoring and shortness of breath, somnolence, and both sleep problem indices. Recent evidence shows that lower sleep quality lowers the threshold of pain and increases the pain intensity in patients with RA [9,16,19].

The relationship between RA therapy and medication used for sleep quality is ambivalent. Some studies have reported the use of biological medication as having a positive effect on sleep quality, with longitudinal observations of anti-TNF substances also reporting greater sleep quality improvements in patients on abatacept in comparison to methotrexate. A trial investigating the effectiveness of indomethacin on sleep quality showed indomethacin to be superior to placebo in a questionnaire-based study. However, polysomnographic studies investigating sleep patterns in patients using NSAIDs showed no changes in sleep patterns or sleep quality in patients with RA. In our study, as presented in Table 1, patients who reported optimal sleep duration were found to more often use disease-modifying drugs and NSAIDs, which is probably connected to their analgesic effect. More research, especially blinded longitudinal studies, should be done to investigate the effects of medication on sleep quality of RA patients, as most cross-sectional studies have reported no connection [8,30,33].

Functional disability was found to be associated with sleep quality, as patients with RA often experience difficulties with the activities of daily living, which was found to be associated with fatigue and sleep disturbance. In addition, disability often leads to greater depression, which in turn leads to sleep disturbance. A relationship between pain, depression, sleep, and functional disability has been shown in numerous studies, which may mean that there is a casual relationship, as pain, fatigue, and depression inhibit normal daily productivity, causing sleep disorders and disability, which then contribute to pain, fatigue, depression, and disability [8,9,33]. In our study, patients who were categorized as having functional disability reported significantly non-optimal sleep duration, as seen in Table 1. However, the HAQ-DI score showed no association with optimal sleep in the multivariate logistic regression model and, interestingly, was found to have a positive relationship with sleep duration. Furthermore, functional disability was found to be significantly correlated with somnolence, shortness of breath, sleep adequacy, sleep disturbance, and both sleep problem indices as shown in Table 3.

The relationship between age and sleep quality in patients with RA is unclear, but some studies have reported lower sleep quality in older patients [30,33]. Our study showed only a small positive correlation with age and snoring, but no correlation with other dimensions of the MOS-SS as seen in Table 3. Other studies have often failed to report an association between age and sleep problems in patients with RA [8,19]. This was confirmed by our logistic regression model, where there was no significant association found between optimal sleep duration and age.

Finally, the study limitations need to be addressed. The cross-sectional study design does not allow for causal conclusions on the relationships between variables. Longitudinal studies need to be performed in order to examine the possible casual associations. Secondly, although the MOS-SS is recommended for use in RA, it refers to a time frame of the previous 4 weeks, which may affect the results due to recall bias. Additionally, we haven't reported on the body mass index (BMI) which is also a potential confounder. Finally, as patients were recruited to the study by their physicians, it is possible that the results are an underestimation due to reporting bias. The relatively small sample size might prevent the generalizability of the study results, as well as the higher proportion of women; however, this is to be expected in a RA patient population. Furthermore, our population consisted of men and women of working age, which may also contribute to the reduced sleep problems.

Given our results and the noted associations of pain and non-optimal sleep in patients with RA it is important to alert the clinical community working with RA patients. Sleep as well as pain assessments should be systematically included in the clinical assessments [34]. However, such monitoring will not be effective in reducing the burden of pain and sleep problems in RA patients, unless appropriate treatment is also not provided. Albeit research indicates the associations of pain and sleep disturbances, pharmacotherapy for these comorbidities receives little attention, and there is yet to be a consensus or evidence based treatment algorithms [35]. Additionally, a recent meta-analysis indicated that non-pharmacological sleep treatments (including physiotherapy, meditation, massage, sleep restriction therapy and sleep scheduling, imagery exercises, and others) were associated with large improvements in sleep quality [36]. In conclusion, there is a high frequency of non-optimal sleep duration in patients with RA of working age; however, these patients are mostly satisfied with their overall sleep quality. Our study further shows the association between higher pain levels and non-optimal sleep. Physicians working with RA patients need to be aware of the sleep issues in this population and include pharmacological and psychological interventions as these may have a positive effect on sleep quality, and in turn on psychological wellbeing, physical wellbeing, and functional disability. Future studies could focus on sleep quality in newly diagnosed patients, as well as longitudinal studies need to be implemented in order to see if improvements in sleep contribute to reduction of depression, pain, and functional disability.

Author Contributions: Conceptualization: C.B., K.H.F., L.E. and T.E.D. Methodology: C.B., K.H.F., L.E. and T.E.D. Investigation and data curation: C.B., T.L., K.H.F. and M.Q. Formal analysis: I.G., S.H. and T.E.D. Writing-original draft preparation: I.G., S.H. and T.E.D. Writing-final review and editing: all authors. Funding acquisition: C.B., K.H.F., M.Q. and L.E.

Acknowledgments: The authors would like to thank Mark Ackerley for the professional proofreading.

References

1. McInnes, I.B.; Schett, G. The pathogenesis of rheumatoid arthritis. *N. Engl. J. Med.* **2011**, *365*, 2205–2219. [CrossRef] [PubMed]
2. Scott, D.L.; Wolfe, F.; Huizinga, T.W. Rheumatoid arthritis. *Lancet* **2010**, *376*, 1094–1108. [CrossRef]
3. Gibofsky, A. Overview of epidemiology, pathophysiology, and diagnosis of rheumatoid arthritis. *Am. J. Manag. Care* **2012**, *18*, S295–S302. [PubMed]
4. Kiltz, U.; van der Heijde, D. Health-related quality of life in patients with rheumatoid arthritis and in patients with ankylosing spondylitis. *Clin. Exp. Rheumatol.* **2009**, *27*, S108–S111. [PubMed]
5. Hirsch, M.; Carlander, B.; Verge, M.; Tafti, M.; Anaya, J.M.; Billiard, M.; Sany, J. Objective and subjective sleep disturbances in patients with rheumatoid arthritis. *Arthritis Rheum.* **1994**, *37*, 41–49. [CrossRef] [PubMed]
6. Kirwan, J.; Heiberg, T.; Hewlett, S.; Hughes, R.; Kvien, T.; Ahlmen, M.; Boers, M.; Minnock, P.; Saag, K.; Shea, B.; et al. Outcomes from the patient perspective workshop at OMERACT 6. *J. Rheumatol.* **2003**, *30*, 868–872. [PubMed]
7. Luyster, F.S.; Chasens, E.R.; Wasko, M.C.; Dunbar-Jacob, J. Sleep quality and functional disability in patients with rheumatoid arthritis. *J. Clin. Sleep Med.* **2011**, *7*, 49–55. [PubMed]
8. Wolfe, F.; Michaud, K.; Li, T. Sleep disturbance in patients with rheumatoid arthritis: Evaluation by medical outcomes study and visual analog sleep scales. *J. Rheumatol.* **2006**, *33*, 1942–1951. [PubMed]
9. Mahowald, M.W.; Mahowald, M.L.; Bundlie, S.R.; Ytterberg, S.R. Sleep fragmentation in rheumatoid arthritis. *Arthritis Rheum.* **1989**, *32*, 974–983. [CrossRef] [PubMed]
10. Kripke, D.F.; Garfinkel, L.; Wingard, D.L.; Klauber, M.R.; Marler, M.R. Mortality associated with sleep duration and insomnia. *Arch. Gen. Psychiatry* **2002**, *59*, 131–136. [CrossRef] [PubMed]
11. Hewlett, S.; Cockshott, Z.; Byron, M.; Kitchen, K.; Tipler, S.; Pope, D.; Hehir, M. Patients' perceptions of fatigue in rheumatoid arthritis: Overwhelming, uncontrollable, ignored. *Arthritis Rheum.* **2005**, *53*, 697–702. [CrossRef] [PubMed]
12. Loppenthin, K.; Esbensen, B.A.; Jennum, P.; Ostergaard, M.; Tolver, A.; Thomsen, T.; Midtgaard, J. Sleep quality and correlates of poor sleep in patients with rheumatoid arthritis. *Clin. Rheumatol.* **2015**, *34*, 2029–2039. [CrossRef] [PubMed]
13. Pollard, L.C.; Choy, E.H.; Gonzalez, J.; Khoshaba, B.; Scott, D.L. Fatigue in rheumatoid arthritis reflects pain, not disease activity. *Rheumatology (Oxford)* **2006**, *45*, 885–889. [CrossRef] [PubMed]
14. Cakirbay, H.; Bilici, M.; Kavakci, O.; Cebi, A.; Guler, M.; Tan, U. Sleep quality and immune functions in rheumatoid arthritis patients with and without major depression. *Int. J. Neurosci.* **2004**, *114*, 245–256. [CrossRef] [PubMed]

15. Lee, Y.C.; Chibnik, L.B.; Lu, B.; Wasan, A.D.; Edwards, R.R.; Fossel, A.H.; Helfgott, S.M.; Solomon, D.H.; Clauw, D.J.; Karlson, E.W. The relationship between disease activity, sleep, psychiatric distress and pain sensitivity in rheumatoid arthritis: A cross-sectional study. *Arthritis Res. Ther.* **2009**, *11*, R160. [CrossRef] [PubMed]
16. Power, J.D.; Perruccio, A.V.; Badley, E.M. Pain as a mediator of sleep problems in arthritis and other chronic conditions. *Arthritis Rheum.* **2005**, *53*, 911–919. [CrossRef] [PubMed]
17. Vgontzas, A.N.; Zoumakis, E.; Lin, H.M.; Bixler, E.O.; Trakada, G.; Chrousos, G.P. Marked decrease in sleepiness in patients with sleep apnea by etanercept, a tumor necrosis factor-alpha antagonist. *J. Clin. Endocrinol. Metab.* **2004**, *89*, 4409–4413. [CrossRef] [PubMed]
18. Nicassio, P.M.; Wallston, K.A. Longitudinal relationships among pain, sleep problems, and depression in rheumatoid arthritis. *J. Abnorm. Psychol.* **1992**, *101*, 514–520. [CrossRef] [PubMed]
19. Westhovens, R.; Van der Elst, K.; Matthys, A.; Tran, M.; Gilloteau, I. Sleep problems in patients with rheumatoid arthritis. *J. Rheumatol.* **2014**, *41*, 31–40. [CrossRef] [PubMed]
20. Zamarron, C.; Maceiras, F.; Mera, A.; Gomez-Reino, J.J. Effect of the first infliximab infusion on sleep and alertness in patients with active rheumatoid arthritis. *Ann. Rheum. Dis.* **2004**, *63*, 88–90. [CrossRef] [PubMed]
21. Wells, G.; Li, T.; Tugwell, P. Investigation into the impact of abatacept on sleep quality in patients with rheumatoid arthritis, and the validity of the mos-sleep questionnaire sleep disturbance scale. *Ann. Rheum. Dis.* **2010**, *69*, 1768–1773. [CrossRef] [PubMed]
22. Berner, C.; Erlacher, L.; Quittan, M.; Fenzl, K.H.; Dorner, T.E. Workability and muscle strength in patients with seropositive rheumatoid arthritis: Survey study protocol. *JMIR Res. Protoc.* **2017**, *6*, e36. [CrossRef] [PubMed]
23. Aletaha, D.; Neogi, T.; Silman, A.J.; Funovits, J.; Felson, D.T.; Bingham, C.O.; Birnbaum, N.S.; Burmester, G.R.; Bykerk, V.P.; Cohen, M.D.; et al. 2010 rheumatoid arthritis classification criteria: An american college of rheumatology/european league against rheumatism collaborative initiative. *Arthritis Rheum.* **2010**, *62*, 2569–2581. [CrossRef] [PubMed]
24. Fries, J.F.; Spitz, P.; Kraines, R.G.; Holman, H.R. Measurement of patient outcome in arthritis. *Arthritis Rheum.* **1980**, *23*, 137–145. [CrossRef] [PubMed]
25. Smith, M.T.; Wegener, S.T. Measures of sleep: The insomnia severity index, medical outcomes study (MOS) sleep scale, pittsburgh sleep diary (PSD), and pittsburgh sleep quality index (PSQI). *Arthritis Rheum.* **2003**, *49*, S184–S196. [CrossRef]
26. Anderson, J.; Caplan, L.; Yazdany, J.; Robbins, M.L.; Neogi, T.; Michaud, K.; Saag, K.G.; O'Dell, J.R.; Kazi, S. Rheumatoid arthritis disease activity measures: American college of rheumatology recommendations for use in clinical practice. *Arthritis Care Res.* **2012**, *64*, 640–647. [CrossRef] [PubMed]
27. Hawker, G.A.; Mian, S.; Kendzerska, T.; French, M. Measures of adult pain: Visual analog scale for pain (VAS pain), numeric rating scale for pain (NRS pain), mcgill pain questionnaire (MPQ), short-form McGill pain questionnaire (SF-MPQ), chronic pain grade scale (CPGS), short form-36 bodily pain scale (SF-36 BPS), and measure of intermittent and constant osteoarthritis pain (ICOAP). *Arthritis Care Res. (Hoboken)* **2011**, *63*, S240–S252. [PubMed]
28. Drewes, A.M.; Nielsen, K.D.; Hansen, B.; Taagholt, S.J.; Bjerregard, K.; Svendsen, L. A longitudinal study of clinical symptoms and sleep parameters in rheumatoid arthritis. *Rheumatology (Oxford)* **2000**, *39*, 1287–1289. [CrossRef]
29. Crosby, L.J. Factors which contribute to fatigue associated with rheumatoid arthritis. *J. Adv. Nurs.* **1991**, *16*, 974–981. [CrossRef] [PubMed]
30. Son, C.N.; Choi, G.; Lee, S.Y.; Lee, J.M.; Lee, T.H.; Jeong, H.J.; Jung, C.G.; Kim, J.M.; Cho, Y.W.; Kim, S.H. Sleep quality in rheumatoid arthritis, and its association with disease activity in a Korean population. *Korean J. Intern. Med.* **2015**, *30*, 384–390. [CrossRef] [PubMed]
31. Wells, G.; Li, T.; Maxwell, L.; Maclean, R.; Tugwell, P. Responsiveness of patient reported outcomes including fatigue, sleep quality, activity limitation, and quality of life following treatment with abatacept for rheumatoid arthritis. *Ann. Rheum. Dis.* **2008**, *67*, 260–265. [CrossRef] [PubMed]
32. Keilani, M.; Crevenna, R.; Dorner, T.E. Sleep quality in subjects suffering from chronic pain. *Wien. Klin. Wochenschr.* **2018**, *130*, 31–36. [CrossRef] [PubMed]

33. Sariyildiz, M.A.; Batmaz, I.; Bozkurt, M.; Bez, Y.; Cetincakmak, M.G.; Yazmalar, L.; Ucar, D.; Celepkolu, T. Sleep quality in rheumatoid arthritis: Relationship between the disease severity, depression, functional status and the quality of life. *J. Clin. Med. Res.* **2014**, *6*, 44–52. [PubMed]
34. Stubbs, B.; Vancampfort, D.; Thompson, T.; Veronese, N.; Carvalho, A.F.; Solmi, M.; Mugisha, J.; Schofield, P.; Matthew Prina, A.; Smith, L.; et al. Pain and severe sleep disturbance in the general population: Primary data and meta-analysis from 240,820 people across 45 low- and middle-income countries. *Gen. Hosp. Psychiatry* **2018**, *53*, 52–58. [CrossRef] [PubMed]
35. Doufas, A.G.; Panagiotou, O.A.; Ioannidis, J.P. Concordance of sleep and pain outcomes of diverse interventions: An umbrella review. *PLoS ONE* **2012**, *7*, e40891. [CrossRef] [PubMed]
36. Tang, N.K.; Lereya, S.T.; Boulton, H.; Miller, M.A.; Wolke, D.; Cappuccio, F.P. Nonpharmacological treatments of insomnia for long-term painful conditions: A systematic review and meta-analysis of patient-reported outcomes in randomized controlled trials. *Sleep* **2015**, *38*, 1751–1764. [CrossRef] [PubMed]

5

The Potential Role of Genomic Medicine in the Therapeutic Management of Rheumatoid Arthritis

Marialbert Acosta-Herrera *, David González-Serna and Javier Martín

Institute of Parasitology and Biomedicine López-Neyra, CSIC, Av. del Conocimiento 17. Armilla, 18016 Granada, Spain; sna.david@ipb.csic.es (D.G.-S.); javiermartin@ipb.csic.es (J.M.)
* Correspondence: m.acostaherrera@ipb.csic.es

Abstract: During the last decade, important advances have occurred regarding understanding of the pathogenesis and treatment of rheumatoid arthritis (RA). Nevertheless, response to treatment is not universal, and choosing among different therapies is currently based on a trial and error approach. The specific patient's genetic background influences the response to therapy for many drugs: In this sense, genomic studies on RA have produced promising insights that could help us find an effective therapy for each patient. On the other hand, despite the great knowledge generated regarding the genetics of RA, most of the investigations performed to date have focused on identifying common variants associated with RA, which cannot explain the complete heritability of the disease. In this regard, rare variants could also contribute to this missing heritability as well as act as biomarkers that help in choosing the right therapy. In the present article, different aspects of genetics in the pathogenesis and treatment of RA are reviewed, from large-scale genomic studies to specific rare variant analyses. We also discuss the shared genetic architecture existing among autoimmune diseases and its implications for RA therapy, such as drug repositioning.

Keywords: rheumatoid arthritis; pharmacogenomics; methotrexate; anti-TNF; personalized medicine

---

1. Introduction

Human diversity includes, among other things, differential responses to environmental stimuli and stress and differential drug metabolism and responses to treatments [1]. This diversity has been in part revealed since the completion of the Human Genome Project, which has improved our knowledge on the underlying biology of disease and its impact on healthcare. Since the completion of this project, a developing field called "personalized medicine" has aimed to adapt medical care to the genetic background of individuals, including diagnosis, therapeutic decision-making, health outcomes, and policy implications of clinical use (National Human Genome Research Institute (NHGRI), https://www.genome.gov/).

The most common variations in human DNA are single-nucleotide polymorphisms (SNPs), which are simple substitutions of one nucleotide for another at a given position [2]. These variants can map into gene coding or noncoding sequences of the genome, and the most studied to date have been biallelic SNPs [3]. These genome variations have been the objects of study of personalized medicine, which has revealed how subtle variations on the genome are responsible for large differences in health outcomes [1]. The main goal of these studies has been to detect associations between genetic variants and a trait or disease [4]. Under the common disease/common variant hypothesis, where common diseases are likely influenced by common genetic variants in the population, traditionally these studies have been focused on candidate gene association studies by comparing the allele frequency of the SNPs in affected and unaffected individuals. If the observed differences were not due to random chance, then they were considered to be associated with the disease or trait. Gene selection was based on the plausible mechanisms involved in disease pathogenesis [1]. At present and thanks to advances in genotyping technology and information on the haplotype structure of the genome, these studies are now directed toward the entire genome in so-called genome-wide association studies (GWAS). These studies are hypothesis-free (where no prior knowledge of the biological pathways is needed) and hypothesis-generating, as the new associations may pinpoint new molecular mechanisms never anticipated before. However, larger sample sizes are needed to fulfill the stringent threshold for statistical significance due to multiple testing adjustments (p-value $< 5 \times 10^{-8}$).

Since the completion of the first GWAS in 2005 [5], human genetic research has been a key player in the discovery of new biological pathways underlying complex diseases. Furthermore, genomic information may allow for the identification of patients with differential abilities to metabolize drugs, assess drug reactions, and eventually develop individualized treatments [6,7], which is the aim of the "treat-to-target" approach, where the therapeutic goal is to reach a state of disease remission or at least lower disease activity [8]. Many challenges continue to exist in the interpretation of GWAS findings. However, it has become fairly clear that drug development with genetic support from GWAS data is twice as likely to reach approval for its use as without this support (from phase I to approval in the different phases of drug development) [9]. In a recent paper by Nelson et al., the authors assessed publicly available GWAS results and combined them with the commercial Informa Pharmaprojects database. They found that those genes associated with a broad spectrum of human diseases were enriched in target genes for drugs approved in the United States or the European Union, highlighting the importance of the provided genetic knowledge in different drug mechanisms. The authors commented that this correlation may be explained by genes with prominent phenotypic changes that might be the most responsive to drug-induced alterations [9].

Interestingly, there have been several cases of genes associated with diseases that were effective drug targets. The most recognized examples have come from cholesterol metabolism: For instance, the gene *HMGCR*, which is associated with serum cholesterol levels [10], is a known target for statins. Additionally, loss of function mutations on the gene *PCSK9* have been described [11], and drugs targeting this gene have been developed to lower cholesterol levels [12,13].

2. Genetics and Therapy Development in Rheumatoid Arthritis

In the largest genetic study of rheumatoid arthritis (RA) conducted to date [14], the authors performed a three-stage transethnic meta-analysis in a total of 100,000 subjects of European and Asian ancestry by evaluating ~10,000,000 SNPs. Stage 1 revealed 57 associated loci, including 17 that had never been associated with the disease before. Afterward, the authors conducted a two-stage replication study for the suggestive loci (p-value $< 5 \times 10^{-6}$), and in a combined analysis of the three stages, they were able to identify 42 novel loci in the transethnic meta-analysis, increasing the total number of RA risk loci to 101. These loci represented a total of 377 associated genes, which were then prioritized. Interestingly, the authors assessed if the associated loci were useful for drug target validation and how approved drugs for other diseases could be linked to RA risk genes, evaluating not only the protein products of the RA-associated genes but also the protein that directly interacts with them in a protein–protein interaction network. From this assessment, the authors found a significant overlap among approved drugs for the treatment of RA that targeted genes that were considered RA risk genes in genetic studies. Additionally, the authors assessed if approved drugs for other diseases might be linked to RA risk genes for drug repurposing and found, for instance, the cases of *CDK4* and *CDK6*, which are targets for different types of cancer treatment [15] and have been shown to weaken disease activity in animal models of RA [15]. All of the above evidence has shown how human genetic data have the potential to be integrated with other biological information to enable personalized treatments.

3. Pharmacogenomic Studies in Rheumatoid Arthritis

Personalized medicine offers fully customized drugs for each person, attending to different conditions (such as genetics), and pharmacogenomics may identify the individual patient's signature, which could help guide treatment selection mostly based on an assessment of genomic variants associated with drug response [16]. In the case of RA, even though routine compounds are suitable for most patients, some of them may not have the desired effect when taking these drugs [17], and patients may remain with high disease activity and irreversible joint damage as a possible consequence [18]. Thus, biomarkers are needed that help us differentiate between good and bad responses to a specific treatment. Although great progress has been made in this field, the objective of finding predictive genetic biomarkers that clearly define the grade of response to specific treatments is still far away. The use of genetic variants as biomarkers that could predict the response to a specific treatment has several advantages, as these variants are stable and would remain unaltered, unlike changes in gene expression and epigenetics, which are highly dependent on the environment.

3.1. Genomic Predictors of Methotrexate

Methotrexate (MTX) is a disease-modifying antirheumatic drug (DMARD) used as first-line therapy in RA [19], and great efforts have been directed toward finding predictive biomarkers of MTX response. These investigations have been centered on analyzing genes involved in the key molecular pathways affecting MTX absorption and metabolism, such as cytokine production, drug transport, or nucleotide synthesis. Most of these studies have been carried out in common variants, and the strongest and most replicated association discovered was for the solute carrier family 19 member 1 (*SLC19A1*) gene, a transport carrier that allows MTX to enter cells. In this sense, several studies have reported the association of rs1051266 with intracellular MTX levels. Indeed, a recent meta-analysis that included 12 studies confirmed the association of this polymorphism with MTX treatment response [20]. The methylene tetrahydrofolate reductase (*MTHFR*) gene has also been one of the most studied genes, as the encoded enzyme is key in the MTX pathway (C677T and A1298C are the most commonly studied SNPs associated with MTX response and toxicity [21,22]): However, there were conflicting results in two meta-analyses [23,24]. Another commonly studied polymorphism is the 347 C/G in the 5-aminoimidazole-4-carboxamide ribonucleotide formyltransferase (*ATIC*) gene, which was recently meta-analyzed in six studies that confirmed its association with responses to and the toxicity of MTX [23]. Although many other SNPs have been associated with MTX response and toxicity in RA patients, most of them could not be replicated, and the studies had a low sample size.

To date, two GWAS have been performed involving MTX activity: Senapati et al. [25] suggested multiple novel risk loci involved in thymidylate synthase (*TYMS*) regulation, and Taylor et al. [26] conducted the largest GWAS on MTX response, including 1424 early RA patients and finding a suggestive association in neuregulin 3 (*NRG3*). However, the authors were not able to replicate their findings. Thus, the existence of predictive models, including several SNPs from different genes associated with MTX response, could help in the creation of specific treatments associated with pharmacogenomics. In this regard, the clinical pharmacogenetics model of response to MTX (CP-MTX) combined clinical data and genotypes from four SNPs in MTX-relevant genes (*MTHF1D rs2236225, ATIC rs2372536, AMPD1 rs17602729*, and *ITPA rs1127354*). This model has been validated in independent samples, and its benefits and costs have been addressed in informing MTX prescription [27–30]. However, it is expected that many more genes and many more variants with modest effects contribute to response to treatment, and therefore the model could be further improved by including other clinical variables and updating the list of associated genetic variants.

The major RA susceptibility region corresponds to the human leukocyte antigen (HLA) locus, concretely the *HLA-DRB1* shared epitope, which is associated with a more severe disease [31]. In this regard, there have been conflicting results regarding the association of the shared epitope with a lower MTX efficacy in monotherapy [32,33]. An additional *HLA-DR* locus, *HLA-DRB4*, is present in nearly all haplotypes containing the strongest associated *HLA-DRB1* alleles [34]. In this sense, a recent study compared MTX responders and nonresponders after stratification for *HLA-DRB4* expression, highlighting that response to MTX is characterized by preponderant innate and adaptive immune activation, respectively [35].

3.2. Genomic Predictors of Tumor Necrosis Factor (TNF) Inhibitors

Biomarkers able to predict responses to biological drugs have received lots of attention. In this line, tumor necrosis factor inhibitors (TNFis) remain the most commonly prescribed first-line biologics, even when these drugs are ineffective in up to 30% of patients [36]. Thus, more than 40 candidate gene studies and 6 GWAS regarding the response to TNFi have been performed to date [37,38]. One of the most commonly studied SNPs is G308A in the tumor necrosis factor (*TNFA*) gene, which has been associated with increased efficacy of adalimumab, infliximab, and etanercept [39,40]. In addition, Krintel et al. [41] suggested an association with *PDE3A–SLCO1C1*, and their results were replicated in a Spanish independent sample, reaching genome-wide significance [42]. Other SNPs linked to clinical responses in anti-TNF therapy are located on protein tyrosine phosphatase receptor type C (*PTPRC*): This has been consistently replicated in independent study samples [43–45]. Other studies have assessed the involvement of the fragment C gamma receptor (*FCGR*) [46], the TNF receptor superfamily 1B (*TNFRSF1B*) [47], and mitogen-activated protein kinase 14 (*MAPK14*) [40] in associations with TNFi response.

There have been many research efforts regarding the HLA region and its implication for TNFi therapies, as it happens with MTX response. One of the first associations observed involved two *HLA-DRB1* alleles encoding the shared epitope, including * 0101 and * 0404, in response to etanercept [48]. Subsequent studies confirmed the association of this locus with anti-TNF treatments, specifically with amino acid positions 11, 71, and 74 [31]. Furthermore, another study identified polymorphisms within the nonclassical *HLA-E* gene associated with clinical outcomes of anti-TNF therapy in female RA patients [49]. Unfortunately, the majority of studies that have been performed to date regarding pharmacogenetics of anti-TNF therapies have revealed inconsistent results, and very few of them have been robustly replicated [50,51]. This lack of replicability might be due to a lack of consensus on the criteria to differentiate the good versus bad responders [51].

Interestingly, a recent study by Sieberts et al. [52] showed that common SNP information did not improve significantly predictive models in contrast to other clinical information. They performed a community-based open assessment and tested a wide range of state-of-the-art modeling methodologies. However, the authors acknowledged some limitations when the number of risk loci was in the order of hundreds or when heritability was better explained by rare variations or copy number variants, which could be the case for TNFi response.

3.3. Other Genomic Predictors

DMARDs such as MTX and biologic agents are the drugs mainly used to treat RA. Nevertheless, there are other concomitant therapies used to reduce inflammation and relieve pain, including steroids and nonsteroidal anti-inflammatory drugs (NSAIDs). In this regard, two studies observed a better response to the combination therapy of MTX and glucocorticoids in RA patients carrying the mutant allele of the C3435T SNP of the multidrug-resistance 1 (*MDR1*) gene [53,54]. In addition, a subsequent study observed that carrying the SNP G2677A/T of the *MDR1* gene was significantly associated with response to glucocorticoid treatment [55].

On the other hand, like other DMARDs, one-third of patients fail to respond to MTX treatment, either because of inefficiency or adverse events. In those cases, leflunomide represents a potential drug to replace MTX as a treatment [19]. Pharmacogenetic studies have indicated an impact of the CYP1A2*1F mutation of the cytochrome P450 family 1 subfamily A member 2 (*CYP1A2*) gene in leflunomide toxicity [56]. Another study observed that rs3213422 of the dihydroorotate dehydrogenase (*DHODH*) gene was associated with leflunomide toxicity and therapeutic effects [57]. Finally, estrogen receptor gene SNPs could influence the response to leflunomide therapy in females [58].

4. Genetic Studies and Rare Variants

International collaborative efforts have enabled the recruitment of unprecedented sizes of study participants: However, despite the increase in statistical power, today many challenges still exist in the interpretation of findings from GWAS, which cannot account for much of the heritability of diseases (the "missing heritability" paradigm) [59]. The possible contribution of rare variants (minor allele frequency (MAF) < 0.5%) with larger effects on this missing heritability has been much discussed, and this may require composite association tests of overall "mutational load" in cases and controls. These genetic variations are not well captured by genotyping arrays. Therefore, whole-exome (WES) and whole-genome sequencing (WGS) is the technology of choice: It generates millions of sequence reads in parallel, increasing the speed and generated volume of data [59]. This technology will provide a deeper characterization of genetic variants within the entire frequency spectrum and their relationship to disease susceptibility.

The impact of rare human variations on complex diseases is still limited, but for most traits, there is an inverse relationship between allele frequency and effect size, with the rarer alleles being those with a higher odds ratio, resembling those in Mendelian disorders [6]. A limited number of studies have assessed these rare genetic variations with success in RA. Li et al. [60] performed a WES study on 124 subjects from an Asian population. The authors identified genes enriched in deleterious variants using a gene burden test that were involved in innate immunity pathways and contributed to the risk of RA in a Han Chinese population. In the case of Bowes et al. [61], the authors utilized an interesting approach by exploiting low-frequency GWAS data by partitioning the data into gene-centric bins and collapsing their genotypes into a single count. The authors were able to prioritize signals mapping to *TNFAIP3*, a known RA risk gene, with replicable results in independent study samples. This study highlighted a previously known hypothesis where genes harboring common variants also harbored rarer variants with larger effects that had not been captured in previous GWAS [59]. To further confirm this hypothesis, Diogo et al. [62] assessed the contribution of rare and common variants in candidate genes from GWAS on RA by deep-sequencing their protein-coding regions. The authors exome-sequenced 25 RA risk genes from GWAS and found an aggregation of rare variants in *IL2RA* and *IL2RB*. They additionally assessed the aggregate contribution of low-frequency and common coding variants and observed an enrichment of coding variants with a nominal signal of association. The authors finally acknowledged the need for increased sample sizes to comprehensively identify variants distributed across the allele frequency spectrum associated with RA.

Interestingly, Eyre et al. [63] evaluated if previously associated linkage peaks were enriched with rare variants. They found that the distributions of rare variants differed significantly among regions showing linkage evidence, but that this effect depended on associations in the HLA region. Along the same line, Bang et al. [64] performed targeted exome sequencing in Korean RA patients. They comprehensively analyzed 10,588 variants of 398 genes and identified 13 nonsynonymous variants with nominal associations and 17 genes with nominal burden signals. However, the authors did not find a significant enrichment of coding variants associated with RA. As mentioned before, there has been little success in confidently identifying rare variants associated with RA, and in the majority of cases, studies have been performed on biological candidate genes. Only completely resequencing the whole exome or genome will eventually pinpoint novel genes harboring rare variants and significantly contribute to the proper assessment of RA heritability.

Interestingly, rare variants have also been evaluated in responses to treatment, as in the case of TNFi. Cui et al. [65] sequenced the coding region of 750 genes in 1,094 RA patients treated with anti-TNF. The authors applied single-variant association, gene-based associations, and gene set analyses in TNF pathway genes: However, they were not able to identify rare and low-frequency protein-coding variants that significantly contributed to anti-TNF treatment response.

5. Shared Genetics in Autoimmunity and Drug Repurposing

Autoimmune disorders, such as RA, are very heterogeneous and share symptoms, risk genes, comorbidities, and familial aggregation, suggesting a common genetic architecture that is extensively recognized in autoimmunity [66,67]. Several studies have revealed these shared genetics through simple comparisons of the associated genes [68], as was the case in a study conducted by our group, where González-Serna et al. [69] considered the association of a rare variant in the *TNFSF13B* gene with RA and replicated this association in systemic lupus erythematosus (SLE) patients. *TNFSF13B* encodes the (B-cell activating factor) BAFF cytokine, which is essential for B-cell homeostasis and the regulation of B-cell maturation, differentiation, and survival [70]. The assessed risk variant is functional and results in a shorter transcript that escapes microRNA inhibition, leading to an increase in the production of the BAFF cytokine. Additionally, it has been observed that this variant is strongly associated with high levels of total IgG and IgM and with reduced monocyte counts [71]. Our reported association with RA highlights the BAFF variant as a common genetic risk factor in autoimmunity. Interestingly, belimumab is a monoclonal antibody targeting human BAFF and was the first targeted therapy approved for SLE [72–74], highlighting the potential for drug repurposing for genetically related conditions.

Recently, a combination of large-scale studies including different phenotypes has proven to be a very useful tool in the identification of shared genetic risk variants and shared pathways involved in these diseases in a systematic fashion [75–77]. The first example is a meta-GWAS that combined 10 pediatric autoimmune diseases and revealed new shared loci with immunoregulatory functions [78]. Another big study by Ellinghaus et al. [79] combined immunochip data from five chronic inflammatory diseases and also found shared genetic loci in seronegative conditions, such as ankylosing spondylitis, psoriasis, primary sclerosing cholangitis, Crohn's disease, and ulcerative colitis. Furthermore, two recent studies by Marquez et al. [80] and Acosta-Herrera et al. [81] assessed the genetic overlap in autoimmune diseases by combining Immunochip and GWAS data, respectively. The authors identified shared risk variants in autoimmunity and common biological mechanisms and suggested novel genes as drug targets as well as promising candidates for drug repurposing. These studies highlighted how a combination of different related phenotypes can contribute to the determination of causal variants in disease and might help in the establishment of personalized treatments.

6. Future Perspectives

Most RA treatments are nonspecific and are based on a trial-and-error approach. Ineffective treatments affect the quality of life of patients, increasing the probability of adverse events and the eventual development of greater disabilities. It is therefore crucial to develop mechanisms to deliver the right drug to the right patients, which is the ultimate goal of precision medicine. In this sense, a small number of associated loci have been consistently replicated regarding treatment response: One of the reasons might be the lack of statistical power of these assessments. RA is a complex and heterogeneous disease, and therefore the response to treatment in RA patients might be influenced by multiple effects of many genetic variants with moderate effect sizes. Thus, larger studies with proper statistical power and more homogeneous classifications of phenotypes are needed to validate previous findings.

Moreover, response to treatment is normally measured with several composite scores, including the disease activity score (DAS-28), American College of Rheumatology, or EULAR response criteria, hindering the possibility of validating the results. Well-described and homogenous measures of responses are critical in pharmacogenetic studies. Additionally, most studies have investigated common genetic variations in treatment response, and a broader assessment of the frequency spectrum might be necessary.

Establishing the association of genes should continue with discoveries of the functional implications of such associations. As commented before, genetic variants alone do not fully explain the risk of suffering the disease, making complementary strategies necessary, including transcriptomic and epigenomics approaches: For example, Plant et al. [82] identified differentially methylated positions on DNA as biomarkers of response to TNFi therapy. Additionally, Spiliopoulou et al. [83] showed that the CD39 and CD40 pathways could be relevant to targeted drug therapy by evaluating the relations of TNFi responses with locus-specific scores, constructed from GWAS data.

Finally, the integration of all of this information with clinical and environmental data will eventually help us to identify the biological mechanisms underlying the development of the disease, to establish accurate biomarkers for patient stratification, and to tailor treatment to genetic architecture, increasing the probability of obtaining an adequate response to a particular drug and eventually achieving disease remission.

Author Contributions: Conceptualization: M.A.-H., D.G.-S., J.M.; original draft preparation: M.A.H., D.G.-S.; review and editing: M.A.-H., J.M. All authors read and approved the final manuscript.

References

1. Subramanian, G.; Adams, M.D.; Venter, J.C.; Broder, S. Implications of the human genome for understanding human biology and medicine. *JAMA* **2001**, *286*, 2296–2307. [CrossRef] [PubMed]
2. Lander, E.S.; Linton, L.M.; Birren, B.; Nusbaum, C.; Zody, M.C.; Baldwin, J.; Devon, K.; Dewar, K.; Doyle, M.; FitzHugh, W.; et al. Initial sequencing and analysis of the human genome. *Nature* **2001**, *409*, 860–921. [PubMed]
3. 1000 Genomes Project Consortium; Abecasis, G.R.; Auton, A.; Brooks, L.D.; DePristo, M.A.; Durbin, R.M.; Handsaker, R.E.; Kang, H.M.; Marth, G.T.; McVean, G.A. An integrated map of genetic variation from 1092 human genomes. *Nature* **2012**, *491*, 56–65. [PubMed]
4. Timpson, N.J.; Greenwood, C.M.T.; Soranzo, N.; Lawson, D.J.; Richards, J.B. Genetic architecture: the shape of the genetic contribution to human traits and disease. *Nat. Rev. Genet.* **2018**, *19*, 110–124. [CrossRef] [PubMed]
5. Klein, R.J.; Zeiss, C.; Chew, E.Y.; Tsai, J.Y.; Sackler, R.S.; Haynes, C.; Henning, A.K.; SanGiovanni, J.P.; Mane, S.M.; Mayne, S.T.; et al. Complement factor H polymorphism in age-related macular degeneration. *Science* **2005**, *308*, 385–389. [CrossRef] [PubMed]
6. Bomba, L.; Walter, K.; Soranzo, N. The impact of rare and low-frequency genetic variants in common disease. *Genome Biol.* **2017**, *18*, 77. [CrossRef] [PubMed]
7. Lauschke, V.M.; Milani, L.; Ingelman-Sundberg, M. Pharmacogenomic biomarkers for improved drug therapy-recent progress and future developments. *AAPS J.* **2017**, *20*, 4. [CrossRef] [PubMed]
8. Burmester, G.R.; Pope, J.E. Novel treatment strategies in rheumatoid arthritis. *Lancet* **2017**, *389*, 2338–2348. [CrossRef]
9. Nelson, M.R.; Tipney, H.; Painter, J.L.; Shen, J.; Nicoletti, P.; Shen, Y.; Floratos, A.; Sham, P.C.; Li, M.J.; Wang, J.; et al. The support of human genetic evidence for approved drug indications. *Nat. Genet.* **2015**, *47*, 856–860. [CrossRef]
10. Kathiresan, S. Lp(a) lipoprotein redux–from curious molecule to causal risk factor. *N. Engl. J. Med.* **2009**, *361*, 2573–2574. [CrossRef]
11. Youngblom, E.; Pariani, M.; Knowles, J.W. Familial Hypercholesterolemia. In *GeneReviews®*; Adam, M.P., Ardinger, H.H., Pagon, R.A., Wallace, S.E., Bean, L.J.H., Stephens, K., Amemiya, A., Eds.; University of Washington: Seattle, WA, USA, 1993.
12. Lopez, D. Inhibition of PCSK9 as a novel strategy for the treatment of hypercholesterolemia. *Drug News Perspect.* **2008**, *21*, 323–330. [CrossRef] [PubMed]
13. Steinberg, D.; Witztum, J.L. Inhibition of PCSK9: A powerful weapon for achieving ideal LDL cholesterol levels. *Proc. Natl. Acad. Sci. USA* **2009**, *106*, 9546–9547. [CrossRef] [PubMed]

14. Okada, Y.; Wu, D.; Trynka, G.; Raj, T.; Terao, C.; Ikari, K.; Kochi, Y.; Ohmura, K.; Suzuki, A.; Yoshida, S.; et al. Genetics of rheumatoid arthritis contributes to biology and drug discovery. *Nature* **2014**, *506*, 376–381. [CrossRef] [PubMed]
15. Sekine, C.; Sugihara, T.; Miyake, S.; Hirai, H.; Yoshida, M.; Miyasaka, N.; Kohsaka, H. Successful treatment of animal models of rheumatoid arthritis with small-molecule cyclin-dependent kinase inhibitors. *J. Immunol.* **2008**, *180*, 1954–1961. [CrossRef] [PubMed]
16. Kurko, J.; Besenyei, T.; Laki, J.; Glant, T.T.; Mikecz, K.; Szekanecz, Z. Genetics of rheumatoid arthritis—A comprehensive review. *Clin. Rev. Allergy Immunol.* **2013**, *45*, 170–179. [CrossRef] [PubMed]
17. Cronstein, B.N. Pharmacogenetics in the rheumatic diseases, from prêt-à-porter to haute couture. *Nat. Clin. Pract. Rheumatol.* **2006**, *2*, 2–3. [CrossRef] [PubMed]
18. Finckh, A.; Liang, M.H.; van Herckenrode, C.M.; de Pablo, P. Long-term impact of early treatment on radiographic progression in rheumatoid arthritis: A meta-analysis. *Arthritis Rheum.* **2006**, *55*, 864–872. [CrossRef]
19. Smolen, J.S.; Landewe, R.; Breedveld, F.C.; Buch, M.; Burmester, G.; Dougados, M.; Emery, P.; Gaujoux-Viala, C.; Gossec, L.; Nam, J.; et al. EULAR recommendations for the management of rheumatoid arthritis with synthetic and biological disease-modifying antirheumatic drugs: 2013 update. *Ann. Rheum. Dis.* **2014**, *73*, 492–509. [CrossRef]
20. Li, X.; Hu, M.; Li, W.; Gu, L.; Chen, M.; Ding, H.; Vanarsa, K.; Du, Y. The association between reduced folate carrier-1 gene 80G/A polymorphism and methotrexate efficacy or methotrexate related-toxicity in rheumatoid arthritis: A meta-analysis. *Int. Immunopharmacol.* **2016**, *38*, 8–15. [CrossRef]
21. Van Ede, A.E.; Laan, R.F.; Blom, H.J.; Huizinga, T.W.; Haagsma, C.J.; Giesendorf, B.A.; de Boo, T.M.; van de Putte, L. The C677T mutation in the methylenetetrahydrofolate reductase gene: a genetic risk factor for methotrexate-related elevation of liver enzymes in rheumatoid arthritis patients. *Arthritis Rheum.* **2001**, *44*, 2525–2530. [CrossRef]
22. Berkun, Y.; Levartovsky, D.; Rubinow, A.; Orbach, H.; Aamar, S.; Grenader, T.; Abou Atta, I.; Mevorach, D.; Friedman, G.; Ben-Yehuda, A. Methotrexate related adverse effects in patients with rheumatoid arthritis are associated with the A1298C polymorphism of the MTHFR gene. *Ann. Rheum. Dis.* **2004**, *63*, 1227–1231. [CrossRef] [PubMed]
23. Lee, Y.H.; Bae, S.C. Association of the ATIC 347 C/G polymorphism with responsiveness to and toxicity of methotrexate in rheumatoid arthritis: a meta-analysis. *Rheumatol. Int.* **2016**, *36*, 1591–1599. [CrossRef] [PubMed]
24. Owen, S.A.; Lunt, M.; Bowes, J.; Hider, S.L.; Bruce, I.N.; Thomson, W.; Barton, A. MTHFR gene polymorphisms and outcome of methotrexate treatment in patients with rheumatoid arthritis: analysis of key polymorphisms and meta-analysis of C677T and A1298C polymorphisms. *Pharmacogenom. J.* **2013**, *13*, 137–147. [CrossRef] [PubMed]
25. Senapati, S.; Singh, S.; Das, M.; Kumar, A.; Gupta, R.; Kumar, U.; Jain, S.; Juyal, R.C.; Thelma, B.K. Genome-wide analysis of methotrexate pharmacogenomics in rheumatoid arthritis shows multiple novel risk variants and leads for TYMS regulation. *Pharmacogenet. Genomics* **2014**, *24*, 211–219. [CrossRef] [PubMed]
26. Taylor, J.C.; Bongartz, T.; Massey, J.; Mifsud, B.; Spiliopoulou, A.; Scott, I.C.; Wang, J.; Morgan, M.; Plant, D.; Colombo, M.; et al. Genome-wide association study of response to methotrexate in early rheumatoid arthritis patients. *Pharmacogenom. J.* **2018**, *18*, 528–538. [CrossRef]
27. Wessels, J.A.; van der Kooij, S.M.; le Cessie, S.; Kievit, W.; Barerra, P.; Allaart, C.F.; Huizinga, T.W.; Guchelaar, H.J.; Pharmacogenetics Collaborative Research Group. A clinical pharmacogenetic model to predict the efficacy of methotrexate monotherapy in recent-onset rheumatoid arthritis. *Arthritis Rheum.* **2007**, *56*, 1765–1775. [CrossRef]
28. Kooloos, W.M.; Wessels, J.A.; van der Kooij, S.M.; Allaart, C.F.; Huizinga, T.W.; Guchelaar, H.J. Optimalization of the clinical pharmacogenetic model to predict methotrexate treatment response: the influence of the number of haplotypes of MTHFR 1298A-677C alleles on probability to respond. *Ann. Rheum. Dis.* **2009**, *68*, 1371. [CrossRef]
29. Fransen, J.; Kooloos, W.M.; Wessels, J.A.; Huizinga, T.W.; Guchelaar, H.J.; van Riel, P.L.; Barrera, P. Clinical pharmacogenetic model to predict response of MTX monotherapy in patients with established rheumatoid arthritis after DMARD failure. *Pharmacogenomics* **2012**, *13*, 1087–1094. [CrossRef]

30. Lopez-Rodriguez, R.; Ferreiro-Iglesias, A.; Lima, A.; Bernardes, M.; Pawlik, A.; Paradowska-Gorycka, A.; Swierkot, J.; Slezak, R.; Gonzalez-Alvaro, I.; Narvaez, J.; et al. Evaluation of a clinical pharmacogenetics model to predict methotrexate response in patients with rheumatoid arthritis. *Pharmacogenom. J.* **2018**, *18*, 539–545. [CrossRef]
31. Viatte, S.; Plant, D.; Han, B.; Fu, B.; Yarwood, A.; Thomson, W.; Symmons, D.P.; Worthington, J.; Young, A.; Hyrich, K.L.; et al. Association of HLA-DRB1 haplotypes with rheumatoid arthritis severity, mortality, and treatment response. *JAMA* **2015**, *313*, 1645–1656. [CrossRef]
32. Saruhan-Direskeneli, G.; Inanc, M.; Fresko, I.; Akkoc, N.; Dalkilic, E.; Erken, E.; Karaaslan, Y.; Kinikli, G.; Oksel, F.; Pay, S.; et al. The role of HLA-DRB1 shared epitope alleles in predicting short-term response to leflunomide in rheumatoid arthritis. *Rheumatology (Oxford)* **2007**, *46*, 1842–1844. [CrossRef] [PubMed]
33. Hider, S.L.; Silman, A.J.; Thomson, W.; Lunt, M.; Bunn, D.; Symmons, D.P. Can clinical factors at presentation be used to predict outcome of treatment with methotrexate in patients with early inflammatory polyarthritis? *Ann. Rheum. Dis.* **2009**, *68*, 57–62. [CrossRef] [PubMed]
34. Heldt, C.; Listing, J.; Sozeri, O.; Blasing, F.; Frischbutter, S.; Muller, B. Differential expression of HLA class II genes associated with disease susceptibility and progression in rheumatoid arthritis. *Arthritis Rheum.* **2003**, *48*, 2779–2787. [CrossRef]
35. Stuhlmuller, B.; Mans, K.; Tandon, N.; Bonin, M.O.; Smiljanovic, B.; Sorensen, T.A.; Schendel, P.; Martus, P.; Listing, J.; Detert, J.; et al. Genomic stratification by expression of HLA-DRB4 alleles identifies differential innate and adaptive immune transcriptional patterns - A strategy to detect predictors of methotrexate response in early rheumatoid arthritis. *Clin. Immunol.* **2016**, *171*, 50–61. [CrossRef] [PubMed]
36. Hetland, M.L.; Christensen, I.J.; Tarp, U.; Dreyer, L.; Hansen, A.; Hansen, I.T.; Kollerup, G.; Linde, L.; Lindegaard, H.M.; Poulsen, U.E.; et al. Direct comparison of treatment responses, remission rates, and drug adherence in patients with rheumatoid arthritis treated with adalimumab, etanercept, or infliximab: results from eight years of surveillance of clinical practice in the nationwide Danish DANBIO registry. *Arthritis Rheum.* **2010**, *62*, 22–32. [PubMed]
37. Bek, S.; Bojesen, A.B.; Nielsen, J.V.; Sode, J.; Bank, S.; Vogel, U.; Andersen, V. Systematic review and meta-analysis: pharmacogenetics of anti-TNF treatment response in rheumatoid arthritis. *Pharmacogenom. J.* **2017**, *17*, 403–411. [CrossRef] [PubMed]
38. Massey, J.; Plant, D.; Hyrich, K.; Morgan, A.W.; Wilson, A.G.; Spiliopoulou, A.; Colombo, M.; McKeigue, P.; Isaacs, J.; Cordell, H.; et al. Genome-wide association study of response to tumour necrosis factor inhibitor therapy in rheumatoid arthritis. *Pharmacogenom. J.* **2018**, *18*, 657–664. [CrossRef] [PubMed]
39. Seitz, M.; Wirthmuller, U.; Moller, B.; Villiger, P.M. The −308 tumour necrosis factor-alpha gene polymorphism predicts therapeutic response to TNFalpha-blockers in rheumatoid arthritis and spondyloarthritis patients. *Rheumatology (Oxford)* **2007**, *46*, 93–96. [CrossRef] [PubMed]
40. Coulthard, L.R.; Taylor, J.C.; Eyre, S.; Biologics in Rheumatoid Arthritis Genetics and Genomics; Robinson, J.I.; Wilson, A.G.; Isaacs, J.D.; Hyrich, K.; Emery, P.; Barton, A.; et al. Genetic variants within the MAP kinase signalling network and anti-TNF treatment response in rheumatoid arthritis patients. *Ann. Rheum. Dis.* **2011**, *70*, 98–103. [CrossRef]
41. Krintel, S.B.; Palermo, G.; Johansen, J.S.; Germer, S.; Essioux, L.; Benayed, R.; Badi, L.; Ostergaard, M.; Hetland, M.L. Investigation of single nucleotide polymorphisms and biological pathways associated with response to TNFalpha inhibitors in patients with rheumatoid arthritis. *Pharmacogenet. Genomics* **2012**, *22*, 577–589. [CrossRef]
42. Acosta-Colman, I.; Palau, N.; Tornero, J.; Fernandez-Nebro, A.; Blanco, F.; Gonzalez-Alvaro, I.; Canete, J.D.; Maymo, J.; Ballina, J.; Fernandez-Gutierrez, B.; et al. GWAS replication study confirms the association of PDE3A-SLCO1C1 with anti-TNF therapy response in rheumatoid arthritis. *Pharmacogenomics* **2013**, *14*, 727–734. [CrossRef] [PubMed]
43. Cui, J.; Saevarsdottir, S.; Thomson, B.; Padyukov, L.; van der Helm-van Mil, A.H.; Nititham, J.; Hughes, L.B.; de Vries, N.; Raychaudhuri, S.; Alfredsson, L.; et al. Rheumatoid arthritis risk allele PTPRC is also associated with response to anti-tumor necrosis factor alpha therapy. *Arthritis Rheum.* **2010**, *62*, 1849–1861. [PubMed]
44. Plant, D.; Prajapati, R.; Hyrich, K.L.; Morgan, A.W.; Wilson, A.G.; Isaacs, J.D.; Biologics in Rheumatoid Arthritis Genetics and Genomics Study Syndicate; Barton, A. Replication of association of the PTPRC gene with response to anti-tumor necrosis factor therapy in a large UK cohort. *Arthritis Rheum.* **2012**, *64*, 665–670. [CrossRef] [PubMed]

45. Ferreiro-Iglesias, A.; Montes, A.; Perez-Pampin, E.; Canete, J.D.; Raya, E.; Magro-Checa, C.; Vasilopoulos, Y.; Sarafidou, T.; Caliz, R.; Ferrer, M.A.; et al. Replication of PTPRC as genetic biomarker of response to TNF inhibitors in patients with rheumatoid arthritis. *Pharmacogenom. J.* **2016**, *16*, 137–140. [CrossRef] [PubMed]
46. Iotchkova, V.; Huang, J.; Morris, J.A.; Jain, D.; Barbieri, C.; Walter, K.; Min, J.L.; Chen, L.; Astle, W.; Cocca, M.; et al. Discovery and refinement of genetic loci associated with cardiometabolic risk using dense imputation maps. *Nat. Genet.* **2016**, *48*, 1303–1312. [CrossRef] [PubMed]
47. Canet, L.M.; Filipescu, I.; Caliz, R.; Lupianez, C.B.; Canhao, H.; Escudero, A.; Segura-Catena, J.; Soto-Pino, M.J.; Ferrer, M.A.; Garcia, A.; et al. Genetic variants within the TNFRSF1B gene and susceptibility to rheumatoid arthritis and response to anti-TNF drugs: a multicenter study. *Pharmacogenet. Genom.* **2015**, *25*, 323–333. [CrossRef]
48. Criswell, L.A.; Lum, R.F.; Turner, K.N.; Woehl, B.; Zhu, Y.; Wang, J.; Tiwari, H.K.; Edberg, J.C.; Kimberly, R.P.; Moreland, L.W.; et al. The influence of genetic variation in the HLA-DRB1 and LTA-TNF regions on the response to treatment of early rheumatoid arthritis with methotrexate or etanercept. *Arthritis Rheum.* **2004**, *50*, 2750–2756. [CrossRef]
49. Iwaszko, M.; Swierkot, J.; Kolossa, K.; Jeka, S.; Wiland, P.; Bogunia-Kubik, K. Polymorphisms within the human leucocyte antigen-E gene and their associations with susceptibility to rheumatoid arthritis as well as clinical outcome of anti-tumour necrosis factor therapy. *Clin. Exp. Immunol.* **2015**, *182*, 270–277. [CrossRef]
50. Ferreiro-Iglesias, A.; Montes, A.; Perez-Pampin, E.; Canete, J.D.; Raya, E.; Magro-Checa, C.; Vasilopoulos, Y.; Caliz, R.; Ferrer, M.A.; Joven, B.; et al. Evaluation of 12 GWAS-drawn SNPs as biomarkers of rheumatoid arthritis response to TNF inhibitors. A potential SNP association with response to etanercept. *PLoS ONE* **2019**, *14*, e0213073. [CrossRef]
51. Bluett, J.; Barton, A. Precision Medicine in Rheumatoid Arthritis. *Rheum. Dis. Clin. North. Am.* **2017**, *43*, 377–387. [CrossRef]
52. Sieberts, S.K.; Zhu, F.; Garcia-Garcia, J.; Stahl, E.; Pratap, A.; Pandey, G.; Pappas, D.; Aguilar, D.; Anton, B.; Bonet, J.; et al. Crowdsourced assessment of common genetic contribution to predicting anti-TNF treatment response in rheumatoid arthritis. *Nat. Commun.* **2016**, *7*, 12460. [CrossRef] [PubMed]
53. Pawlik, A.; Wrzesniewska, J.; Fiedorowicz-Fabrycy, I.; Gawronska-Szklarz, B. The MDR1 3435 polymorphism in patients with rheumatoid arthritis. *Int. J. Clin. Pharmacol. Ther.* **2004**, *42*, 496–503. [CrossRef] [PubMed]
54. Drozdzik, M.; Rudas, T.; Pawlik, A.; Kurzawski, M.; Czerny, B.; Gornik, W.; Herczynska, M. The effect of 3435C>T MDR1 gene polymorphism on rheumatoid arthritis treatment with disease-modifying antirheumatic drugs. *Eur. J. Clin. Pharmacol.* **2006**, *62*, 933–937. [CrossRef] [PubMed]
55. Cuppen, B.V.; Pardali, K.; Kraan, M.C.; Marijnissen, A.C.; Yrlid, L.; Olsson, M.; Bijlsma, J.W.; Lafeber, F.P.; Fritsch-Stork, R.D. Polymorphisms in the multidrug-resistance 1 gene related to glucocorticoid response in rheumatoid arthritis treatment. *Rheumatol. Int.* **2017**, *37*, 531–536. [CrossRef] [PubMed]
56. Bohanec Grabar, P.; Rozman, B.; Tomsic, M.; Suput, D.; Logar, D.; Dolzan, V. Genetic polymorphism of CYP1A2 and the toxicity of leflunomide treatment in rheumatoid arthritis patients. *Eur. J. Clin. Pharmacol.* **2008**, *64*, 871–876. [CrossRef] [PubMed]
57. Pawlik, A.; Herczynska, M.; Kurzawski, M.; Safranow, K.; Dziedziejko, V.; Drozdzik, M. The effect of exon (19C>A) dihydroorotate dehydrogenase gene polymorphism on rheumatoid arthritis treatment with leflunomide. *Pharmacogenomics* **2009**, *10*, 303–309. [CrossRef]
58. Dziedziejko, V.; Kurzawski, M.; Safranow, K.; Chlubek, D.; Pawlik, A. The effect of ESR1 and ESR2 gene polymorphisms on the outcome of rheumatoid arthritis treatment with leflunomide. *Pharmacogenomics* **2011**, *12*, 41–47. [CrossRef] [PubMed]
59. Manolio, T.A.; Collins, F.S.; Cox, N.J.; Goldstein, D.B.; Hindorff, L.A.; Hunter, D.J.; McCarthy, M.I.; Ramos, E.M.; Cardon, L.R.; Chakravarti, A.; et al. Finding the missing heritability of complex diseases. *Nature* **2009**, *461*, 747–753. [CrossRef]
60. Araki, Y.; Mimura, T. The Histone Modification Code in the Pathogenesis of Autoimmune Diseases. *Mediators Inflamm.* **2017**, *2017*, 2608605. [CrossRef]
61. Stahl, E.A.; Raychaudhuri, S.; Remmers, E.F.; Xie, G.; Eyre, S.; Thomson, B.P.; Li, Y.; Kurreeman, F.A.; Zhernakova, A.; Hinks, A.; et al. Genome-wide association study meta-analysis identifies seven new rheumatoid arthritis risk loci. *Nat. Genet.* **2010**, *42*, 508–514. [CrossRef]

62. Diogo, D.; Kurreeman, F.; Stahl, E.A.; Liao, K.P.; Gupta, N.; Greenberg, J.D.; Rivas, M.A.; Hickey, B.; Flannick, J.; Thomson, B.; et al. Rare, low-frequency, and common variants in the protein-coding sequence of biological candidate genes from GWASs contribute to risk of rheumatoid arthritis. *Am. J. Hum. Genet.* **2013**, *92*, 15–27. [CrossRef] [PubMed]
63. Eyre, S.; Ke, X.; Lawrence, R.; Bowes, J.; Panoutsopoulou, K.; Barton, A.; Thomson, W.; Worthington, J.; Zeggini, E. Examining the overlap between genome-wide rare variant association signals and linkage peaks in rheumatoid arthritis. *Arthritis Rheum.* **2011**, *63*, 1522–1526. [CrossRef] [PubMed]
64. Bang, S.Y.; Na, Y.J.; Kim, K.; Joo, Y.B.; Park, Y.; Lee, J.; Lee, S.Y.; Ansari, A.A.; Jung, J.; Rhee, H.; et al. Targeted exon sequencing fails to identify rare coding variants with large effect in rheumatoid arthritis. *Arthritis Res. Ther.* **2014**, *16*, 447. [CrossRef] [PubMed]
65. Cui, J.; Diogo, D.; Stahl, E.A.; Canhao, H.; Mariette, X.; Greenberg, J.D.; Okada, Y.; Pappas, D.A. The role of rare protein-coding variants in anti–tumor necrosis factor treatment response in rheumatoid arthritis. *Arthritis Rheum.* **2017**, *69*, 735–741. [CrossRef] [PubMed]
66. Zhernakova, A.; van Diemen, C.C.; Wijmenga, C. Detecting shared pathogenesis from the shared genetics of immune-related diseases. *Nat. Rev. Genet.* **2009**, *10*, 43–55. [CrossRef] [PubMed]
67. Zhernakova, A.; Withoff, S.; Wijmenga, C. Clinical implications of shared genetics and pathogenesis in autoimmune diseases. *Nat. Rev. Endocrinol.* **2013**, *9*, 646–659. [CrossRef] [PubMed]
68. Wang, N.; Shen, N.; Vyse, T.J.; Anand, V.; Gunnarson, I.; Sturfelt, G.; Rantapaa-Dahlqvist, S.; Elvin, K.; Truedsson, L.; Andersson, B.A.; et al. Selective IgA deficiency in autoimmune diseases. *Mol. Med.* **2011**, *17*, 1383–1396. [CrossRef]
69. Gonzalez-Serna, D.; Ortiz-Fernandez, L.; Vargas, S.; Garcia, A.; Raya, E.; Fernandez-Gutierrez, B.; Lopez-Longo, F.J.; Balsa, A.; Gonzalez-Alvaro, I.; Narvaez, J.; et al. Association of a rare variant of the TNFSF13B gene with susceptibility to rheumatoid arthritis and systemic lupus erythematosus. *Sci. Rep.* **2018**, *8*, 8195. [CrossRef]
70. Woodland, R.T.; Schmidt, M.R.; Thompson, C.B. BLyS and B cell homeostasis. *Semin. Immunol.* **2006**, *18*, 318–326. [CrossRef]
71. Steri, M.; Orru, V.; Idda, M.L.; Pitzalis, M.; Pala, M.; Zara, I.; Sidore, C.; Faa, V.; Floris, M.; Deiana, M.; et al. Overexpression of the Cytokine BAFF and Autoimmunity Risk. *N. Engl. J. Med.* **2017**, *376*, 1615–1626. [CrossRef]
72. Vincent, F.B.; Morand, E.F.; Schneider, P.; Mackay, F. The BAFF/APRIL system in SLE pathogenesis. *Nat. Rev. Rheumatol.* **2014**, *10*, 365–373. [CrossRef] [PubMed]
73. Furie, R.; Petri, M.; Zamani, O.; Cervera, R.; Wallace, D.J.; Tegzova, D.; Sanchez-Guerrero, J.; Schwarting, A.; Merrill, J.T.; Chatham, W.W.; et al. A phase III, randomized, placebo-controlled study of belimumab, a monoclonal antibody that inhibits B lymphocyte stimulator, in patients with systemic lupus erythematosus. *Arthritis Rheum.* **2011**, *63*, 3918–3930. [CrossRef] [PubMed]
74. Navarra, S.V.; Guzman, R.M.; Gallacher, A.E.; Hall, S.; Levy, R.A.; Jimenez, R.E.; Li, E.K.; Thomas, M.; Kim, H.Y.; Leon, M.G.; et al. Efficacy and safety of belimumab in patients with active systemic lupus erythematosus: A randomised, placebo-controlled, phase 3 trial. *Lancet* **2011**, *377*, 721–731. [CrossRef]
75. Lopez-Isac, E.; Martin, J.E.; Assassi, S.; Simeon, C.P.; Carreira, P.; Ortego-Centeno, N.; Freire, M.; Beltran, E.; Narvaez, J.; Alegre-Sancho, J.J.; et al. Cross-disease meta-analysis of genome-wide association studies for systemic sclerosis and rheumatoid arthritis reveals irf4 as a new common susceptibility locus. *Arthritis Rheumatol.* **2016**, *68*, 2338–2344. [CrossRef] [PubMed]
76. Marquez, A.; Vidal-Bralo, L.; Rodriguez-Rodriguez, L.; Gonzalez-Gay, M.A.; Balsa, A.; Gonzalez-Alvaro, I.; Carreira, P.; Ortego-Centeno, N.; Ayala-Gutierrez, M.M.; Garcia-Hernandez, F.J.; et al. A combined large-scale meta-analysis identifies COG6 as a novel shared risk locus for rheumatoid arthritis and systemic lupus erythematosus. *Ann. Rheum. Dis.* **2017**, *76*, 286–294. [CrossRef] [PubMed]
77. Coenen, M.J.; Trynka, G.; Heskamp, S.; Franke, B.; van Diemen, C.C.; Smolonska, J.; van Leeuwen, M.; Brouwer, E.; Boezen, M.H.; Postma, D.S.; et al. Common and different genetic background for rheumatoid arthritis and coeliac disease. *Hum. Mol. Genet.* **2009**, *18*, 4195–4203. [CrossRef] [PubMed]
78. Li, Y.R.; Li, J.; Zhao, S.D.; Bradfield, J.P.; Mentch, F.D.; Maggadottir, S.M.; Hou, C.; Abrams, D.J.; Chang, D.; Gao, F.; et al. Meta-analysis of shared genetic architecture across ten pediatric autoimmune diseases. *Nat. Med.* **2015**, *21*, 1018–1027. [CrossRef] [PubMed]

79. Ellinghaus, D.; Jostins, L.; Spain, S.L.; Cortes, A.; Bethune, J.; Han, B.; Park, Y.R.; Raychaudhuri, S.; Pouget, J.G.; Hubenthal, M.; et al. Analysis of five chronic inflammatory diseases identifies 27 new associations and highlights disease-specific patterns at shared loci. *Nat. Genet.* **2016**, *48*, 510–518. [CrossRef]
80. Marquez, A.; Kerick, M.; Zhernakova, A.; Gutierrez-Achury, J.; Chen, W.M.; Onengut-Gumuscu, S.; Gonzalez-Alvaro, I.; Rodriguez-Rodriguez, L.; Rios-Fernandez, R.; Gonzalez-Gay, M.A.; et al. Meta-analysis of Immunochip data of four autoimmune diseases reveals novel single-disease and cross-phenotype associations. *Genome Med.* **2018**, *10*, 97. [CrossRef]
81. Acosta-Herrera, M.; Kerick, M.; Gonzalez-Serna, D.; Myositis Genetics, C.; Scleroderma Genetics, C.; Wijmenga, C.; Franke, A.; Gregersen, P.K.; Padyukov, L.; Worthington, J.; et al. Genome-wide meta-analysis reveals shared new loci in systemic seropositive rheumatic diseases. *Ann. Rheum. Dis.* **2019**, *78*, 311–319. [CrossRef]
82. Plant, D.; Webster, A.; Nair, N.; Oliver, J.; Smith, S.L.; Eyre, S.; Hyrich, K.L.; Wilson, A.G.; Morgan, A.W.; Isaacs, J.D.; et al. Differential methylation as a biomarker of response to etanercept in patients with rheumatoid arthritis. *Arthritis Rheumatol.* **2016**, *68*, 1353–1360. [CrossRef] [PubMed]
83. Spiliopoulou, A.; Colombo, M.; Plant, D.; Nair, N.; Cui, J.; Coenen, M.J.; Ikari, K.; Yamanaka, H.; Saevarsdottir, S.; Padyukov, L.; et al. Association of response to TNF inhibitors in rheumatoid arthritis with quantitative trait loci for CD40 and CD39. *Ann. Rheum. Dis.* **2019**. (E-pub ahead of print). [CrossRef] [PubMed]

6

Pseudoerosions of Hands and Feet in Rheumatoid Arthritis: Anatomic Concepts and Redefinition

Lena Hirtler [1,*], Claus Rath [1], Hannes Platzgummer [2], Daniel Aletaha [3] and Franz Kainberger [2]

1 Division of Anatomy, Center for Anatomy and Cell Biology, Medical University of Vienna, Vienna 1090, Austria; claus.rath@meduniwien.ac.at
2 Department of Biomedical Imaging and Image-Guided Therapy, Medical University of Vienna, Vienna 1090, Austria; hannes.platzgummer@meduniwien.ac.at (H.P.); franz.kainberger@meduniwien.ac.at (F.K.)
3 Division of Rheumatology, Department of Internal Medicine, Medical University of Vienna, Vienna 1090, Austria; daniel.aletaha@meduniwien.ac.at
* Correspondence: lena.hirtler@meduniwien.ac.at

Abstract: Rheumatoid arthritis is a chronic inflammatory disease characterized by the development of osseous and cartilaginous damage. The correct differentiation between a true erosion and other entities—then often called "pseudoerosions"—is essential to avoid misdiagnosing rheumatoid arthritis and to correctly interpret the progress of the disease. The aims of this systematic review were as follows: to create a definition and delineation of the term "pseudoerosion", to point out morphological pitfalls in the interpretation of images, and to report on difficulties arising from choosing different imaging modalities. A systematic review on bone erosions in rheumatoid arthritis was performed based on the Preferred Reporting Items for Systematic Reviews and Meta-Analyses (PRISMA) guidelines. The following search terms were applied in PubMed and Scopus: "rheumatoid arthritis", "bone erosion", "ultrasonography", "radiography", "computed tomography" and "magnetic resonance imaging". Appropriate exclusion criteria were defined. The systematic review registration number is 138826. The search resulted ultimately in a final number of 25 papers. All indications for morphological pitfalls and difficulties utilizing imaging modalities were recorded and summarized. A pseudoerosion is more than just a negative definition of an erosion; it can be anatomic (e.g., a normal osseous concavity) or artefact-related (i.e., an artificial interruption of the calcified zones). It can be classified according to their configuration, shape, content, and can be described specifically with an anatomical term. "Calcified zone" is a term to describe the deep components of the subchondral, subligamentous and subtendinous bone, and may be applied for all non-cancellous borders of a bone, thus representing a third type of the bone matrix beside the cortical and the trabecular bone.

Keywords: rheumatoid arthritis; pseudoerosions; hand; foot; ultrasonography; radiography; computed tomography; magnetic resonance imaging

---

1. Introduction

Rheumatoid arthritis (RA) manifests with three types of structural joint damage: joint space narrowing, erosions, and capsular abnormalities in the form of synovial proliferation and subluxations [1–4]. The diagnosis of erosions and their quantification as part of radiographic scoring systems is an accepted surrogate biomarker of structural progression of arthritis [4,5]. Erosions in RA have been defined in consensus statements and in studies with high-resolution peripheral quantitative computed tomography (HRpqCT) as cortical defects, breaks, or other discontinuities with underlying trabecular bone loss and characteristic locations that can be identified with imaging [6–12]. On radiographs, according to the 2010 ACR/EULAR (American College of Rheumatology/European

League Against Rheumatism) rheumatoid arthritis classification criteria [13,14], erosions have to be seen at least at three separate joints at the interphalangeal (PIP), metacarpophalangeal (MCP), wrist (counted as one joint), or metatarsophalangeal (MTP) joints [15,16]. For ultrasound (US) and magnetic resonance imaging (MRI), the operational OMERACT (outcome measures in rheumatology) definition requests the abnormality being visible in two planes [17,18].

At the wrist, the most frequent locations are the capitate, ulna, lunate, triquetrum, and scaphoid [19–26], at the ankle the distal fibular notch, the navicular, cuneiform and cuboid bones are often involved, the talus and calcaneus less frequently [27,28]. Why erosions occur at these sites is commonly explained by immunological and anatomical models [29–31]. The latter mainly refer to the thinning of cartilage near capsular insertions at bones (bare areas) and to microdamage [32–36]. Following immunologically-based concepts, erosion formation is explained by increased bone resorption and decreased bone formation at certain locations in the subchondral bone [37]. Werner et al. [32] showed a correlation between cortical micro-channels and the occurrence of bone erosions in bare areas.

Especially in early, preclinical or undifferentiated arthritis with small or no erosions, it is necessary to differentiate a true rheumatic erosion from the various forms of normal erosion-simulating concavities of the bony surface and therefor avoid false-positive statements [38,39]. Such so-called pseudoerosions [40] have been described to be smooth and well demarcated on radiographs, ultrasound, computed tomography (CT) and MRI [41]. The effect of misinterpreting a normal anatomic concavity as an erosion or vice versa may be estimated from the intra- and inter-reader variations of scoring systems and has been directly mentioned for the RAMRIS (rheumatoid arthritis MRI score) [42,43]. The spectrum of MRI "erosion-like" lesions is broad: Ejbjerg et al. [44] observed them in 1.9% of healthy persons, whereas Olech et al. [45] saw them in 65%. Rothschild [46] questioned if such findings should be interpreted as true erosions, old erosions from earlier diseases without clinical significance, or other. For the US, a 30% false-positive rate of erosion detection has been reported [47]. The computer-assisted assessment of erosions was considered helpful, but difficulties in discriminating those from normal bony concavities were observed [48,49].

The aim of this systematic review was (1) to evaluate the frequency of specifically stated difficulties arising in the interpretation of imaging modalitis in search for bone erosions, (2) to define the characteristic anatomic appearances and patterns of pseudoerosions with respect to the potential pitfalls in the diagnosis of RA as reported in the literature and (3) to develop an anatomic concept for improving the accuracy and precision of imaging assessment.

2. Materials and Methods

A systematic review on bone erosions in RA was performed based on the guidelines of the PRISMA (Preferred Reporting Items for Systematic Reviews and Meta-Analyses) statement and was registered accordingly (No. 138826) [50].

2.1. Search Strategy

The search was performed in PubMed (Medline) and Scopus with the following search terms: "rheumatoid arthritis", "bone erosion", "ultrasonography", "radiography", "computed tomography" and "magnetic resonance imaging" (example for search in PubMed: "rheumatoid arthritis" AND bone AND erosion AND (ultrasonography OR radiography OR "computed tomography" OR "magnetic resonance imaging"). No specific date was defined as starting point, the end of search was 31 May 2019. English language was defined as a required criterium.

2.2. Selection Criteria

All original studies investigating the diagnosis of RA with X-ray, sonography, CT or MRI and describing false positive diagnoses of bone erosions and erosion-like changes published before 31 May 2019 were included. Exclusion criteria were animal studies, feasibility studies, other inflammatory diseases, clinical studies comparing therapeutic measurements in RA, studies comparing the sensitivity of imaging modalities without report of false positive diagnosed erosions or erosion-like lesions, surgical procedures or longitudinal studies without direct reference to this topic, case reports and conference papers. Additionally, all papers without full text availability were excluded from the analysis.

Data extraction was performed by using a standardized Excel (Microsoft Corporation, Redmont, WA, USA) data extraction form: first author, year of publication, country, study population, number of patients, imaging modality, joints evaluated, reported sensitivity of imaging modalities, reported false positive or false negative diagnosis of bone erosions, reported limitations in image interpretation with respect to anatomy, the differential diagnosis to other erosive diseases, artifacts and signal-to-noise reduction.

3. Results

The search with the defined terms resulted in a total of 1487 results. An additional number of 59 papers were added after reference-screening. The flow diagram of the literature review may be seen in Figure 1. Ultimately, only 25 papers reported specifically on false-positive results or erosion-like changes.

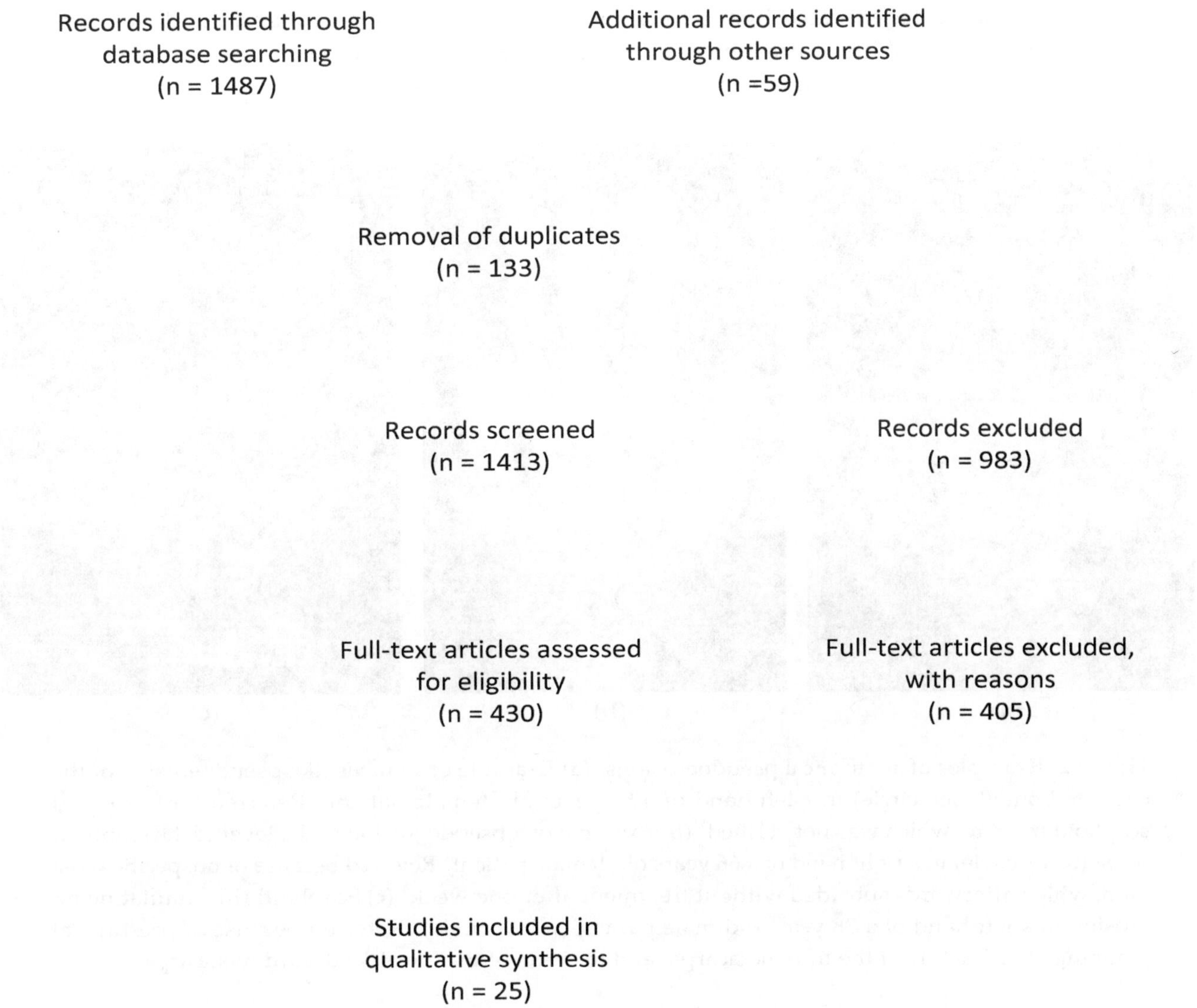

Figure 1. Flow diagram of the literature review.

Based on the information gathered in the remaining papers, the false-positive results were subdivided into anatomic pseudoerosions, if the explanation for the false-positive diagnosis was described as a morphological phenomenon, and into artifact-related pseudoerosions, if the explanation for the false-positive diagnosis was related to the respective imaging technique.

3.1. Anatomic Pseudoerosions

Anatomic pseudoerosions, i.e., normal concavities of a bone with a potential for misinterpreting them as arthritis-related erosions, were described in twelve original papers and reviews and may be classified into four types according to their anatomic form and configuration (Table 1): (1) a groove or notch or its incomplete form, i.e., a jutty, (2) a sulcus as part of an osteofibrous channel, (3) a subcapital neck on long bones, or (4) a nutritional channel or a zonal roughness [3,11,41,51–57]. According to their shape, they may be grouped into (1) shallow or broad concavities and (2) subchondral cysts, if en-face displayed on an image and occasionally with a small opening to the joint space, or (3) channel-like structures (Figure 2a,c) [3,54,55]. The anatomic location of pseudoerosions is predominantly at the carpal bones, the MCP- and the MTP-joints. Almost always they are linked to a ligament insertion (Figure 2b), a mucosal fold fixation or the hood of a tendon sheath, and occur at the noncortical bone, also known calcified zones (i.e., borders of the subchondral and enthesial calcified bone with the adjacent underlying trabecular structures). The content of pseudoerosions is visible with US and MRI and may be normal or degenerated ligament tissue, or blood vessels [44,56] and the development of edematous changes [58]. With contrast media, a slight enhancement can be observed, however, in one publication rare cases of strong enhancement was documented [56].

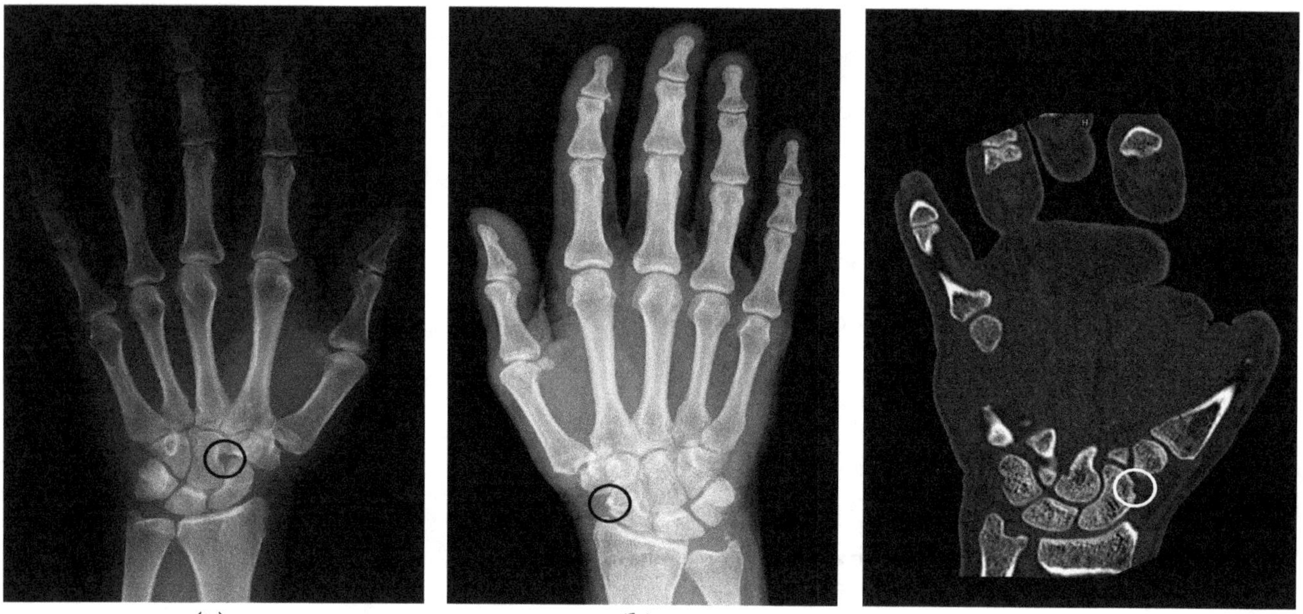

(a) (b) (c)

Figure 2. Examples of anatomical pseudoerosions. (**a**) Example of a sulcus like pseudoerosion of the capitate bone (black circle) in a left hand of a 52 years old female patient. Referred for suspected scaphoid fracture, which was not verified. (**b**) Example of a pseudoerosion at the level of the scaphoid waist (black circle) in a right hand of a 66 years old female patient. Referred because of unspecific wrist pain, which afterwards subsided without treatment after one week. (**c**) Scaphoid rim simulating an erosion in a left hand of a 38 years old male patient (white circle). Referred because of presurgical planning after fracture of the fifth metacarpal and luxation of the fourth and third metacarpal.

Table 1. Pseudoerosions.

Citation	Type of Article	Imaging Modality	Reported Pseudoerosion	Explanation
Alasaarela et al., 1998 [58]	Original research	Magnetic resonance imaging (MRI) (1.0T T1, T2 and proton density, PD)	False positive interpretation	Pre-erosive oedematous changes in subchondral bone in MRI
Barnabe et al., 2016 [11]	Original research	High-resolution peripheral quantitative computed tomography (HRpqCT)	Carpal pseudoerosions	Arterial foramina
Canella Moraes Carmo et al., 2009 [54]	Original research	Computed tomography (CT)	Carpal pseudoerosions	ligament insertions tendinous sulci
Dohn et al., 2006 [53]	Original research	Sonography	Erosion-like changes	Metacarpophalangeal (MCP) joints
Dohn et al., 2013 [57]	Original research	Sonography	False positive interpretation	Cortical irregularities (osteophytes, notches at the metacarpal neck, subcortical bone cysts)
Ejbjerg et al., 2004 [44]	Original research	MRI (1.0 T1 spin echo, STIR, T2 spin echo fat-suppressed	Erosion-like changes	Capitate, lunate
Martel et al., 1965 [3]	Original research	Plain radiography	Carpal pseudoerosion	Normal deep groove in the capitate in about 10%
McQueen et al., 2005 [51]	Review article	MRI (T1, T2 fat-saturated)	False positive interpretation	Attachments of interosseous ligaments of the wrist, articular ligaments of the MCP joints, nutrient foramina
Peluso et al., 2015 [52]	Original research	3D sonography	False positive interpretation	Arterial foramina Osteophytes
Robertson et al., 2006 [56]	Original research	MRI (1.5T, T1 spin echo, fat-suppressed FSE, fat-suppressed PD-weighted FSE, 3D SPGR)	Carpal pseudoerosions	ligament insertions
Torshizy et al., 2008 [55]	Original research	CT	Tarsal pseudoerosions	attachment site of joint capsule ligament insertions tendinous sulci
Wawer et al., 2014 [41]	Original research	Plain radiography	Carpal pseudoerosions	ligament insertions

STIR = Short TI Inversion Recovery, FSE = Fast Spin Echo, SPGR = Spoiled Gradient Recalled Echo.

3.2. *Artifact-Related Pesudoerosions*

Artifact-related pseudoerosions were mentioned in 18 original papers and reviews and may be caused due to (1) partial volume artifacts of cross-sectional images or other modality-specific artifacts (ultrasound diffraction or reflection, insufficient fat suppression with MRI), or (2) a low signal-to-noise ratio (Table 2) [1,5,52,57–68].

Table 2. Imaging difficulties.

Citation	Type of Article	Imaging Modality	Reported Problem
Alasaarela et al., 1998 [58]	Original research	CT	Examination of a curvilinear object—the more the reformat plane parallels the z-axis, the more resolution of multiplanar reformats is impaired. The partial volume effect is harmful.
		Plain radiography	Information dependent on projections used
Albrecht et al., 2013 [1]	Original research	Plain radiography	2D character of radiography
		CT	No simultaneous assessment of inflammatory changes of RA

Table 2. *Cont.*

Citation	Type of Article	Imaging Modality	Reported Problem
Amin et al., 2012 [62]	Original research	Plain radiography	Beam has to hit erosion tangentially to show cortical break
Aurell et al., 2018 [63]	Original research	Plain radiography	Possibility of false negative evaluation, if the orifice of the erosion is not hit tangentially
Cimmino et al., 2002 [60]	Original research	MRI (T2 spin echo or gradient echo)	Failed fat suppression can mimic bone marrow edema
Dohn et al., 2013 [57]	Original research	Sonography	Some areas of hand and wrist are inaccessible for ultrasound beam
Dohn et al., 2008 [65]	Original research	MRI (0.6T T1 3D fast field echo)	Overestimation of erosion size due to difficult differentiation between cortical bone and erosion
Ejbjerg et al., 2006 [64]	Original research	Plain radiography	Up to 30% of an MCP joint bone has to be eroded before detection
Emond et al., 2012 [68]	Original research	MRI (1T 3D spoiled gradient echo)	Boundaries of erosions difficult to differentiate
Foley-Nolan et al., 1991 [59]	Original research	Plain radiography	Erosions only visible when large percentage of bone thickness has been destroyed
Forslind et al., 2003 [61]	Original research	Plain radiography	Delineation of erosions difficult in patients with osteoporosis
		MRI (1.0T 3D T2 gradient echo, T1 spin echo with and without fat-saturation)	False negative interpretation due to contiguous looking erosions
Kleyer et al., 2016 [66]	Original research	MRI (1.5T T1)	Small cortical breaks not seen on MRI—validation by HRpqCT
McQueen et al., 1998 [69]	Original research	MRI (1.5T T1 and T2 with and without fat suppression)	Partial volume artefacts may lead to false positive indications of erosions
McQueen et al., 2001 [70]	Original research	Plain radiography	Identification of erosions hampered by poor visibility at the carpus
Peluso et al., 2015 [52]	Original research	Ultrasonography	Due to anatomical structure, multiplanar distribution of bones that restricts the ultrasound beam and alters the correct visualization
Ulas et al., 2019 [67]	Original research	MRI (1.5T): Susceptibility-weighted imaging, SWI T1w	False positive identification of erosions due to motion artefacts, strong susceptibility artefacts at tissue intersections Weak differentiation of cortical bone
Wakefield et al., 2000 [5]	Original research	Plain radiography	Typical anatomical location of bone erosions difficult to see until it lies in the tangential plane of the radiographic beam.
		Plain radiography	Periarticular osteoporosis
Wawer et al., 2014 [41]	Original research	Plain radiography	Less density in subcortical cancellous bone due to synovial and bony hyperemia, overlapping of carpal bones, presence of osteophytes

4. Discussion

From the viewpoint of imaging anatomy, a misinterpretation of erosions in RA may occur due to (1) anatomic pseudoerosions, or (2) artifact-related pseudoerosions as a result of an inadequate investigation technique. Pseudoerosions and erosions are commonly located at certain areas of the surface outline of the calcified bone, also known as calcified zones. These may therefore, besides cortical bone and trabecular bone, be regarded as a third type of organization of the bone matrix.

The term "calcified zones" (Figure 3) in this context is therefore proposed to describe the borders of the subchondral and enthesial calcified bone with the adjacent underlying trabecular structures. It may be extended for describing all parts of intraarticular bone apart from the cortex. With its overlying tissue of hyaline cartilage, synovium or capsule-ligamentous structures it forms anatomic units. The relationship between these zones and the adjacent tissues is so tight that the fibrous layers of tendon sheaths, bursae, periosteum or the cartilaginous zones of entheses or hyaline cartilage are in direct continuation with the subjacent bone, thus providing direct contact with synovial tissue. The concept of the subchondral zone was used by Dihlmann [71] to describe the mineralized zone of hyaline cartilage as part of the subchondral bone. It may be extended to describe a subligamentous, subtendinous or subbursal zone of the bone. Utilizing sub-millimeter spatial resolution CT, these calcified zones can be displayed. Differentiating the normal calcified zone from erosional changes, i.e., irregular margins and sclerotic reaction, is the main challenge in differentiating true erosions from pseudoerosions [72].

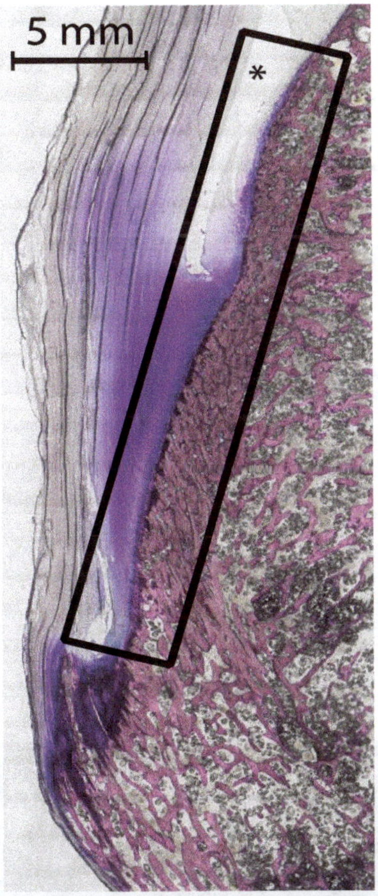

Figure 3. Example of a calcified zone. Thin ground section of the calcaneal tuberosity, the calcaneal tendon and the calcaneal bursa—also a frequent location of bone erosions. The described calcified zone as subchondral and enthesial calcified bone with adjacent underlying trabecular structures including the overlying tissues is marked by the rectangle. The asterix marks the calcaneal bursa. A 5 mm scale is included, the tissue was stained with Giemsa.

Pseudoerosions have to be differentiated from other pathologies as ganglion cysts, crystal-induced arthropathies, tuberculosis or other infections, and from degenerative lesions in the form of erosions, subchondral (pseudo)cysts or beak-shaped osteophytes as there are so many similarities in location [38,60]. Intraosseous ganglion cysts are common and almost always have a continuity with a ligament which underwent mucous degeneration [73,74]. Especially in the elderly population, the more prevalent degenerative changes of the bone may be difficult to be differentiated from RA-related erosions [38,75]. However, in children interpretational problems may arise. There, normal concavities simulating erosions have been referred to as "bony depressions" at certain locations in the wrist [76–78]. Such pseudoerosions in children may be big, indicating that size is not a reliable feature for differentiating normal variants from true erosions.

4.1. Anatomic Pseudoerosions

An anatomic pseudoerosion can be defined as a normal concavity of a bone outlined by a smooth and thin calcified zone with the potential for a false-positive misinterpretation of an erosion. In this form, the term pseudoerosion is more precise than "notch" or "bony depression" and may be preferred as it contains a prognostic impact for the imaging assessment of arthritis. Such clinically oriented annotations, examples are the scaphoid waist and the metacarpal neck as typical sites for fractures, have been in use in traumatology and may be of help in the assessment of arthritis-related erosions, too (list of described pseudoerosions in Table 3, an overview of anatomical pseudoerosions in the hand may also be found in Figure 4).

Table 3. List of pseudoerosions with anatomic description.

Location	Name	Description
Scaphoid waist, palmar aspect	Scaphoid waist	Tendon hood of radial-sided carpal tunnel with radio-scapho-capitate ligament
Scaphoid, radial aspect of midpart		Scapho-capsular ligament or mucosal fold insertions
Capitate, distal ulnar portion [41]	Ulnar capitate notch	Intercarpal ligaments
Capitate, radial portion	Radial capitate notch	Intercarpal ligaments
Lunate, radial aspect		Scapholuntate ligament
Hamate, distal radial portion [41]		Insertion of capitatohamate ligament and carpometacarpal ligaments
Hamate, distal ulnar portion [41]		Insertion of carpometacarpal ligaments
Triquetrum, radial and dorsal aspect	Radial triquetral notch	Insertion of the radiotriquetral ligament
Triquetrum, ulnar and proximal aspect		Insertion of the ulnotriquetral ligament
Metacarpal bases	metacarpal base notches	Insertion of intercarpal ligaments
Metacarpal or metatarsal neck and heads	metacarpal or metatarsal head notch	Insertion of metacarpophalangeal ligaments or joint capsule
5th metatarsal head		Slight normal varus angulation of metatarsal head
Achilles tendon insertion		Insertion jutty

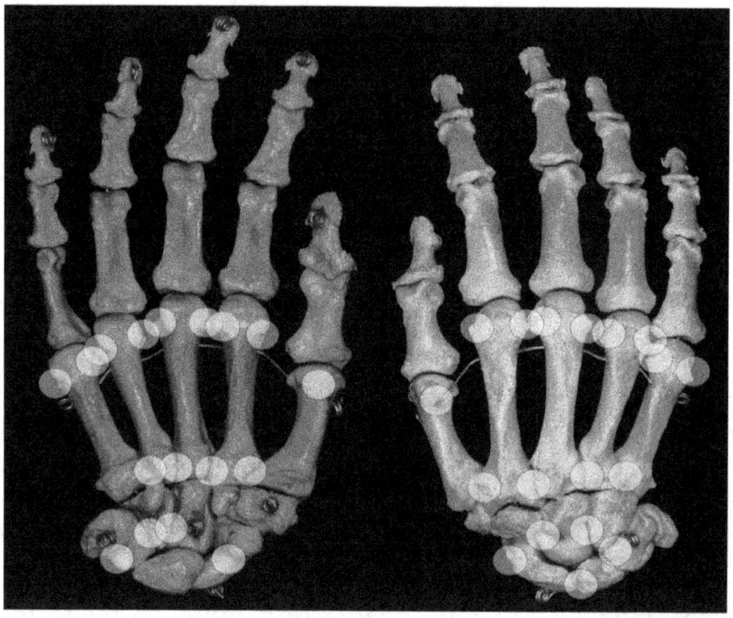

Figure 4. Locations of anatomical pseudoerosions. Overview on possible locations of anatomical pseudoerosions as summarized in Table 3. Right skeletal hand, on the left view from palmar, on the right view from dorsal.

Grooves due to ligament or tendon insertions have a varying appearance as described in the enthesis concept by Benjamin and McGonagle [79]. Such prominent grooves can cause the appearance of a pseudoerosion (Figure 2a). A groove may occur in three forms: (1) at a non-apophyseal direct tendon or ligament attachment where the uncalcified components of the enthesis enters the bone, (2) at an apophysis with overhanging edges, or (3) at an incomplete apophysis, a jutty, at the indirect attachments of a tendon or ligament with a tangential transition into the periosteum. For example, pseudoerosions resulting from the first form are the metacarpal ligament insertions at the bases of the metacarpal bones [80]. At the dorsal aspect of the triquetral bone, such a pseudoerosion may be formed by the distal insertion of the radiotriquetral ligament along with other components of the dorsal radiocarpal ligament. On the capitate, on which several strong carpal ligaments have their insertion, and many other carpal bones, intercarpal ligaments may cause pseudoerosions [51]. Examples for the second form may be the non-spherical form of metacarpal and metatarsal heads, which can be explained by the collateral ligament complexes running laterally and medially with smoothly outlined shallow metacarpal grooves containing these structures. At the metacarpals, these grooves are bordered by little tubercles for the proximal attachment of the collateral ligaments (Figure 4) [81]. Moraes do Carmo et al. [54] identified three concavities in the first metacarpal head (intersesamoid, ulnar, and radial) and two in those of the fingers (ulnar and radial). They described dorsal depressions of the metacarpal heads due to the extensor digitorum tendons in one third of their anatomic specimens which correlated with observations with ultrasound made by Boutry et al. [82,83]. A similar study was done for defining pseudoerosions of the metatarsal heads by Torshizy et al. [55] who described anatomic variations in the normal osseous concavities of the lateral and medial aspects of each metatarsal head. Typical jutties, i.e., examples for the third form of grooves, are the small round or oval subcapsular notches at the proximal phalangeal bases [80,84]. At the Achilles tendon insertion, proximal to its jutty shallow irregularities beneath the calcaneal bursa may represent true erosions [85].

Osseous sulci are commonly roofed with a ligament, fascia or other fibrous tissue, thus forming an osteofibrous channel for a tendon within a synovial tendon sheath. A subcapital neck of the distal metacarpal and the metatarsal bones is a small metaphyseal narrowing that may cause a pseudoerosion on projection radiographs, ultrasound or MRI [86]. At the distal fifth metacarpal bone, due to its slight varus angulation this neck may be more prominent.

Nutritional channels may appear as pseudoerosion on MR if their orifice is displayed as a little T2-weighted hyperintense spot [51]. Their superficial orifice is often located at a roughness of the calcified zones which as a whole may simulate an erosion [11,34,87]. Some of these iuxtaarticular surface roughnesses may be specified as crests or ridges that correspond to attachment sites for redundant joint capsule [55]. Others, especially on carpal bones, may be due to indentations of innominate ligamentous attachments or synovial folds [51]. Such typical structures visible between the radial aspect of the scaphoid and the radial carpal collateral ligament may be called scapho-capsular ligaments (Figure 2C). Roughness of the calcified zones may be visible at various sites and should be differentiated from shallow extensive true erosions and from advanced cartilage degeneration [88].

4.2. Artefact-Related Pseudoerosions

Artefact-related pseudoerosions are defined as an interruption of the sharp outline of the calcified zones. Important causes are a low signal-to-noise ratio, a partial volume artefact, or in case of ultrasound irregular backscattering with artefacts on an incongruent or rough surface. A low signal-to-noise ratio could be caused by over-penetration of the X-ray beam through the bone or due to insufficient spatial or contrast resolution. This effect is more severe in cases with low calcium content in the calcified zones or the subjacent trabecular bone, previously referred to as subchondral osteoporosis or as pre-erosions, and may be enhanced by swelling of the overlying soft tissue. With ultrasound, diffraction or a complex backscattering of the waves on a curved or irregular surface may cause various pseudo-effects on the retrieved image [51,69,89].

Although X-ray is most commonly used in the diagnosis of RA it is CT which can be regarded as the best imaging modality for differentiating pseudoerosions from true erosions [53,62,63,90–94]. Several studies [34,95–98] describe a significant decrease of trabecular volume and number and an increased trabecular heterogeneity in patients with rheumatoid arthritis by using HRpqCT. This trabecular bone loss as the intramedullary component of bone erosions may contribute the largest part and may therefore be a reason for misinterpretation of erosions or pseudoerosions in radiographs as this imaging method is relatively insensitive to trabecular bone loss [60,99].

In addition, MRI and US are reported to be more sensitive than plain radiography [53,62,90–94], but this especially seems to be dependent on the location investigated [88,100]. In some cases, radiography may even be superior to MRI in detecting bony erosions despite its lack of three dimensionality [1,3,5,58,99,101,102]. Through its high spatial resolution it can differentiate smaller erosions which otherwise would present themselves as continuous on MRI [61,65].

Thus, it is important to recognize several parameters to achieve a decrease of cognitive diagnostic errors especially in early arthritis. These include slight variations in the respective projection technique and individual ligament laxity or postinflammatory scarring of ligaments. In addition, the roughness of a calcified zone, and the transitional changes between normal bone and true inflammatory erosions are until now not or only scarcely addressed. Even the projection of the joints, even if the relevant anatomic landmarks are displayed according to the standards, is highly variable. One has also to keep in mind that discrete forms of malalignment due to ulnar deviations or other forms of arthritic subluxation, ligament laxity with a slight rotation of bones, and variations in their arrangement may cause a more prominent appearance of a pseudoerosion [3,51,57,102].

4.3. *Erosions-in-Pseudoerosions*

Both anatomic and artefact-related pseudoerosions are located at sites with direct or indirect contact to inflammatory tissue in arthritis, and therefore, are at higher risk for destruction. Areas of the articular bone without any cartilage covering are more prone to erosive destructions by synovial tissue and effusion [3,32]. Hence, in an anatomically preformed concavity a true inflammatory erosion may develop. McQueen et al. [51] described these erosions-in-pseudoerosions (Figure 5) for the attachment sites of the intercarpal ligaments. It may be observed at the site of ligamentous attachments covered by synovial folds at the metacarpal or metatarsal heads or at the wrist. On the other hand, true erosions may be classified as normal variants. It remains unclear whether these are incidental findings or subclinical erosions [3,57,102].

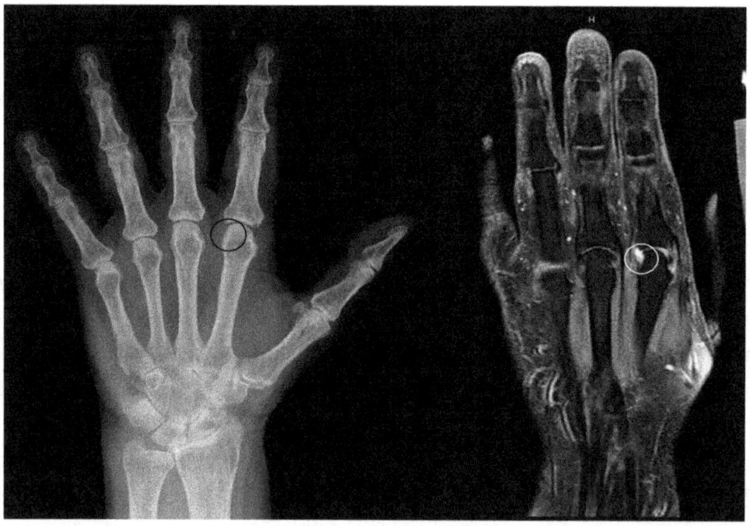

Figure 5. Erosions within pseudoerosions. Example of the development of an erosion within a pseudoerosion (black/white circle) in a left hand of a 65 years old female patient with longstanding mild seropositive rheumatoid arthritis. Left: radiograph, right: MRI.

4.4. Limitations

A limitation of this study was that the defined search terms resulted in a large quantity of papers, which had to be screened. However, generally accepted terms for mimickers of true erosions do not exist, are described in various forms and additionally with more equivocal definitions than expected at the beginning of this project. Nonetheless, this wide search net allowed for the inclusion of all relevant sources describing the phenomenon of pseudoerosions and minimized the possibility of excluding the respective publications.

5. Conclusions

In conclusion, a pseudoerosion is more than just a negative definition of an erosion. It can be defined as a normal osseous concavity (anatomic pseudoerosion) and/or an artefactual interruption of the calcified zones (artefact-related pseudoerosion). It can be classified according to their configuration, shape, content, and can be directly anatomically named. "Calcified zone" is a term to describe the deep components of the subchondral, subligamentous and subtendinous bone and may be applied for all non-cancellous borders of a bone, thus representing a third type of the bone matrix beside the cortical and the trabecular bone. Anatomic pseudoerosions are almost always related to a ligament insertion or the osteo-fibrous channel of a tendon sheath, therefore, being of high risk for microdamage and the development of a "true" arthritic erosion. Understanding these peculiar aspects of the bony surface with relation to ligament insertions and osteofibrous channels may be of help in improving the assessment of erosions and for reducing over- and underdiagnosis of true erosions.

6. Take Home Message

1. Pseudoerosions may be subclassified into anatomic (normal osseous cavity) and artefact-related (artefactual interruption of the calcified zone).
2. The term "calcified zone" describes the deep components of the subchondral, subligamentous and subtendinous bone and may be applied for all non-cancellous borders of a bone.
3. Pseudoerosions can be regarded as anatomic sites at risk for the development of "true" arthritic erosions.

Author Contributions: Conceptualization, L.H. and F.K.; methodology, L.H.; software, L.H.; validation, L.H., C.R. and F.K.; formal analysis, L.H. and F.K.; investigation, L.H.; resources, L.H.; data curation, L.H.; writing—original draft preparation, L.H. and F.K.; writing—review and editing, L.H., H.P., D.A., C.R. and F.K.; visualization, L.H.; supervision, F.K.

References

1. Albrecht, A.; Finzel, S.; Englbrecht, M.; Rech, J.; Hueber, A.; Schlechtweg, P.; Uder, M.; Schett, G. The structural basis of MRI bone erosions: An assessment by microCT. *Ann. Rheum. Dis.* **2013**, *72*, 1351–1357. [CrossRef] [PubMed]
2. Hetland, M.L.; Ejbjerg, B.; Horslev-Petersen, K.; Jacobsen, S.; Vestergaard, A.; Jurik, A.G.; Stengaard-Pedersen, K.; Junker, P.; Lottenburger, T.; Hansen, I.; et al. MRI bone oedema is the strongest predictor of subsequent radiographic progression in early rheumatoid arthritis. Results from a 2-year randomised controlled trial (CIMESTRA). *Ann. Rheum. Dis.* **2009**, *68*, 384–390. [CrossRef] [PubMed]
3. Martel, W.; Hayes, J.T.; Duff, I.F. The Pattern of Bone Erosion in the Hand and Wrist in Rheumatoid Arthritis. *Radiology* **1965**, *84*, 204–214. [CrossRef] [PubMed]
4. Buckland-Wright, J.C. Microfocal radiographic examination of erosions in the wrist and hand of patients with rheumatoid arthritis. *Ann. Rheum. Dis.* **1984**, *43*, 160–171. [CrossRef]
5. Wakefield, R.J.; Gibbon, W.W.; Conaghan, P.G.; O'Connor, P.; McGonagle, D.; Pease, C.; Green, M.J.; Veale, D.J.; Isaacs, J.D.; Emery, P. The value of sonography in the detection of bone erosions in patients with rheumatoid arthritis: A comparison with conventional radiography. *Arthritis Rheum.* **2000**, *43*, 2762–2770. [CrossRef]

6. Kellgren, J.H.; Lawrence, J.S. Radiological assessment of rheumatoid arthritis. *Ann. Rheum. Dis.* **1957**, *16*, 485–493. [CrossRef]
7. Larsen, A.; Dale, K.; Eek, M. Radiographic evaluation of rheumatoid arthritis and related conditions by standard reference films. *Acta Radiol. Diagn.* **1977**, *18*, 481–491. [CrossRef]
8. Larsen, A. Radiological grading of rheumatoid arthritis. An interobserver study. *Scand. J. Rheumatol.* **1973**, *2*, 136–138. [CrossRef]
9. van der Heijde, D.M. Plain X-rays in rheumatoid arthritis: Overview of scoring methods, their reliability and applicability. *Baillieres Clin. Rheumatol.* **1996**, *10*, 435–453. [CrossRef]
10. van der Heijde, D.; Dankert, T.; Nieman, F.; Rau, R.; Boers, M. Reliability and sensitivity to change of a simplification of the Sharp/van der Heijde radiological assessment in rheumatoid arthritis. *Rheumatology* **1999**, *38*, 941–947. [CrossRef]
11. Barnabe, C.; Toepfer, D.; Marotte, H.; Hauge, E.M.; Scharmga, A.; Kocijan, R.; Kraus, S.; Boutroy, S.; Schett, G.; Keller, K.K.; et al. Definition for Rheumatoid Arthritis Erosions Imaged with High Resolution Peripheral Quantitative Computed Tomography and Interreader Reliability for Detection and Measurement. *J. Rheumatol.* **2016**, *43*, 1935–1940. [CrossRef] [PubMed]
12. Ibrahim-Nasser, N.; Marotte, H.; Valery, A.; Salliot, C.; Toumi, H.; Lespessailles, E. Precision and sources of variability in the assessment of rheumatoid arthritis erosions by HRpQCT. *Jt. Bone Spine* **2018**, *85*, 211–217. [CrossRef] [PubMed]
13. Aletaha, D.; Neogi, T.; Silman, A.J.; Funovits, J.; Felson, D.T.; Bingham, C.O.; Birnbaum, N.S.; Burmester, G.R.; Bykerk, V.P.; Cohen, M.D.; et al. 2010 rheumatoid arthritis classification criteria: An American College of Rheumatology/European League Against Rheumatism collaborative initiative. *Ann. Rheum. Dis.* **2010**, *69*, 1580–1588. [CrossRef] [PubMed]
14. Funovits, J.; Aletaha, D.; Bykerk, V.; Combe, B.; Dougados, M.; Emery, P.; Felson, D.; Hawker, G.; Hazes, J.M.; Huizinga, T.; et al. The 2010 American College of Rheumatology/European League Against Rheumatism classification criteria for rheumatoid arthritis: Methodological report phase I. *Ann. Rheum. Dis.* **2010**, *69*, 1589–1595. [CrossRef]
15. van der Heijde, D.; van der Helm-van Mil, A.H.; Aletaha, D.; Bingham, C.O.; Burmester, G.R.; Dougados, M.; Emery, P.; Felson, D.; Knevel, R.; Kvien, T.K. EULAR definition of erosive disease in light of the 2010 ACR/EULAR rheumatoid arthritis classification criteria. *Ann. Rheum. Dis.* **2013**, *72*, 479–481. [CrossRef]
16. Siddle, H.J.; Hensor, E.M.; Hodgson, R.J.; Grainger, A.J.; Redmond, A.C.; Wakefield, R.J.; Helliwell, P.S. Anatomical location of erosions at the metatarsophalangeal joints in patients with rheumatoid arthritis. *Rheumatology* **2014**, *53*, 932–936. [CrossRef]
17. Alcalde, M.; D'Agostino, M.A.; Bruyn, G.A.; Moller, I.; Iagnocco, A.; Wakefield, R.J.; Naredo, E.; Force, O.U.T. A systematic literature review of US definitions, scoring systems and validity according to the OMERACT filter for tendon lesion in RA and other inflammatory joint diseases. *Rheumatology* **2012**, *51*, 1246–1260. [CrossRef]
18. Ostergaard, M.; Peterfy, C.; Conaghan, P.; McQueen, F.; Bird, P.; Ejbjerg, B.; Shnier, R.; O'Connor, P.; Klarlund, M.; Emery, P.; et al. OMERACT Rheumatoid Arthritis Magnetic Resonance Imaging Studies. Core set of MRI acquisitions, joint pathology definitions, and the OMERACT RA-MRI scoring system. *J. Rheumatol.* **2003**, *30*, 1385–1386.
19. Ostergaard, M.; Moller Dohn, U.; Duer-Jensen, A.; Hetland, M.L.; Horslev-Petersen, K.; Stengaard-Pedersen, K.; Junker, P.; Podenphant, J.; Ejbjerg, B. Patterns of magnetic resonance imaging bone erosion in rheumatoid arthritis–which bones are most frequently involved and show the most change? *J. Rheumatol.* **2011**, *38*, 2014–2017. [CrossRef]
20. Hammer, H.B.; Haavardsholm, E.A.; Boyesen, P.; Kvien, T.K. Bone erosions at the distal ulna detected by ultrasonography are associated with structural damage assessed by conventional radiography and MRI: A study of patients with recent onset rheumatoid arthritis. *Rheumatology* **2009**, *48*, 1530–1532. [CrossRef]
21. Resnick, D.; Gmelich, J.T. Bone fragmentation in the rheumatoid wrist: Radiographic and pathologic considerations. *Radiology* **1975**, *114*, 315–321. [CrossRef]
22. Boutry, N.; Morel, M.; Flipo, R.M.; Demondion, X.; Cotten, A. Early rheumatoid arthritis: A review of MRI and sonographic findings. *AJR Am. J. Roentgenol.* **2007**, *189*, 1502–1509. [CrossRef]
23. Leak, R.S.; Rayan, G.M.; Arthur, R.E. Longitudinal radiographic analysis of rheumatoid arthritis in the hand and wrist. *J. Hand Surg. Am. Vol.* **2003**, *28*, 427–434. [CrossRef]

24. Lee, K.A.; Min, S.H.; Kim, T.H.; Lee, S.H.; Kim, H.R. Magnetic resonance imaging-assessed synovial and bone changes in hand and wrist joints of rheumatoid arthritis patients. *Korean J. Intern. Med.* **2019**, *34*, 651–659. [CrossRef]
25. Kitamura, T.; Murase, T.; Hashimoto, J.; Tomita, T.; Arimitsu, S.; Yoshikawa, H.; Sugamoto, K. Radiographic study on the pattern of wrist joint destruction in rheumatoid arthritis. *Clin. Rheumatol.* **2011**, *30*, 353–359. [CrossRef]
26. Taleisnik, J. Rheumatoid synovitis of the volar compartment of the wrist joint: Its radiological signs and its contribution to wrist and hand deformity. *J. Hand Surg. Am. Vol.* **1979**, *4*, 526–535. [CrossRef]
27. Karasick, D.; Schweitzer, M.E.; O'Hara, B.J. Distal fibular notch: A frequent manifestation of the rheumatoid ankle. *Skelet. Radiol.* **1997**, *26*, 529–532.
28. Baan, H.; Bezooijen, R.; Avenarius, J.K.; Dubbeldam, R.; Drossaers-Bakker, W.K.; van de Laar, M.A. Magnetic resonance imaging of the rheumatic foot according to the RAMRIS system is reliable. *J. Rheumatol.* **2011**, *38*, 1003–1008. [CrossRef]
29. Lee, D.M.; Weinblatt, M.E. Rheumatoid arthritis. *Lancet* **2001**, *358*, 903–911. [CrossRef]
30. Tan, A.L.; Tanner, S.F.; Conaghan, P.G.; Radjenovic, A.; O'Connor, P.; Brown, A.K.; Emery, P.; McGonagle, D. Role of metacarpophalangeal joint anatomic factors in the distribution of synovitis and bone erosion in early rheumatoid arthritis. *Arthritis Rheum.* **2003**, *48*, 1214–1222. [CrossRef]
31. Schett, G.; Gravallese, E. Bone erosion in rheumatoid arthritis: Mechanisms, diagnosis and treatment. *Nat. Rev. Rheumatol.* **2012**, *8*, 656–664. [CrossRef]
32. Werner, D.; Simon, D.; Englbrecht, M.; Stemmler, F.; Simon, C.; Berlin, A.; Haschka, J.; Renner, N.; Buder, T.; Engelke, K.; et al. Early Changes of the Cortical Micro-Channel System in the Bare Area of the Joints of Patients with Rheumatoid Arthritis. *Arthritis Rheumatol.* **2017**, *69*, 1580–1587. [CrossRef]
33. McQueen, F.; Clarke, A.; McHaffie, A.; Reeves, Q.; Williams, M.; Robinson, E.; Dong, J.; Chand, A.; Mulders, D.; Dalbeth, N. Assessment of cartilage loss at the wrist in rheumatoid arthritis using a new MRI scoring system. *Ann. Rheum. Dis.* **2010**, *69*, 1971–1975. [CrossRef]
34. Peters, M.; van Tubergen, A.; Scharmga, A.; Driessen, A.; van Rietbergen, B.; Loeffen, D.; Weijers, R.; Geusens, P.; van den Bergh, J. Assessment of Cortical Interruptions in the Finger Joints of Patients with Rheumatoid Arthritis Using HR-pQCT, Radiography, and MRI. *J. Bone Miner. Res.* **2018**, *33*, 1676–1685. [CrossRef]
35. Conaghan, P.G.; O'Connor, P.; McGonagle, D.; Astin, P.; Wakefield, R.J.; Gibbon, W.W.; Quinn, M.; Karim, Z.; Green, M.J.; Proudman, S.; et al. Elucidation of the relationship between synovitis and bone damage: A randomized magnetic resonance imaging study of individual joints in patients with early rheumatoid arthritis. *Arthritis Rheum.* **2003**, *48*, 64–71. [CrossRef]
36. Schleich, C.; Muller-Lutz, A.; Sewerin, P.; Ostendorf, B.; Buchbender, C.; Schneider, M.; Antoch, G.; Miese, F. Intra-individual assessment of inflammatory severity and cartilage composition of finger joints in rheumatoid arthritis. *Skelet. Radiol.* **2015**, *44*, 513–518. [CrossRef]
37. Favalli, E.G.; Becciolini, A.; Biggioggero, M. Structural integrity versus radiographic progression in rheumatoid arthritis. *RMD Open* **2015**, *1*, e000064. [CrossRef]
38. Boeters, D.M.; Nieuwenhuis, W.P.; van Steenbergen, H.W.; Reijnierse, M.; Landewe, R.B.M.; van der Helm-van Mil, A.H.M. Are MRI-detected erosions specific for RA? A large explorative cross-sectional study. *Ann. Rheum. Dis.* **2018**, *77*, 861–868. [CrossRef]
39. Felloni, P.; Larkman, N.; Dunca, R.; Cotton, A. Inflammatory Arthritides: Imaging Pitfalls. In *Pitfalls in Musculoskeletal Radiology*; Peh, W., Ed.; Springer: Berlin/Heidelberg, Germany, 2017; pp. 697–712.
40. Dihlmann, W.; Bandick, J. *Die Gelenksilhouette: Das Informationspotential der Röntgenstrahlen*; Springer: Berlin/Heidelberg, Germany, 1995.
41. Wawer, R.; Budzik, J.F.; Demondion, X.; Forzy, G.; Cotten, A. Carpal pseudoerosions: A plain X-ray interpretation pitfall. *Skelet. Radiol.* **2014**, *43*, 1377–1385. [CrossRef]
42. Sharp, J.T.; Wolfe, F.; Lassere, M.; Boers, M.; Van Der Heijde, D.; Larsen, A.; Paulus, H.; Rau, R.; Strand, V. Variability of precision in scoring radiographic abnormalities in rheumatoid arthritis by experienced readers. *J. Rheumatol.* **2004**, *31*, 1062–1072.

43. McQueen, F.M.; Benton, N.; Perry, D.; Crabbe, J.; Robinson, E.; Yeoman, S.; McLean, L.; Stewart, N. Bone edema scored on magnetic resonance imaging scans of the dominant carpus at presentation predicts radiographic joint damage of the hands and feet six years later in patients with rheumatoid arthritis. *Arthritis Rheum.* **2003**, *48*, 1814–1827. [CrossRef]
44. Ejbjerg, B.; Narvestad, E.; Rostrup, E.; Szkudlarek, M.; Jacobsen, S.; Thomsen, H.S.; Ostergaard, M. Magnetic resonance imaging of wrist and finger joints in healthy subjects occasionally shows changes resembling erosions and synovitis as seen in rheumatoid arthritis. *Arthritis Rheum.* **2004**, *50*, 1097–1106. [CrossRef] [PubMed]
45. Olech, E.; Crues, J.V.; Yocum, D.E.; Merrill, J.T. Bone marrow edema is the most specific finding for rheumatoid arthritis (RA) on noncontrast magnetic resonance imaging of the hands and wrists: A comparison of patients with RA and healthy controls. *J. Rheumatol.* **2010**, *37*, 265–274. [CrossRef] [PubMed]
46. Rothschild, B.M. Significance of "Erosion-like Lesions" in "Healthy Controls". *J. Rheumatol.* **2010**, *37*, 1964. [CrossRef] [PubMed]
47. Finzel, S.; Ohrndorf, S.; Englbrecht, M.; Stach, C.; Messerschmidt, J.; Schett, M.; Backhaus, G. A detailed comparative study of high-resolution ultrasound and micro-computed tomography for detection of arthritic bone erosions. *Arthritis Rheum.* **2011**, *63*, 1231–1236. [CrossRef]
48. Langs, G.; Peloschek, P.; Bischof, H.; Kainberger, F. Model-based erosion spotting and visualization in rheumatoid arthritis. *Acad. Radiol.* **2007**, *14*, 1179–1188. [CrossRef]
49. Yang, H.; Rivoire, J.; Hoppe, M.; Srikhum, W.; Imboden, J.; Link, T.M.; Li, X. Computer-aided and manual quantifications of MRI synovitis, bone marrow edema-like lesions, erosion and cartilage loss in rheumatoid arthritis of the wrist. *Skelet. Radiol.* **2015**, *44*, 539–547. [CrossRef]
50. Liberati, A.; Altman, D.G.; Tetzlaff, J.; Mulrow, C.; Gotzsche, P.C.; Ioannidis, J.P.; Clarke, M.; Devereaux, P.J.; Kleijnen, J.; Moher, D. The PRISMA statement for reporting systematic reviews and meta-analyses of studies that evaluate health care interventions: Explanation and elaboration. *J. Clin. Epidemiol.* **2009**, *62*, e1-34. [CrossRef]
51. McQueen, F.; Ostergaard, M.; Peterfy, C.; Lassere, M.; Ejbjerg, B.; Bird, P.; O'Connor, P.; Genant, H.; Shnier, R.; Emery, P.; et al. Pitfalls in scoring MR images of rheumatoid arthritis wrist and metacarpophalangeal joints. *Ann. Rheum. Dis.* **2005**, *64*, i48–i55. [CrossRef]
52. Peluso, G.; Bosello, S.L.; Gremese, E.; Mirone, L.; Di Gregorio, F.; Di Molfetta, V.; Pirronti, T.; Ferraccioli, G. Detection of bone erosions in early rheumatoid arthritis: 3D ultrasonography versus computed tomography. *Clin. Rheumatol.* **2015**, *34*, 1181–1186. [CrossRef]
53. Dohn, U.M.; Ejbjerg, B.J.; Court-Payen, M.; Hasselquist, M.; Narvestad, E.; Szkudlarek, M.; Moller, J.M.; Thomsen, H.S.; Ostergaard, M. Are bone erosions detected by magnetic resonance imaging and ultrasonography true erosions? A comparison with computed tomography in rheumatoid arthritis metacarpophalangeal joints. *Arthritis Res. Ther.* **2006**, *8*, R110. [CrossRef]
54. Canella Moraes Carmo, C.; Cruz, G.P.; Trudell, D.; Hughes, T.; Chung, C.; Resnick, D. Anatomical features of metacarpal heads that simulate bone erosions: Cadaveric study using computed tomography scanning and sectional radiography. *J. Comput. Assist. Tomogr.* **2009**, *33*, 573–578. [CrossRef]
55. Torshizy, H.; Hughes, T.H.; Trudell, D.; Resnick, D. Anatomic features of metatarsal heads that simulate erosive disease: Cadaveric study using CT, radiography, and dissection with special emphasis on cross-sectional characterization of osseous anatomy. *AJR Am. J. Roentgenol.* **2008**, *190*, W175–W181. [CrossRef]
56. Robertson, P.L.; Page, P.J.; McColl, G.J. Inflammatory arthritis-like and other MR findings in wrists of asymptomatic subjects. *Skelet. Radiol.* **2006**, *35*, 754–764. [CrossRef]
57. Dohn, U.M.; Terslev, L.; Szkudlarek, M.; Hansen, M.S.; Hetland, M.L.; Hansen, A.; Madsen, O.R.; Hasselquist, M.; Moller, J.; Ostergaard, M. Detection, scoring and volume assessment of bone erosions by ultrasonography in rheumatoid arthritis: Comparison with CT. *Ann. Rheum. Dis.* **2013**, *72*, 530–534. [CrossRef]
58. Alasaarela, E.; Suramo, I.; Tervonen, O.; Lahde, S.; Takalo, R.; Hakala, M. Evaluation of humeral head erosions in rheumatoid arthritis: A comparison of ultrasonography, magnetic resonance imaging, computed tomography and plain radiography. *Br. J. Rheumatol.* **1998**, *37*, 1152–1156. [CrossRef]
59. Foley-Nolan, D.; Stack, J.P.; Ryan, M.; Redmond, U.; Barry, C.; Ennis, J.; Coughlan, R.J. Magnetic resonance imaging in the assessment of rheumatoid arthritis—A comparison with plain film radiographs. *Br. J. Rheumatol.* **1991**, *30*, 101–106. [CrossRef]

60. Cimmino, M.A.; Bountis, C.; Silvestri, E.; Garlaschi, G.; Accardo, S. An appraisal of magnetic resonance imaging of the wrist in rheumatoid arthritis. *Semin. Arthritis Rheum.* **2000**, *30*, 180–195. [CrossRef]
61. Forslind, K.; Johanson, A.; Larsson, E.M.; Svensson, B. Magnetic resonance imaging of the fifth metatarsophalangeal joint compared with conventional radiography in patients with early rheumatoid arthritis. *Scand. J. Rheumatol.* **2003**, *32*, 131–137. [CrossRef]
62. Amin, M.F.; Ismail, F.M.; el Shereef, R.R. The role of ultrasonography in early detection and monitoring of shoulder erosions, and disease activity in rheumatoid arthritis patients; comparison with MRI examination. *Acad. Radiol.* **2012**, *19*, 693–700. [CrossRef]
63. Aurell, Y.; Andersson, M.; Forslind, K. Cone-beam computed tomography, a new low-dose three-dimensional imaging technique for assessment of bone erosions in rheumatoid arthritis: Reliability assessment and comparison with conventional radiography—A BARFOT study. *Scand. J. Rheumatol.* **2018**, *47*, 173–177. [CrossRef]
64. Ejbjerg, B.J.; Vestergaard, A.; Jacobsen, S.; Thomsen, H.; Ostergaard, M. Conventional radiography requires a MRI-estimated bone volume loss of 20% to 30% to allow certain detection of bone erosions in rheumatoid arthritis metacarpophalangeal joints. *Arthritis Res. Ther.* **2006**, *8*, R59. [CrossRef]
65. Dohn, U.M.; Ejbjerg, B.J.; Hasselquist, M.; Narvestad, E.; Moller, J.; Thomsen, H.S.; Ostergaard, M. Detection of bone erosions in rheumatoid arthritis wrist joints with magnetic resonance imaging, computed tomography and radiography. *Arthritis Res. Ther.* **2008**, *10*, R25. [CrossRef]
66. Kleyer, A.; Krieter, M.; Oliveira, I.; Faustini, F.; Simon, D.; Kaemmerer, N.; Cavalcante, A.; Tabosa, T.; Rech, J.; Hueber, A.; et al. High prevalence of tenosynovial inflammation before onset of rheumatoid arthritis and its link to progression to RA-A combined MRI/CT study. *Semin. Arthritis Rheum.* **2016**, *46*, 143–150. [CrossRef]
67. Ulas, S.T.; Diekhoff, T.; Hermann, K.G.A.; Poddubnyy, D.; Hamm, B.; Makowski, M.R. Susceptibility-weighted MR imaging to improve the specificity of erosion detection: A prospective feasibility study in hand arthritis. *Skelet. Radiol.* **2019**, *48*, 721–728. [CrossRef]
68. Emond, P.D.; Inglis, D.; Choi, A.; Tricta, J.; Adachi, J.D.; Gordon, C.L. Volume measurement of bone erosions in magnetic resonance images of patients with rheumatoid arthritis. *Magn. Reson. Med.* **2012**, *67*, 814–823. [CrossRef]
69. McQueen, F.M.; Stewart, N.; Crabbe, J.; Robinson, E.; Yeoman, S.; Tan, P.L.; McLean, L. Magnetic resonance imaging of the wrist in early rheumatoid arthritis reveals a high prevalence of erosions at four months after symptom onset. *Ann. Rheum. Dis.* **1998**, *57*, 350–356. [CrossRef]
70. McQueen, F.M.; Benton, N.; Crabbe, J.; Robinson, E.; Yeoman, S.; McLean, L.; Stewart, N. What is the fate of erosions in early rheumatoid arthritis? Tracking individual lesions using X rays and magnetic resonance imaging over the first two years of disease. *Ann. Rheum. Dis.* **2001**, *60*, 859–868.
71. Dihlmann, W. A early sign of arthritis. The loss of subchondral marginal lamellae. *Z. Rheumaforsch.* **1968**, *27*, 129–132.
72. Regensburger, A.; Rech, J.; Englbrecht, M.; Finzel, S.; Kraus, S.; Hecht, K.; Kleyer, A.; Haschka, J.; Hueber, A.J.; Cavallaro, A.; et al. A comparative analysis of magnetic resonance imaging and high-resolution peripheral quantitative computed tomography of the hand for the detection of erosion repair in rheumatoid arthritis. *Rheumatology* **2015**, *54*, 1573–1581. [CrossRef]
73. Schrank, C.; Meirer, R.; Stabler, A.; Nerlich, A.; Reiser, M.; Putz, R. Morphology and topography of intraosseous ganglion cysts in the carpus: An anatomic, histopathologic, and magnetic resonance imaging correlation study. *J. Hand Surg. Am.* **2003**, *28*, 52–61. [CrossRef]
74. Paparo, F.; Fabbro, E.; Piccazzo, R.; Revelli, M.; Ferrero, G.; Muda, A.; Cimmino, M.A.; Garlaschi, G. Multimodality imaging of intraosseous ganglia of the wrist and their differential diagnosis. *Radiol. Med.* **2012**, *117*, 1355–1373. [CrossRef]
75. Mangnus, L.; van Steenbergen, H.W.; Lindqvist, E.; Brouwer, E.; Reijnierse, M.; Huizinga, T.W.; Gregersen, P.K.; Berglin, E.; Rantapaa-Dahlqvist, S.; van der Heijde, D.; et al. Studies on ageing and the severity of radiographic joint damage in rheumatoid arthritis. *Arthritis Res. Ther.* **2015**, *17*, 222. [CrossRef]
76. Avenarius, D.M.; Ording Muller, L.S.; Eldevik, P.; Owens, C.M.; Rosendahl, K. The paediatric wrist revisited—Findings of bony depressions in healthy children on radiographs compared to MRI. *Pediatr. Radiol.* **2012**, *42*, 791–798. [CrossRef]

77. Boavida, P.; Hargunani, R.; Owens, C.M.; Rosendahl, K. Magnetic resonance imaging and radiographic assessment of carpal depressions in children with juvenile idiopathic arthritis: Normal variants or erosions? *J. Rheumatol.* **2012**, *39*, 645–650. [CrossRef]
78. Boavida, P.; Lambot-Juhan, K.; Muller, L.S.; Damasio, B.; de Horatio, L.T.; Malattia, C.; Owens, C.M.; Rosendahl, K. Carpal erosions in children with juvenile idiopathic arthritis: Repeatability of a newly devised MR-scoring system. *Pediatr. Radiol.* **2015**, *45*, 1972–1980. [CrossRef]
79. Benjamin, M.; McGonagle, D. The anatomical basis for disease localisation in seronegative spondyloarthropathy at entheses and related sites. *J. Anat.* **2001**, *199*, 503–526. [CrossRef]
80. Platzer, W. *Taschenatlas Anatomie 01. Bewegungsapparat*; Thieme Georg Verlag: New York, NY, USA, 2009.
81. Standring, S. *Gray's Anatomy: The Anatomical Basis of Clinical Practice*; Elsevier: Amsterdam, The Netherlands, 2008.
82. Boutry, N.; Larde, A.; Demondion, X.; Cortet, B.; Cotten, H.; Cotten, A. Metacarpophalangeal joints at US in asymptomatic volunteers and cadaveric specimens. *Radiology* **2004**, *232*, 716–724. [CrossRef]
83. Fanghänel, J.; Pera, F.; Anderhuber, F.; Nitsch, R. *Waldeyer—Anatomie des Menschen*, 18th ed.; Walter de Gruyter: Berlin, Germany, 2009.
84. Manaster, B.J.; Crim, J.R. *Imaging Anatomy: Musculoskeletal*; Elsevier: Amsterdam, The Netherlands, 2016.
85. Eshed, I.; Bollow, M.; McGonagle, D.G.; Tan, A.L.; Althoff, C.E.; Asbach, P.; Hermann, K.G. MRI of enthesitis of the appendicular skeleton in spondyloarthritis. *Ann. Rheum. Dis.* **2007**, *66*, 1553–1559. [CrossRef]
86. Boutry, N.; Hachulla, E.; Flipo, R.M.; Cortet, B.; Cotten, A. MR imaging findings in hands in early rheumatoid arthritis: Comparison with those in systemic lupus erythematosus and primary Sjogren syndrome. *Radiology* **2005**, *236*, 593–600. [CrossRef]
87. Boutroy, S.; Chapurlat, R.; Vanden-Bossche, A.; Locrelle, H.; Thomas, T.; Marotte, H. Erosion or vascular channel? *Arthritis Rheum.* **2015**, *67*, 2956. [CrossRef]
88. Hoving, J.L.; Buchbinder, R.; Hall, S.; Lawler, G.; Coombs, P.; McNealy, S.; Bird, P.; Connell, D. A comparison of magnetic resonance imaging, sonography, and radiography of the hand in patients with early rheumatoid arthritis. *J. Rheumatol.* **2004**, *31*, 663–675.
89. Wang, B.; Overgaard, S.; Chemnitz, J.; Ding, M. Cancellous and Cortical Bone Microarchitectures of Femoral Neck in Rheumatoid Arthritis and Osteoarthritis Compared with Donor Controls. *Calcif. Tissue Int.* **2016**, *98*, 456–464. [CrossRef] [PubMed]
90. Perry, D.; Stewart, N.; Benton, N.; Robinson, E.; Yeoman, S.; Crabbe, J.; McQueen, F. Detection of erosions in the rheumatoid hand; a comparative study of multidetector computerized tomography versus magnetic resonance scanning. *J. Rheumatol.* **2005**, *32*, 256–267. [PubMed]
91. Dohn, U.M.; Ejbjerg, B.J.; Hasselquist, M.; Narvestad, E.; Court-Payen, M.; Szkudlarek, M.; Moller, J.; Thomsen, H.S.; Ostergaard, M. Rheumatoid arthritis bone erosion volumes on CT and MRI: Reliability and correlations with erosion scores on CT, MRI and radiography. *Ann. Rheum. Dis.* **2007**, *66*, 1388–1392. [CrossRef] [PubMed]
92. Hermann, K.G.; Backhaus, M.; Schneider, U.; Labs, K.; Loreck, D.; Zuhlsdorf, S.; Schink, T.; Fischer, T.; Hamm, B.; Bollow, M. Rheumatoid arthritis of the shoulder joint: Comparison of conventional radiography, ultrasound, and dynamic contrast-enhanced magnetic resonance imaging. *Arthritis Rheum.* **2003**, *48*, 3338–3349. [CrossRef]
93. Hodler, J.; Terrier, B.; von Schulthess, G.K.; Fuchs, W.A. MRI and sonography of the shoulder. *Clin. Radiol.* **1991**, *43*, 323–327. [CrossRef]
94. Klarlund, M.; Ostergaard, M.; Jensen, K.E.; Madsen, J.L.; Skjodt, H.; Lorenzen, I. Magnetic resonance imaging, radiography, and scintigraphy of the finger joints: One year follow up of patients with early arthritis. The TIRA Group. *Ann. Rheum. Dis.* **2000**, *59*, 521–528. [CrossRef]
95. Yang, H.; Yu, A.; Burghardt, A.J.; Virayavanich, W.; Link, T.M.; Imboden, J.B.; Li, X. Quantitative characterization of metacarpal and radial bone in rheumatoid arthritis using high resolution-peripheral quantitative computed tomography. *Int. J. Rheum. Dis.* **2017**, *20*, 353–362. [CrossRef]
96. Fouque-Aubert, A.; Boutroy, S.; Marotte, H.; Vilayphiou, N.; Bacchetta, J.; Miossec, P.; Delmas, P.D.; Chapurlat, R.D. Assessment of hand bone loss in rheumatoid arthritis by high-resolution peripheral quantitative CT. *Ann. Rheum. Dis.* **2010**, *69*, 1671–1676. [CrossRef]

97. Feehan, L.; Buie, H.; Li, L.; McKay, H. A customized protocol to assess bone quality in the metacarpal head, metacarpal shaft and distal radius: A high resolution peripheral quantitative computed tomography precision study. *BMC Musculoskelet. Disord.* **2013**, *14*, 367. [CrossRef] [PubMed]
98. Kocijan, R.; Finzel, S.; Englbrecht, M.; Engelke, K.; Rech, J.; Schett, G. Decreased quantity and quality of the periarticular and nonperiarticular bone in patients with rheumatoid arthritis: A cross-sectional HR-pQCT study. *J. Bone Miner. Res.* **2014**, *29*, 1005–1014. [CrossRef] [PubMed]
99. Guermazi, A.; Taouli, B.; Lynch, J.A.; Peterfy, C.G. Imaging of bone erosion in rheumatoid arthritis. *Semin. Musculoskelet. Radiol.* **2004**, *8*, 269–285. [CrossRef] [PubMed]
100. Zayat, A.S.; Ellegaard, K.; Conaghan, P.G.; Terslev, L.; Hensor, E.M.; Freeston, J.E.; Emery, P.; Wakefield, R.J. The specificity of ultrasound-detected bone erosions for rheumatoid arthritis. *Ann. Rheum. Dis.* **2015**, *74*, 897–903. [CrossRef] [PubMed]
101. Buckland-Wright, J.C. X-ray assessment of activity in rheumatoid disease. *Br. J. Rheumatol.* **1983**, *22*, 3–10. [CrossRef]
102. Canella, C.; Philippe, P.; Pansini, V.; Salleron, J.; Flipo, R.M.; Cotten, A. Use of tomosynthesis for erosion evaluation in rheumatoid arthritic hands and wrists. *Radiology* **2011**, *258*, 199–205. [CrossRef]

7

Regulation of Th17 Cytokine-Induced Osteoclastogenesis via SKI306X in Rheumatoid Arthritis

Hae-Rim Kim [1,†], Kyoung-Woon Kim [2,†], Bo-Mi Kim [2], Ji-Yeon Won [2], Hong-Ki Min [1], Kyung-Ann Lee [3], Tae-Young Kim [4] and Sang-Heon Lee [1,*]

1 Division of Rheumatology, Department of Internal Medicine, Research Institute of Medical Science, School of Medicine, Konkuk University, Seoul 05030, Korea
2 Conversant Research Consortium in Immunologic Disease, Seoul St. Mary's Hospital, The Catholic University of Korea, Seoul 06591, Korea
3 Division of Rheumatology, Department of Internal Medicine, Soonchunhyang University Hospital, Seoul 04401, Korea
4 Department of Orthopedic Surgery, School of Medicine, Konkuk University, Seoul 05030, Korea
* Correspondence: shlee@kuh.ac.kr
† These authors contributed equally to this work.

Abstract: This study aimed to investigate the regulatory effect of SKI306X, a mixed extract of three herbs, in T helper (Th)17 cytokine-induced inflammation and joint destruction in rheumatoid arthritis (RA). Synovial fibroblasts were isolated from RA patients and cultured with Th17 cytokines including interleukin (IL)-17, IL-21, and IL-22 and SKI306X, and tumor necrosis factor (TNF)-α, IL-1β, and receptor activator of nuclear factor kappa-B ligand (RANKL) expression and production were investigated using real-time PCR and ELISA of culture media. After peripheral blood (PB) cluster of differentiation (CD)14$^+$ monocytes were cultured in media supplemented with Th17 cytokines and SKI306X, tartrate-resistant acid phosphatase positive (TRAP$^+$) multinucleated giant cells (mature osteoclasts) were enumerated and gene expression associated with osteoclast maturation was assessed via real-time PCR analysis. After PB monocytes were co-cultured with IL-17-stimulated RA synovial fibroblasts in the presence of SKI306X, osteoclast differentiation was assessed. When RA synovial fibroblasts were cultured with IL-17, IL-21, and IL-22, TNF-α, IL-1β, and RANKL expression and production were increased; however, SKI306X reduced cytokine expression and production. When PB monocytes were cultured in media supplemented with Th17 cytokines, osteoclast differentiation was stimulated; however, SKI306X decreased osteoclast differentiation and osteoclast maker expression. When PB monocytes were co-cultured with IL-17-stimulated RA synovial fibroblasts, osteoclast differentiation was increased; however, SKI306X decreased osteoclast differentiation and osteoclast maker expression. SKI306X reduced Th17 cytokine-induced TNF-α, IL-1β, and RANKL expression and osteoclast differentiation, providing novel insights into adjuvant therapy for regulating inflammation and joint destruction in RA.

Keywords: rheumatoid arthritis; synovial fibroblasts; cytokine; osteoclast; herbal medicine

1. Introduction

A few decades ago, Korean patients with rheumatoid arthritis (RA) received herbal medication and acupuncture before they visited rheumatologic clinics. They believed the herbal therapies could cure RA without any adverse effects. By the time these patients visited rheumatologists, they already had joint destruction and disability because of delayed treatment with disease-modifying antirheumatic drugs (DMARDs). RA is currently considered an autoimmune inflammatory disease requiring treatment with DMARDs, which has led to an increase in rheumatologic consultations. However, DMARDs do not always have therapeutic effects in RA, they can display adverse effects and are highly expensive [1]. Hence, some patients prefer complementary and alternative medication, primarily including herbal medication [1,2]. According to the Korean RA registry (KORONA), 10.5% of patients received complementary and alternative medicines de novo and among them, 17% received herbal medication and 55% received acupuncture [3].

SKI306X, a mixed extract of three herbs, is a purified extract prepared from a mixture of three Oriental herbal plants, *Clematis mandshurica*, *Trichosanthes kirilowii*, and *Prunella vulgaris* [4]. According to the Donguibogam, i.e., 'Principles and Practice of Eastern Medicine' written in 1610, *Clematis mandshurica* effectively reduces lower back and knee pain, *Trichosanthes kirilowii* reduces febrile sensations and dry mouth, and *Prunella vulgaris* effectively reduces lymphadenitis, abscess, and ulcers. The anti-inflammatory effects of SKI306X have been reported previously.

SKI306X inhibits tumor necrosis factor (TNF)-α, leukotriene B4, and nitric oxide (NO) production in macrophages and cyclooxygenase-2 expression [5]. It inhibits TNF-α, prostaglandin E2, and interleukin (IL)-1β production by stimulated peripheral blood (PB) mononuclear cells [6] and is commonly used to treat osteoarthritis owing to its chondroprotective effects. SKI306X inhibits the IL-1β-induced production of proteoglycans, NO, matrix metalloproteinases (MMPs) and degradation of glycosaminoglycan by cartilage [4,6]. A preclinical animal study reported that SKI306X protects against osteoarthritis. Collagenase injection at the knee joint of rabbits led to osteoarthritis-like degeneration of articular cartilage and development of synovial tissues; however, SKI306X reduces osteoarthritis-like histological changes [4]. In chondrocytes cultured in media supplemented with IL-1α, the cumulative activity of MMP-3 and MMP-13 increased; however, SKI306X significantly reduced their activities and inhibited the activation of the proenzyme MMP-3 to the active MMP-3 [7]. In clinical trials of knee osteoarthritis, SKI306X treatment resulted in greater changes in pain and function than the placebo [8,9]. The change in cartilage volume and thickness of the lateral tibia were reportedly greater after treatment with SKI306X than the placebo [8].

Two studies have reported that SKI306X has similar effects in controlling for pain and disease activity and has greater cardiovascular safety than celecoxib in RA. When SKI306X was compared with celecoxib among RA patients, SKI306X was not inferior to celecoxib with regards to pain score (visual analog scale), American College of Rheumatology (ACR) 20 response rate, frequency of rescue medication, and drug-related adverse effects [10]. Unlike celecoxib, SKI306X does not have a higher risk of cardiovascular events in patients with RA and osteoarthritis [11]. However, the limitation of this clinical study was that celecoxib is not a DMARD and it cannot prevent joint destruction. Thus far, no study has investigated the anti-inflammatory and joint protective effects of SKI306X in RA. Therefore, this study aimed to investigate the regulatory effect of SKI306X in T helper (Th)17 cytokine-induced inflammation and bone destruction in RA.

2. Methods

2.1. Patients

Informed consent was obtained from all patients, and the experimental protocol was approved by the Institutional Review Board for Human Research, Konkuk University Hospital (KUH1010186, approved on January 22nd 2010). Synovial tissues were isolated from eight RA patients (mean age 63.4 ± 4.6 years, range 38–76 years) undergoing total knee and hip replacement surgery.

2.2. Isolation of Synovial Fibroblasts

Synovial fibroblasts were isolated by enzymatic digestion of synovial tissues, as described previously [12,13]. Synovial fibroblast cell lines were prepared from synovectomized tissue of RA patients undergoing joint replacement surgery. To set up cell lines, synovial tissues were minced into 2–3 mm pieces and treated for 4 h with 4 mg/mL type 1 collagenase (Worthington Biochemicals, Freehold,

NJ, USA) in Dulbecco's modified Eagle's medium (DMEM) at 37 °C in 5% CO_2. Dissociated cells were centrifuged at 500× *g* and were resuspended in DMEM supplemented with 10% fetal calf serum (FCS), 2 mM L-glutamine, 100 U/mL penicillin, and 100 μg/mL streptomycin. Suspended cells were plated in 75 cm^2 culture flasks and cultured at 37 °C in 5% CO_2. Medium was replaced every 3 days, and once the primary culture reached confluence, cells were split weekly. Cells at passages 5 to 8 contained a homogeneous population of synovial fibroblasts (<2.5% CD14 positive, <1% CD3 positive, and <1% CD19 positive in flow cytometric analysis).

2.3. Reagents

Recombinant human IL-17 (20 ng/mL), IL-21 (20 ng/mL), IL-22 (20 ng/mL), and macrophage colony-stimulating factor (M-CSF) (25 ng/mL) were purchased from R&D Systems (Minneapolis, MN, USA). SKI306X (at 0 μg/mL, 1 μg/mL, 5 μg/mL and 10 μg/mL) were generously provided by the Life Science R&D Center of SK Chemicals (Seongnam, Korea). Anti-TNF-α, anti-IL-1β and anti-RANKL antibodies were purchased from R&D Systems.

2.4. Real-Time PCR

Synovial fibroblasts were stimulated with IL-17, IL-21, or IL-22. Synovial fibroblasts were incubated in the presence or absence of SKI306X for 3 h before the addition of IL-17, IL-21, or IL-22. After incubation for 72 h, mRNA was extracted using RNAzol B (Biotex Laboratories, Houston, TX, USA) according to the manufacturer's instructions.

2.5. Enzyme-Linked Immunosorbent Assay (ELISA)

TNF-α, IL-1β, IL-8 and soluble receptor activator of nuclear factor kappa-B ligand (sRANKL) levels in the culture supernatants from RA synovial fibroblasts were measured using a sandwich ELISA according to R&D System's instructions.

2.6. Osteoclast Formation

PB monocytes were prepared from heparinized blood by Ficoll–Hypaque (GE Healthcare, Pittsburgh, PA, USA) density gradient centrifugation. Monocytes were added to the IL-17-pretreated RA synovial fibroblasts with fresh media. Monocytes were co-cultured for 3 weeks in α-minimal essential medium and 10% fetal bovine serum (FBS) in the presence of 25 ng/mL recombinant human macrophage-colony stimulating factor (rhM-CSF). On day 21, tartrate-resistant acid phosphatase (TRAP)-positive cells were identified using a leukocyte acid phosphatase kit according to Sigma-Aldrich's protocol [14].

2.7. Statistical Analysis

The data are expressed as means ± standard deviation (SD). Statistical difference was assessed using Mann–Whitney *U* test for analyzing two groups or one-way analysis of variance (ANOVA) with Bonferroni's multiple comparison post-hoc test for analyzing more than three groups. A p value < 0.05 was considered statistically significant.

3. Results

3.1. Regulatory Effect of SKI306X on Th17 Cytokine-Induced TNF-α Expression and Production in RA Synovial Fibroblasts

When RA synovial fibroblasts were cultured in media supplemented with IL-17, IL-21, or IL-22, TNF-α was upregulated; however, SKI306X reduced Th17 cytokine-induced TNF-α expression (Figure 1A), TNF-α production was increased upon IL-17 stimulation in culture media, and SKI306X reduced TNF-α production (Figure 1B).

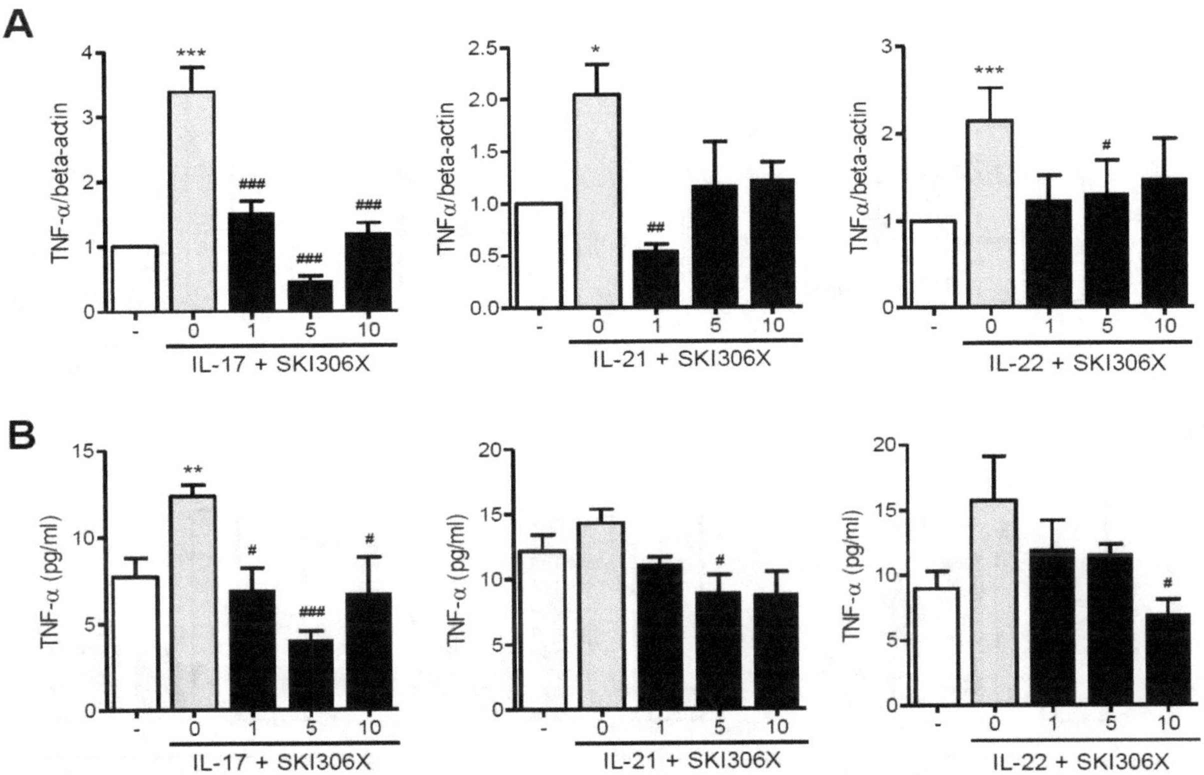

Figure 1. The inhibitory effect of SKI306X, a mixed extract of three herbs, in T helper (Th)17 cytokine-induced tumor necrosis factor (TNF)-α expression and production by synovial fibroblasts in rheumatoid arthritis (RA). (**A**) RA synovial fibroblasts were cultured in media supplemented with interleukin (IL)-17, IL-21, and IL-22 in the presence of various doses of SKI306X, and TNF-α was examined using real-time PCR, normalized to that of beta-actin and reported in relative expression units. (**B**) RA synovial fibroblasts were cultured with IL-17, IL-21, and IL-22 in the presence of various concentrations of SKI306X, and TNF-α production in culture media was determined using ELISA. The data represent the mean ± standard deviation (SD) values from six independent experiments. * $p < 0.05$, ** $p < 0.01$ and *** $p < 0.001$ compared with the nil condition (white bars). # $p < 0.05$, ## $p < 0.01$ and ### $p < 0.001$ compared with the Th17 cytokine stimulating condition (gray bars).

3.2. The Regulatory Effect of SKI306X on Th17 Cytokine-Induced IL-1β Expression and Production in RA Synovial Fibroblasts

When RA synovial fibroblasts were cultured in media supplemented with IL-17 or IL-22, IL-1β was upregulated; however, SKI306X reduced Th17 cytokine-induced IL-1β expression. Stimulation with IL-21 resulted in a similar, albeit non-significant, effect (Figure 2A). Furthermore, IL-1β production was increased after IL-17 or IL-21 supplementation in culture media, and SKI306X reduced IL-1β production (Figure 2B).

However, IL-21 and IL-22 did not promote IL-8 expression and production. Although IL-17 induced IL-8 expression and production, SKI306X inhibited IL-17-induced IL-8 production in RA synovial fibroblasts but did not affect IL-17-induced IL-8 expression.

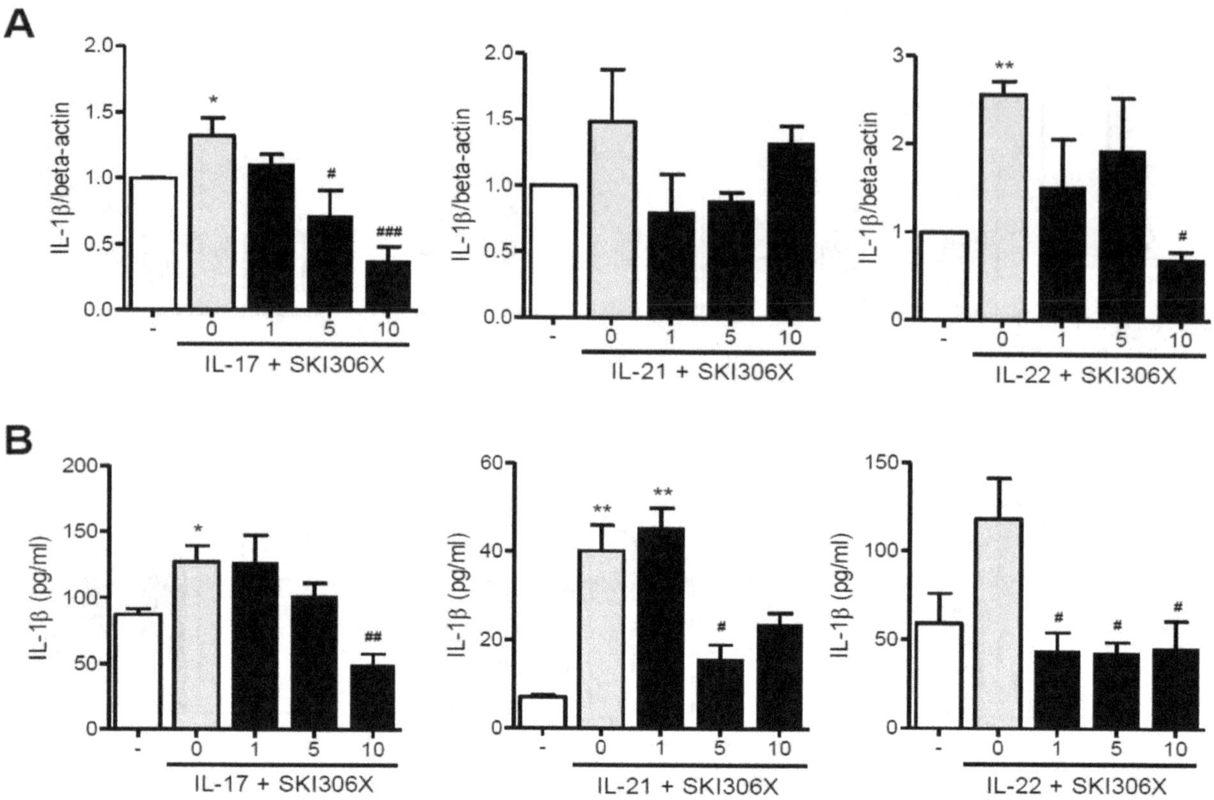

Figure 2. The inhibitory effect of SKI306X in Th17 cytokine-induced IL-1β expression and production in synovial fibroblasts in RA. (**A**) RA synovial fibroblasts were cultured in medium supplemented with IL-17, IL-21, and IL-22 with various concentrations of SKI306X, and IL-1β expression was examined using real-time PCR, normalized to beta-actin and reported in relative expression units. (**B**) RA synovial fibroblasts were cultured in medium supplemented with IL-17, IL-21, and IL-22 in the presence of various doses of SKI306X, and IL-1β production in the culture media was determined via ELISA. The data represent mean ± SD values from six independent experiments. * $p < 0.05$ and ** $p < 0.01$ compared with the nil condition (white bars). # $p < 0.05$, ## $p < 0.01$ and ### $p < 0.001$ compared with the Th17 cytokine stimulating condition (gray bars).

3.3. Regulatory Effect of SKI306X on Th17 Cytokine-Induced RANKL Expression and Production in RA Synovial Fibroblasts

On culturing RA synovial fibroblasts in media supplemented with IL-17 or IL-22, RANKL was upregulated; however, SKI306X reduced Th17 cytokine-induced RANKL expression (Figure 3A). Furthermore, RANKL production was increased upon IL-17 supplementation in culture media, and SKI306X reduced IL-17-induced RANKL production (Figure 3B).

3.4. Regulatory Effect of SKI306X on Th17 Cytokine-Induced Osteoclast Differentiation from PB Monocytes

When $CD14^+$ monocytes isolated from the PB of healthy donors were cultured in media supplemented with IL-17 and monocyte colony stimulating factor (M-CSF), TRAP-positive multinucleated osteoclasts were differentiated, and SKI306X reduced osteoclast differentiation in a dose-dependent manner. Osteoclast markers including TRAP, cathepsin K, and dendritic cell specific transmembrane protein (DC-STAMP) were upregulated upon IL-17 stimulation, and SKI306X downregulated these factors (Figure 4A). Monocyte stimulation with IL-21 or IL-22 yielded a similar pattern as IL-17 during osteoclast differentiation. On culturing $CD14^{+}$ monocytes in media supplemented with IL-21 or IL-22 and M-CSF, TRAP-positive multinucleated osteoclasts differentiated, and SKI306X reduced osteoclast differentiation in a dose-dependent manner. Osteoclast markers including TRAP, cathepsin K, DC-STAMP, and ATP6v0d2 were also upregulated upon IL-21 and IL-22 stimulation, and SKI306X reduced their expression (Figure 4B,C).

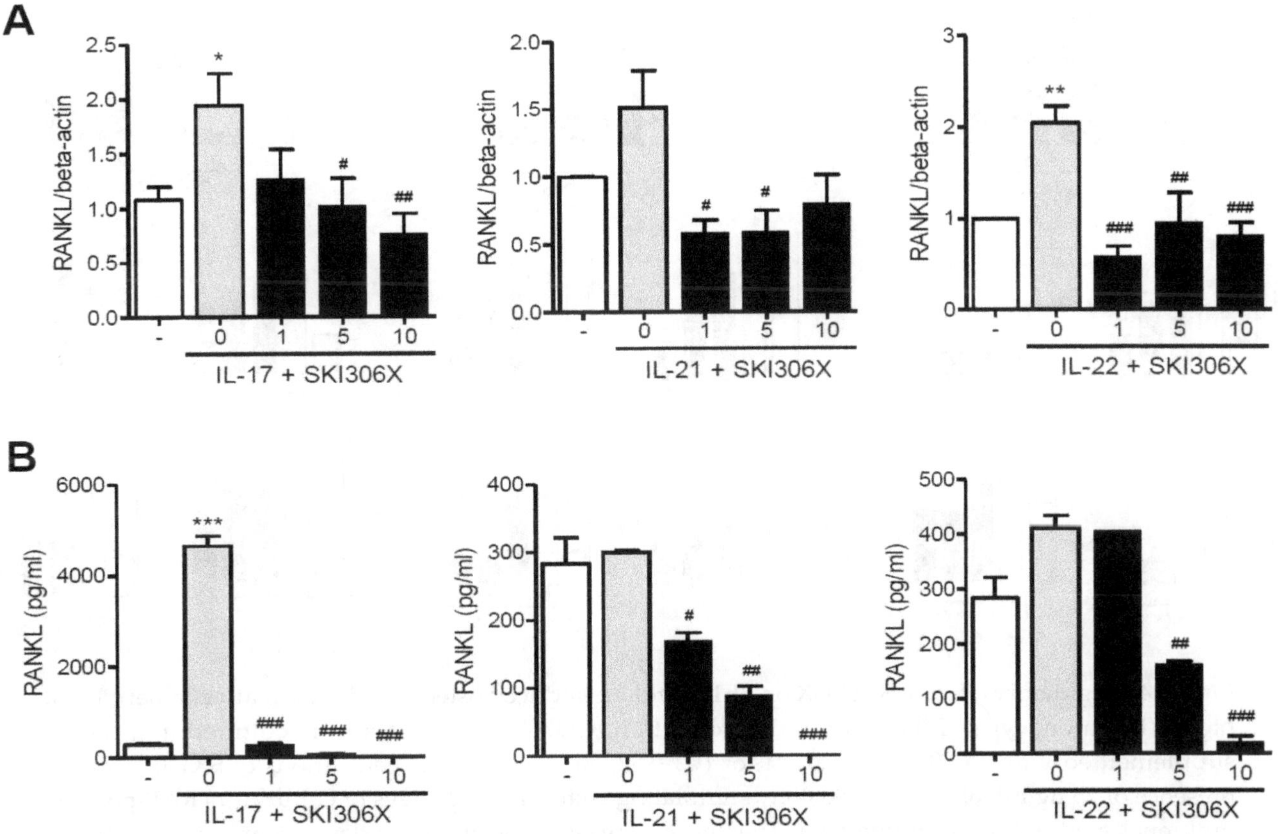

Figure 3. The inhibitory effect of SKI306X in Th17 cytokine-induced receptor activator of nuclear factor kappa-B ligand (RANKL) expression and production in synovial fibroblasts in RA. (**A**) RA synovial fibroblasts were cultured in medium supplemented with IL-17, IL-21, and IL-22 with various concentrations of SKI306X, and RANKL expression was examined using real-time PCR, normalized to beta-actin and reported in relative expression units. (**B**) RA synovial fibroblasts were cultured in medium supplemented with IL-17, IL-21, and IL-22 with various concentrations of SKI306X, and RANKL production in the culture media was examined using ELISA. The data represent mean ± SD values from six independent experiments. * $p < 0.05$, ** $p < 0.01$ and *** $p < 0.001$ compared with the nil condition (white bars). # $p < 0.05$, ## $p < 0.01$ and ### $p < 0.001$ compared with the Th17 cytokine stimulating condition (gray bars).

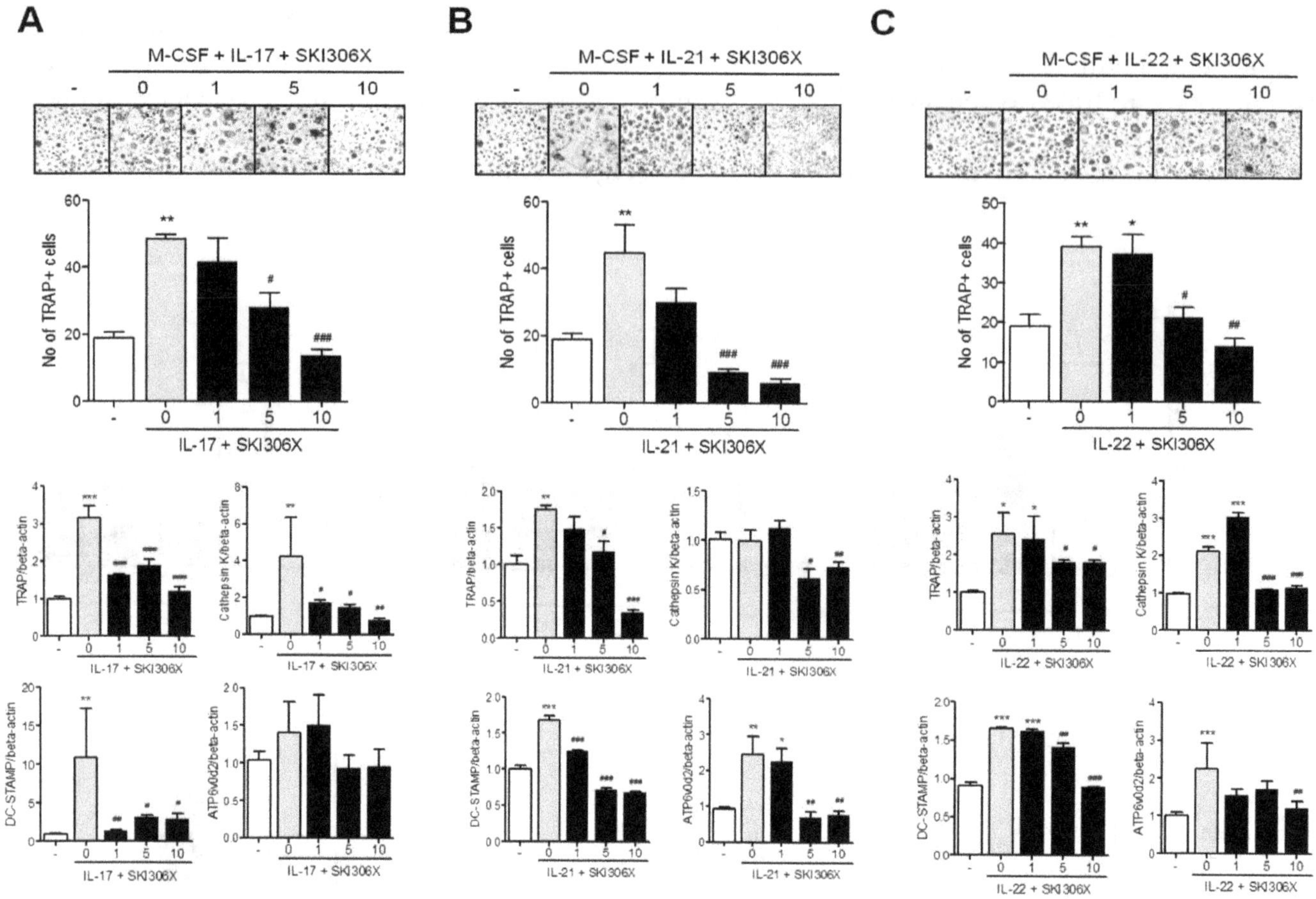

Figure 4. Regulatory effect of SKI306X on Th17 cytokine-induced osteoclast differentiation in peripheral blood (PB) monocytes. PB cluster of differentiation (CD)14^{+} monocytes were cultured in medium supplemented with (**A**) IL-17, (**B**) IL-21, or (**C**) IL-22 and various concentrations of SKI306X in the presence of 25 ng/mL of monocyte colony stimulating factor. After 21 days of culturing, TRAP-positive multinucleated cells were enumerated. The figures represent one of three independent experiments and the bars represent mean ± SD values. The expression of osteoclast markers including tartrate-resistant acid phosphatase (TRAP), cathepsin K, dendritic cell specific transmembrane protein (DC-STAMP), and ATP6v0d2 was quantified using real-time PCR, normalized to beta-actin and reported in relative expression units. * $p < 0.05$, ** $p < 0.01$ and *** $p < 0.001$ compared with the nil condition (white bars). # $p < 0.05$, ## $p < 0.01$ and ### $p < 0.001$ compared with the Th17 cytokine stimulating condition (gray bars).

3.5. Regulatory Effect of SKI306X on Osteoclast Differentiation from PB Monocytes Co-Cultured with IL-17-Stimulated RA Synovial Fibroblasts

CD14^{+} monocytes isolated from PB were co-cultured with IL-17-prestimulated RA synovial fibroblasts in media supplemented with M-CSF, and TRAP-positive multinucleated osteoclasts were differentiated and compared with non-stimulated RA synovial fibroblasts. SKI306X reduced osteoclast differentiation (Figure 5A). Furthermore, osteoclast markers including TRAP, cathepsin K, and nuclear factor of activated T-cells, cytoplasmic 1 (NF-ATc1) were upregulated when osteoclast precursors were co-cultured with IL-17-prestimulated RA synovial fibroblasts, and SKI306X reduced their expression (Figure 5B).

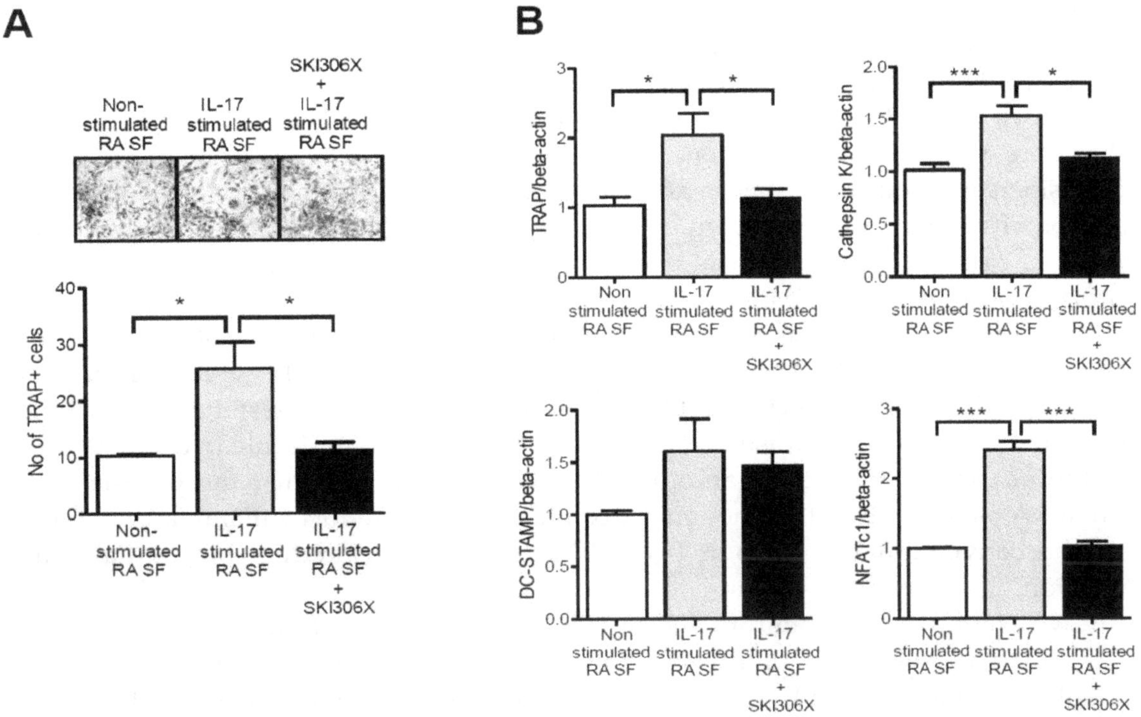

Figure 5. The regulatory effect of SKI306X on osteoclast differentiation in co-cultures of PB monocytes and IL-17-stimulated synovial fibroblasts (SF) in RA. (**A**) After PB monocytes were co-cultured with IL-17 stimulated RA synovial fibroblasts in the presence of monocyte colony stimulating factor and SKI306X for 21 days, the TRAP-positive multinucleated cells were enumerated. The figures represent one of three independent experiments and the bars represent mean ± SD values. (**B**) The expression of osteoclast markers including TRAP, cathepsin K, DC-STAMP, and nuclear factor of activated T-cells, cytoplasmic 1 (NF-ATc1) was quantified using real-time PCR, normalized to beta-actin and reported in relative expression units. * $p < 0.05$ and *** $p < 0.001$.

4. Discussion

In some Asian countries, herbal medicines are commonly used for treating arthritis. Although many patients do not receive prompt diagnosis and treatment for RA, some patients have experienced therapeutic effects using herbal medication [1,3]. SKI306X is widely used to manage osteoarthritis in Korea; however, no study has reported the efficacy of herbal medication in RA. This study aimed to investigate the anti-inflammatory and osteoprotective effects of SKI306X in Th17 cytokine-induced inflammation and osteoclast differentiation in RA.

To determine the anti-inflammatory effect of SKI306X, we examined Th17 cytokine-induced TNF-α and IL-1β expression in RA synovial fibroblasts. We selected synovial fibroblasts and Th17 cytokines in this study because they are primary targets in RA pathogenesis; however, they are very active effector cells, which can induce and aggravate inflammatory processes [15,16]. We previously reported that IL-21, IL-22, and IL-17 stimulate RA synovial fibroblasts to produce inflammatory cytokines [13,17,18]. Moreover, Th17 overproduction and the differentiation of Th17-positive cells are one of the major events in RA pathogenesis; hence, reduction of the Th17 response regulates inflammation and joint destruction in RA [19,20]. IL-17, IL-21, and IL-22 upregulated TNF-α and IL-1β in RA synovial fibroblasts and SKI306X effectively reduced their expression. A previous study reported that SKI306X reduces lipopolysaccharide (LPS)-induced TNF-α and IL-1β production in human peripheral blood mononuclear cells (PBMCs) [20]. Another study reported that SKI306X inhibits TNF-α release from LPS-stimulated human whole blood; however, it does not affect IL-1β release [5]. LPS is a nonspecific stimulant in the inflammatory processes. In this study, we used RA synovial fibroblasts, which represent target cells, and stimulated them with Th17 cytokines as specific stimulators and LPS as a non-specific cellular stimulator. Thus, we replicated pathological conditions in vitro and investigated the therapeutic effect of SKI306X. Reduction of Th17-induced TNF-α and IL-1β expression and production by SKI306X indicates that SKI306X plays a potential anti-inflammatory role in Th17-induced inflammation in RA.

Furthermore, we determined the bone protective role of SKI306X in RA. In RA, loss of cartilage and bone erosion cause joint destruction and subsequent joint disability. Bone erosion is caused by bone resorption of synovial osteoclasts, which in turn are activated by RANKL and other inflammatory cytokines. They originate from synovial tissues, subchondral bone, and circulating monocytes in inflammatory conditions [21]. We examined the dual roles of SKI306X in the reduction of RANKL production from synovial fibroblasts and in the inhibition of osteoclast differentiation. Because synovial fibroblasts are major sources of RANKL [13,22,23], SKI306X inhibited Th17 cytokine-induced RANKL expression and production in RA synovial fibroblasts. These findings suggest that SKI306X potentially ameliorates bone destruction because RANKL is a very important molecule in osteoclast activation. In recent clinical trials, denosumab, an anti-RANKL antibody, inhibited the progression of joint destruction in RA patients [24,25]. Although denosumab does not reduce inflammation, combinatorial treatment with conventional or biologic DMARDs can effectively reduce both inflammation and joint destruction.

Finally, we examined the inhibitory effect of SKI306X in osteoclast differentiation. RA treatment is primarily aimed at preventing joint destruction; hence, inhibition of osteoclastogenesis is critical for treatment. Circulating $CD14^+$ monocytes are precursors of osteoclasts and they upregulate RANK on the cell surface and interact with RANKL that is primarily produced by RA synovial fibroblasts and Th17 cells [26]. Th17 cytokines independently induce osteoclast differentiation from their precursor [17,18,27]. In this study, when PB monocytes were cultured in media supplemented with Th17 cytokines and SKI306X, SKI306X reduced Th17 cytokine-induced osteoclast differentiation. The underlying mechanism of action of this drug is unclear; hence, further studies are required to determine the cell receptors and signaling pathways involved herein.

Monocytes express various chemokine receptors including C-C chemokine receptor type 2 (CCR2) and (C-X3-C motif) chemokine receptor 1 (CX3CR1) and interact with chemokine ligands expressed by synovial fibroblasts. Their interaction promotes cellular activation, migration, and recruitment into the synovium of RA patients [26]. To investigate their interactions, we co-cultured monocytes with RA synovial fibroblasts under osteoclast-differentiating conditions. RA synovial fibroblasts can potentially augment osteoclastogenesis [28], and TNF-α- or IL-17-stimulated synovial fibroblasts are more effective at osteoclastogenesis [17]. Osteoblast differentiation was augmented when RA synovial fibroblasts were stimulated with IL-17 and then co-cultured with monocytes rather than non-stimulation with IL-17. However, SKI306X restored IL-17-augmented osteoclast differentiation in stimulated synovial fibroblasts. These results suggest that SKI306X reduces osteoclastogenesis through its effects on both osteoclast precursors and cellular interactions with synovial fibroblasts.

There are only two clinical studies of SKI306X in RA; however, the studies have limitations regarding the assessment of the clinical efficacy of SKI306X in RA patients. One study is a six-week, double blinded noninferiority study for assessment of pain relief and tolerability of SK1306X compared with celecoxib. The duration of the study is too short to assess clinical efficacy and protective effect of joint destruction. Because SKI306X is compared with celecoxib rather than DMARDs, the disease modifying effect of SKI306X for RA cannot be assessed [10]. The other study evaluated cardiovascular risk associated with SKI306X use in RA patients which was compared with celecoxib and naproxen. A total of 27,253 patients were studied and the incidence of major cardiovascular events was highest for celecoxib (15.4%), followed by SKI306X (8.6%) and naproxen (8%). SKI306X did not have a higher risk of cardiovascular events than naproxen. This study is a retrospective observational study using data from National Health Insurance Service–National Sample Cohort and it does not assess the therapeutic efficacy of SKI306X. However, this study has a meaningful result because the cardiovascular risk is high in RA patients and it influences their survival [11]. RA is associated with high cardiovascular risk, affecting patient survival, and inflammation and atherosclerosis are closely linked; the pathological features are similar in both disease states and they share common risk factors [29]. Furthermore, the overall risk of metabolic syndrome is higher in patients with RA than in healthy controls and RA is associated with body weight changes, dyslipidemia, adipokine profile changes and insulin resistance in metabolic syndrome [30]. Although IL-17 has a double-sided effect in atherosclerosis, IL-17 could be involved in the process of atherosclerosis of RA. It induces the release of chemokines and their ligands (chemokine (C-X-C motif) ligand (CXCL)1, CXCL2, CXCL8 and CXCL10), which recruit neutrophils and monocytes to the atherosclerotic lesion. IL-17 simulates monocytes to produce IL-6, TNF-α and IL-1β, which enhance plaque instability [31,32]. In early atherosclerosis, increased carotid intima-media thickness is associated with the IL-17-related chemokine eotaxin [33], and in RA patients, IL-17 is the main predictor of microvascular function and arterial compliance, suggesting a significant role for IL-17 in increased cardiovascular risk in RA [34].

This study is the first to report that SKI306X regulates RANKL production and osteoclast differentiation in RA. The mechanism of action of SKI306X is unclear, unlike that of conventional DMARDs. Recently, targeted or biologic DMARDs have been preferred in treating active RA; however, their usage in combination with SKI306X potentially results in in additional therapeutic effects. There have been no clinical or experimental studies of the comparison between SKI306X and other DMARDs such as methotrexate or hydroxychloroquine. There are only comparative clinical studies of SKI306X for assessment of pain relief, tolerability and cardiovascular risk. Based upon the results of this study, a comparison study of the therapeutic effects of SKI306X versus DMARDs and the assessment of combination effects of SKI306X with DMARDs in RA patients should be performed in the future.

5. Conclusions

SKI306X reduced both inflammation and osteoclast differentiation in RA, reducing Th17 cytokine-induced TNFα and IL-1β expression and production in RA synovial fibroblasts during inflammation. SKI306X ameliorated RANKL production in synovial fibroblasts and osteoclast differentiation in circulating monocytes. SKI306X is thus a potential novel therapeutic agent to prevent inflammation and joint destruction in RA.

Author Contributions: Conceptualization: S.-H.L.; Data curation: H.-R.K., K.-W.K.; Formal analysis: H.-R.K., K.-W.K.; Funding acquisition: H.-R.K., K.-W.K., S.-H.L.; Investigation: H.-R.K., K.-W.K., B.-M.K., J.-Y.W., H.-K.M., K.-A.L., T.-Y.K.; Methodology: H.-R.K., K.-W.K., S.-H.L.; Resources: B.-M.K., J.-Y.W., H.-K.M., K.-A.L., T.-Y.K.; Validation: B.-M.K., J.-Y.W., H.-K.M., K.-A.L., T.-Y.K.; Visualization: H.-R.K., K.-W.K.; Writing—Original draft: H.-R.K., K.-W.K., S.-H.L.; Writing—Review and editing: K.-W.K., H.-R.K., B.-M.K., J.-Y.W., H.-K.M., K.-A.L., T.-Y.K., S.-H.L.

Abbreviations

Th17	T helper 17
IL-17	interleukin 17
IL-21	interleukin 21
IL-22	interleukin 22
RA	rheumatoid arthritis
FLSs	fibroblast-like synoviocytes
TRAP	tartrate-resistant acid phosphatase
TNF-α	tumor necrosis factor-α
IL-1β	interleukin-1β
M-CSF	macrophage colony-stimulating factor
RANKL	receptor activator of nuclear factor kappa-B ligand

References

1. Rambod, M.; Nazarinia, M.; Raieskarimian, F. The prevalence and predictors of herbal medicines usage among adult rheumatoid arthritis patients: A case-control study. *Complement. Ther. Med.* **2018**, *41*, 220–224. [CrossRef] [PubMed]
2. Teekachunhatean, S.; Kunanusorn, P.; Rojanasthien, N.; Sananpanich, K.; Pojchamarnwiputh, S.; Lhieochaiphunt, S.; Pruksakorn, S. Chinese herbal recipe versus diclofenac in symptomatic treatment of osteoarthritis of the knee: A randomized controlled trial [ISRCTN70292892]. *BMC Complement. Altern. Med.* **2004**, *4*, 19. [CrossRef] [PubMed]
3. Han, M.; Sung, Y.K.; Cho, S.K.; Kim, D.; Won, S.; Choi, C.B.; Bang, S.Y.; Cha, H.S.; Choe, J.Y.; Chung, W.T.; et al. Factors Associated with the Use of Complementary and Alternative Medicine for Korean Patients with Rheumatoid Arthritis. *J. Rheumatol.* **2015**, *42*, 2075–2081. [CrossRef] [PubMed]
4. Choi, J.H.; Kim, D.Y.; Yoon, J.H.; Youn, H.Y.; Yi, J.B.; Rhee, H.I.; Ryu, K.H.; Jung, K.; Han, C.K.; Kwak, W.J.; et al. Effects of SKI 306X, a new herbal agent, on proteoglycan degradation in cartilage explant culture and collagenase-induced rabbit osteoarthritis model. *Osteoarthr. Cartil.* **2002**, *10*, 471–478. [CrossRef] [PubMed]
5. Kim, J.H.; Ryu, K.H.; Jung, K.W.; Han, C.K.; Kwak, W.J.; Cho, Y.B. Effects of SKI306X on arachidonate metabolism and other inflammatory mediators. *Biol. Pharm. Bull.* **2005**, *28*, 1615–1620. [CrossRef] [PubMed]
6. Hartog, A.; Hougee, S.; Faber, J.; Sanders, A.; Zuurman, C.; Smit, H.F.; van der Kraan, P.M.; Hoijer, M.A.; Garssen, J. The multicomponent phytopharmaceutical SKI306X inhibits in vitro cartilage degradation and the production of inflammatory mediators. *Phytomedicine* **2008**, *15*, 313–320. [CrossRef] [PubMed]
7. Kim, J.H.; Ryu, K.H.; Jung, K.W.; Han, C.K.; Kwak, W.J.; Cho, Y.B. SKI306X suppresses cartilage destruction and inhibits the production of matrix metalloproteinase in rabbit joint cartilage explant culture. *J. Pharmacol. Sci.* **2005**, *98*, 298–306. [CrossRef] [PubMed]
8. Kim, J.I.; Choi, J.Y.; Kim, K.G.; Lee, M.C. Efficacy of JOINS on Cartilage Protection in Knee Osteoarthritis: Prospective Randomized Controlled Trial. *Knee Surg. Relat. Res.* **2017**, *29*, 217–224. [CrossRef]
9. Ha, C.W.; Park, Y.B.; Min, B.W.; Han, S.B.; Lee, J.H.; Won, Y.Y.; Park, Y.S. Prospective, randomized, double-blinded, double-dummy and multicenter phase IV clinical study comparing the efficacy and safety of PG201 (Layla) and SKI306X in patients with osteoarthritis. *J. Ethnopharmacol.* **2016**, *181*, 1–7. [CrossRef]
10. Song, Y.W.; Lee, E.Y.; Koh, E.M.; Cha, H.S.; Yoo, B.; Lee, C.K.; Baek, H.J.; Kim, H.; Suh, Y.; Kang, S.W.; et al. Assessment of comparative pain relief and tolerability of SKI306X compared with celecoxib in patients with rheumatoid arthritis: A 6-week, multicenter, randomized, double-blind, double-dummy, phase III, noninferiority clinical trial. *Clin. Ther.* **2007**, *29*, 862–873. [CrossRef]
11. Woo, Y.; Hyun, M.K. Evaluation of cardiovascular risk associated with SKI306X use in patients with osteoarthritis and rheumatoid arthritis. *J. Ethnopharmacol.* **2017**, *207*, 42–46. [CrossRef] [PubMed]
12. Kim, K.W.; Cho, M.L.; Kim, H.R.; Ju, J.H.; Park, M.K.; Oh, H.J.; Kim, J.S.; Park, S.H.; Lee, S.H.; Kim, H.Y. Up-regulation of stromal cell-derived factor 1 (CXCL12) production in rheumatoid synovial fibroblasts through interactions with T lymphocytes: Role of interleukin-17 and CD40L-CD40 interaction. *Arthritis Rheum.* **2007**, *56*, 1076–1086. [CrossRef] [PubMed]
13. Kim, H.R.; Kim, K.W.; Kim, B.M.; Lee, K.A.; Lee, S.H. N-acetyl-l-cysteine controls osteoclastogenesis through regulating Th17 differentiation and RANKL in rheumatoid arthritis. *Korean J. Intern. Med.* **2019**, *34*, 210–219. [CrossRef] [PubMed]
14. Kong, Y.Y.; Yoshida, H.; Sarosi, I.; Tan, H.L.; Timms, E.; Capparelli, C.; Morony, S.; Oliveira-dos-Santos, A.J.; Van, G.; Itie, A.; et al. OPGL is a key regulator of osteoclastogenesis, lymphocyte development and lymph-node organogenesis. *Nature* **1999**, *397*, 315–323. [CrossRef] [PubMed]
15. Lefevre, S.; Meier, F.M.; Neumann, E.; Muller-Ladner, U. Role of synovial fibroblasts in rheumatoid arthritis. *Curr. Pharm. Des.* **2015**, *21*, 130–141. [CrossRef] [PubMed]
16. Neumann, E.; Lefevre, S.; Zimmermann, B.; Gay, S.; Müller-Ladner, U. Rheumatoid arthritis progression mediated by activated synovial fibroblasts. *Trends Mol. Med.* **2010**, *16*, 458–468. [CrossRef] [PubMed]
17. Kim, K.W.; Kim, H.R.; Kim, B.M.; Cho, M.L.; Lee, S.H. Th17 cytokines regulate osteoclastogenesis in rheumatoid arthritis. *Am. J. Pathol.* **2015**, *185*, 3011–3024. [CrossRef] [PubMed]
18. Kim, K.W.; Kim, H.R.; Park JY Park, J.S.; Oh, H.J.; Woo, Y.J.; Park, M.K.; Cho, M.L.; Lee, S.H. Interleukin-22 promotes osteoclastogenesis in rheumatoid arthritis through induction of RANKL in human synovial fibroblasts. *Arthritis Rheum.* **2012**, *64*, 1015–1023. [CrossRef]

19. Roeleveld, D.M.; Koenders, M.I. The role of the Th17 cytokines IL-17 and IL-22 in Rheumatoid Arthritis pathogenesis and developments in cytokine immunotherapy. *Cytokine* **2015**, *74*, 101–107. [CrossRef]
20. Roeleveld, D.M.; van Nieuwenhuijze, A.E.; van den Berg, W.B.; Koenders, M.I. The Th17 pathway as a therapeutic target in rheumatoid arthritis and other autoimmune and inflammatory disorders. *BioDrugs* **2013**, *27*, 439–452. [CrossRef]
21. Amarasekara, D.S.; Yun, H.; Kim, S.; Lee, N.; Kim, H.; Rho, J. Regulation of Osteoclast Differentiation by Cytokine Networks. *Immune Netw.* **2018**, *18*, e8. [CrossRef] [PubMed]
22. Tunyogi-Csapo, M.; Kis-Toth, K.; Radacs, M.; Farkas, B.; Jacobs, J.J.; Finnegan, A.; Mikecz, K.; Glant, T.T. Cytokine-controlled RANKL and osteoprotegerin expression by human and mouse synovial fibroblasts: Fibroblast-mediated pathologic bone resorption. *Arthritis Rheum.* **2008**, *58*, 2397–2408. [CrossRef] [PubMed]
23. Kim, H.R.; Kim, B.M.; Won, J.Y.; Lee, K.A.; Ko, H.M.; Kang, Y.S.; Lee, S.H.; Kim, K.W. Quercetin, a Plant Polyphenol, Has Potential for the Prevention of Bone Destruction in Rheumatoid Arthritis. *J. Med. Food* **2019**, *22*, 152–161. [CrossRef] [PubMed]
24. Takeuchi, T.; Tanaka, Y.; Soen, S.; Yamanaka, H.; Yoneda, T.; Tanaka, S.; Nitta, T.; Okubo, N.; Genant, H.K.; van der Heijde, D. Effects of the anti-RANKL antibody denosumab on joint structural damage in patients with rheumatoid arthritis treated with conventional synthetic disease-modifying antirheumatic drugs (DESIRABLE study): A randomised, double-blind, placebo-controlled phase 3 trial. *Ann Rheum. Dis.* **2019**, *78*, 899–907. [PubMed]
25. Ishiguro, N.; Tanaka, Y.; Yamanaka, H.; Yoneda, T.; Ohira, T.; Okubo, N.; Genant, H.K.; van der Heijde, D.; Takeuchi, T. Efficacy of denosumab with regard to bone destruction in prognostic subgroups of Japanese rheumatoid arthritis patients from the phase II DRIVE study. *Rheumatology (Oxford)* **2019**, *58*, 997–1005. [CrossRef]
26. Rana, A.K.; Li, Y.; Dang, Q.; Yang, F. Monocytes in rheumatoid arthritis: Circulating precursors of macrophages and osteoclasts and, their heterogeneity and plasticity role in RA pathogenesis. *Int. Immunopharmacol.* **2018**, *65*, 348–359. [CrossRef] [PubMed]
27. Kim, K.W.; Kim, B.M.; Lee, K.A.; Lee, S.H.; Firestein, G.S.; Kim, H.R. Histamine and Histamine H4 Receptor Promotes Osteoclastogenesis in Rheumatoid Arthritis. *Sci. Rep.* **2017**, *7*, 1197. [CrossRef] [PubMed]
28. Takayanagi, H. New developments in osteoimmunology. *Nat. Rev. Rheumatol.* **2012**, *8*, 684–689. [CrossRef] [PubMed]
29. Skeoch, S.; Bruce, I.N. Atherosclerosis in rheumatoid arthritis: Is it all about inflammation? *Nat. Rev. Rheumatol.* **2015**, *11*, 390–400. [CrossRef]
30. Kerekes, G.; Nurmohamed, M.T.; Gonzalez-Gay, M.A.; Seres, I.; Paragh, G.; Kardos, Z.; Baráth, Z.; Tamási, L.; Soltész, P.; Szekanecz, Z. Rheumatoid arthritis and metabolic syndrome. *Nat. Rev. Rheumatol.* **2014**, *10*, 691–696. [CrossRef]
31. Lu, X. The Impact of IL-17 in Atherosclerosis. *Curr. Med. Chem.* **2017**, *24*, 2345–2358. [CrossRef] [PubMed]
32. Ryu, H.; Chung, Y. Regulation of IL-17 in atherosclerosis and related autoimmunity. *Cytokine* **2015**, *74*, 219–227. [CrossRef] [PubMed]
33. Tarantino, G.; Costantini, S.; Finelli, C.; Capone, F.; Guerriero, E.; La Sala, N.; Gioia, S.; Castello, G. Is serum Interleukin-17 associated with early atherosclerosis in obese patients? *J. Transl. Med.* **2014**, *12*, 214. [CrossRef] [PubMed]
34. Marder, W.; Khalatbari, S.; Myles JD Hench, R.; Yalavarthi, S.; Lustig, S.; Brook, R.; Kaplan, M.J. Interleukin 17 as a novel predictor of vascular function in rheumatoid arthritis. *Ann. Rheum. Dis.* **2011**, *70*, 1550–1555. [CrossRef] [PubMed]

8

Infliximab Induced a Dissociated Response of Severe Periodontal Biomarkers in Rheumatoid Arthritis Patients

Mélanie Rinaudo-Gaujous [1], Vincent Blasco-Baque [2], Pierre Miossec [3], Philippe Gaudin [4], Pierre Farge [5], Xavier Roblin [6], Thierry Thomas [7,8], Stephane Paul [1,†] and Hubert Marotte [7,8,†,*]

1 GIMAP EA3064, Laboratory of Immunology and Immunomonitoring, CIC CIE3 Inserm Vaccinology, Hôpital Nord, CHU Saint-Etienne, 42270 Saint-Priest-en-Jarez, France; melanie.rinaudogaujous@chpg.mc (M.R.-G.); stephane.paul@chu-st-etienne.fr (S.P.)

2 Institute of Cardiovascular and Metabolic Diseases, CHU Rangueil, 31400 Toulouse, France; vincent.blasco@inserm.fr

3 Clinical Immunology Unit, Departments of Immunology and Rheumatology, Hôpital Edouard Herriot, CHU Lyon, 69003 Lyon, France; pierre.miossec@univ-lyon1.fr

4 Department of Rheumatology, CHU Grenoble, 38130 Échirolles, France; pgaudin@chu-grenoble.fr

5 Faculty of Odontology, University Lyon I., 69622 Villeurbanne, France; pierre.farge@univ-lyon1.fr

6 Department of Gastroenterology, Hôpital Nord, CHU Saint-Etienne, 42270 Saint-Priest-en-Jarez, France; xavier.roblin@chu-st-etienne.fr

7 Department of Rheumatology, Hôpital Nord, CHU Saint-Etienne, 42055 Saint-Etienne, France; thierry.thomas@chu-st-etienne.fr

8 INSERM U1059, Université de Lyon–Université Jean Monnet, 42023 Saint-Etienne, France

* Correspondence: hubert.marotte@chu-st-etienne.fr

† These authors contribute equally to this work.

Abstract: Objective: Rheumatoid arthritis and periodontal disease are associated together, but the effect of therapy provided for one disease to the second one remained under-investigated. This study investigated effect of infliximab therapy used to treat rheumatoid arthritis (RA) on various biomarkers of periodontal disease (PD) severity including serologies of *Porphyromonas gingivalis* and *Prevotella intermedia* and matrix metalloproteinase 3. Methods: Seventy nine RA patients were enrolled at the time to start infliximab therapy and the 28 joint disease activity score (DAS28), anti-cyclic citrullinated petides 2nd generation (anti-CCP2), anti-*P. gingivalis* antibody, and Matrix metalloproteinase 3 (MMP-3) were monitored before and at 6 months of infliximabtherapy. Joint damage and severe periodontal disease were assessed at baseline. Anti-CCP2, anti-*P. gingivalis* antibody, and MMP-3 weredetermined by enzyme-linked immunosorbent assay (ELISA). Results: At baseline, anti-CCP2 titers were associated with anti-*P. gingivalis* lipopolysaccharide (LPS)-specific antibodies titers ($p < 0.05$). Anti-*P. gingivalis* antibodies were not significantly correlated with clinical, biological, or destruction parameters of RA disease. At 6 months of infliximab therapy, MMP-3 level decreased (from 119 ± 103 ng/mL to 62.44 ± 52 ng/mL; $p < 0.0001$), whereas *P. gingivalis* antibody levels remained at the same level. DAS28 and inflammation markers C-reactive protein (CRP) and Erythrocyte sedimentation rate (ESR) also decreased significantly during infliximab therapy ($p < 0.05$) as anti-CCP2 levels ($p < 0.001$). Only high MMP-3 level at baseline was associated with infliximab efficacy ($p < 0.01$). Conclusion: MMP-3 level can be a useful marker of the efficacy of infliximab in RA patients. The treatment did not affect anti-*P. gingivalis* antibodies.

Keywords: Rheumatoid arthritis; *Porphyromonas gingivalis*; periodontal disease; matrix metalloproteinase 3; infliximab

1. Introduction

Rheumatoid arthritis (RA) is the most frequently chronic inflammatory joint disease characterized by synovial hypertrophy and inflammation with joint and subchondral bone destruction, which correlates with disability and loss of function [1]. Epidemiological studies suggest an association between RA and periodontal disease (PD) and confirmed by a recent meta-analysis [2]. Both diseases (RA and PD) share important similarities in their pathogenesis involving similar genetic background [3] or production of large amount of proinflammatory cytokines such as tumor necrosis factor alpha (TNF) [4]. In, P.D., inflammation is initiated and perpetuated by a subset of bacteria, including *Porphyromonas gingivalis* (*P. gingivalis*) and *Prevotella intermedia* (*P. intermedia*), two specific gram-negative anaerobic bacteria, which colonize the gingival sulcus and proliferate in the gingival plaque. The resulting chronic inflammatory response by the host induces destruction of the supporting structures of the teeth defining severe PD. *P. gingivalis* presence seems to be specific of severe PD. This was reinforced by recent data from an experimental rat model confirming the specific involvement of *P. gingivalis* in arthritis onset [5]. Furthermore, bacterial colonization was also described in the gut of RA patients [6].

Anti-citrullinated protein antibodies (ACPA) are the highest specific biomarker for RA diagnosis or prognosis and are now included in the new RA criteria [1]. Endogenous or exogenous peptidyl-arginine deiminases (PADs) induced citrullinated proteins by conversion of peptidyl-arginine to peptidyl-citrulline. This is part of many physiological processes [7]. However, smoking or *P. gingivalis* infection could induce excess of citrullination in some conditions [8]. Since ACPA occurred some years before RA clinical onset [9], *P. gingivalis* infection could precede RA onset and be a key player for initiation and maintenance of the autoimmune inflammatory responses in RA [10]. *P. gingivalis* is the unique known pathogen to have a specific enzyme PAD (PPAD) [11], which induce citrullination of proteins [12] and could provide a rupture of tolerance with ACPA induction.

Indirect presence of *P. gingivalis* by serology demonstrated that high concentrations of anti-*P. gingivalis* antibody in established [12] or early RA patients [13]. This indirect biomarker of *P. gingivalis* correlated with the gingival bacteria load assessed by polymerase chain reaction [13,14]. PD is related to many other anaerobic periodontal pathogens including *P. intermedia*, which was also detected in both the serum and synovial fluids of RA patients [15].

Matrix metalloproteinase 3 (MMP-3) is one of the major MMPs expressed in rheumatoid synovial tissue [16]. MMP-3 is mainly involved in bone and cartilage degradation in RA or bone destruction in PD [17]. Thus, MMP-3 is already considered as a biomarker for RA and PD destruction [18]. In, P.D., a MMP-3 polymorphism was described as associated to PD [19]. Furthermore, strategy based on MMP-3 monitoring improved clinical response and reduced joint destruction in RA [20]. In both PD and, R.A., production of proinflammatory cytokines, as TNF., is increased and specific blocking of TNF improves two-third of RA patients [21]. Only few studies have reported predictive factors of response to infliximab in RA [21], but no relevant clinical or biological markers can be used in the daily practice. In only one previous study, PD was related to be a predictive factor for a non-response to TNF blocker therapy in RA patients [22]. Persistence of *P. gingivalis* in gingival tissue could participate to maintain local and systemic inflammation in relation with treatment resistance [23]. Only few studies explored therapeutic effect for PD on RA [24] and *vice versa* [25].

Since both diseases are associated at the susceptibility and severity level [24], therapy from one disease should be efficient to the second one. This concept was recently reinforce by the first demonstration of PD severity on RA activity [26]. We already reviewed previously [24] impact of some biologic disease modifying anti-rheumatic drugs (bDMARDs) on PD. Infliximab treatment worsened the gingival inflammation, but decreased the gingival destruction of bone [25]. A the opposite, rituximab [27] or tocilizumab [28] decreased gingival inflammation or gingival bone destruction related to the PD. Accordingly, in case of severe PD B-cell blocker or IL-6 receptor blockers could be considered preferentially compared to TNF blocker. At the opposite, some non-surgical PD therapy reported decreased of anti-*P. gingivalis* antibodies without effect on ACPA level [29].

Thus, our aim in this study was to correlate marker of PD severity (MMP-3, anti-*P. gingivalis* and anti-*P. intermedia* antibodies) and to assess effect of infliximab therapy on PD severe biomarkers in RA patients. In addition, the usefulness of these biomarkers was assessed for prediction of clinical response to infliximab therapy.

2. Patients and methods

2.1. Patients and Controls

Seventy nine RA patients treated with methotrexate with active disease and starting infliximab therapy were included consecutively. Following clinical parameters were recorded: Age, sex, disease duration, patient's global assessment of disease activity, 28 tender and swollen joint counts, and the 28 joint disease activity score (DAS28). Joint damage and severe PD were defined by a right Larsen wrist score ≥ 2 and Hugoson and Jordan criteria, respectively as previously used [3]. Wrist X-rays were examined by the same reader (HM) as panoramic X-rays (PF). Clinical response to infliximab was defined by a decrease of DAS28 > 1.2. Blood samples were collected before and at 6 months of infliximab therapy to assess anti-cyclic citrullinated peptide second generation (CCP2), rheumatoid factor (RF), MMP-3, and antibodies against *P. gingivalis* and *P. intermedia.* Sera from two control groups were used in this study. We enrolled 27 healthy blood donors as control healthy volunteers and 28 patients with inflammatory bowel disease (IBD) and 35 patients with systemic lupus erythematosus (SLE), as inflammatory disorders controls. Local clinical ethics committee approved the protocol and all patients gave their written informed consent.

2.2. Methods

Determination of anti-*P. gingivalis* and anti-*Escherichia coli* LPS-specific antibodies by enzyme-linked immunosorbent assay (ELISA). To optimise our evaluation anti-*P. gingivalis* antibody assessed by ELISA., we performed two standardised ways for coating: Whole extract or lipopolysaccharide (LPS) components. LPS from *P. gingivalis* (InvivoGen, Toulouse, France) was coated on 96-well plates (Nunc, Dominique Dutscher, Brumath, France) at 10 μg/mL (diluted in carbonate buffer, pH 9.6) and incubated overnight at 4 °C. We used LPS from *Escherichia coli* (*E. coli*, InvivoGen, Toulouse, France) as control with the same dilution. Wells were washed three times with phosphate buffered saline (PBS)-Tween (0.005%). Plasma were diluted to 1:600 in PBS containing 1% of bovine serum albumin (BSA) and incubated (in duplicate) for 2 h at room temperature. Plates were washed as described above and incubated with peroxidase-conjugated goat anti-human IgG H + L (Jackson ImmunoResearch, West Grove, PA, USA) (diluted 1:50 000 in PBS) for 2 h at room temperature. After a final wash, detection was made by tetramethylbenzidine substrate (R&D Systems, Minneapolis, MN., USA). The reaction was stopped by the addition of H_2SO_4 (1M) solution and absorbances were measured at 450 nm.

2.2.1. Determination of Anti-P. gingivalis and Anti-P. intermedia Whole Extract Antibodies by ELISA

P. gingivalis strain ATCC 33277 and *P. intermedia* CIP 103607 were grown on sterile non-selective agar containing defibrinated sheep blood, supplemented with 0.0002% menadione sodium bisulfite and 0.4% hemin chloride. Cultures were then placed in an anaerobic chamber for 7 days at 37 °C. Then, colonies were recovered in a sterile water solution and centrifuged for 20 min at 5000× *g*. Pellets were diluted in sterile PBS at 50 mg/mL and were frozen at −20 °C until use. *P. gingivalis* or *P. intermedia* solution was then washed twice with carbonate buffer (pH 9.6) and diluted in the same buffer to obtain a solution of 1 McFarland (DensiCHEK plus, Biomérieux, Craponne, France). The solution was heated to 60 °C for 45 min, filtered (0.22 μm), diluted 1:10, coated on a 96-well plate and then incubated overnight at 4 °C. Plasma were diluted to 1:900 in PBS containing 1% BSA. Following steps are identical to those described for the LPS-specific ELISA. Cut-off values for seropositivity to *P. gingivalis* (LPS and whole extract) and *P. intermedia* were determined by concentrations higher than the 95th percentile in 27 healthy blood donors.

A calibration curve was systematically done for each plate with dilutions of a pool of positive plasma diluted six times from 1:100 to 1:16200 to correct for plate-to-plate variation. Two plasma controls (high and low positives) were included on all plates. All intra assay coefficients of variation (CV) were below 6.5%. Inter assay CV for the high positive control were 13%, 8%, and 28% for *P. gingivalis* whole extract, LPS assay and *P. intermedia* assay, respectively. Results are expressed in Arbitrary Units (AU) defined by the pool dilution (10 AU = 1:16200 to 2430 AU = 1:100).

Furthermore, determination of citrullinated proteins in *P. gingivalis* whole extract or LPS was assessed by using the specific anti-CCP2 detection antibody (Phadia, Thermo Fisher Scientific, Uppsala, Sweden).

2.2.2. Assessments of ACPA, R.F., and MMP-3

MMP-3 blood concentrations were determined by a commercial ELISA method (AESKU.diagnostics, Wendelsheim, Germany). ACPA was assessed by anti-CCP2, and RF (IgA and IgM) were measured by ELIA method on ImmunoCap 250 (Phadia, Thermo Fisher Scientific, Uppsala, Sweden). Anti-CCP2 was considered to be positive at a cut off value of 10 U/mL., RF IgA at 14 IU/mL and RF IgM at 3.5 IU/mL, as recommended by the manufacturer.

2.3. Statistical Analysis

Since data were not normally distributed, they were expressed as median and interquartile range 25–75% (IQR 25–75) or number (%). Correlations were performed by Spearman tests. Comparisons between controls and RA patients were performed by Mann Whitney test. Comparisons between baseline and 6 months of infliximab treatment were performed by Wilcoxon test. Statistics were done with the software GraphPad Prism (version 5.0). p values less than 0.05 were considered as statistically significant.

3. Results

3.1. RA Population

Our RA population had the main characteristics of RA patients treated with TNF inhibitors as reported in the Table 1. In this cohort, severe PD was present in 51 RA patients and severe PD was associated with joint damage (χ^2 test = 4.4; p = 0.0276).

Table 1. Characteristics of rheumatoid arthritis (RA) patients at baseline and after infliximab therapy.

	Baseline	6 Months	*p* Values
Sex (female/male)	63/16		
Age, years	52.8 (43.3–59.4)		
Disease duration (years)	9 (5–13)		
No destruction, *n* (%)	12 (15.2%)		
Wrist destruction, *n* (%)	56 (70.9%)		
Periodontal disease, *n* (%)	51 (64.6%)		
DAS28	5.1 (4.1–5.7)	3.5 (2.7–4.3)	<0.0001
ESR (mm/h)	34 (20–49)	18 (10–32)	<0.0001
CRP (mg/L)	18 (7–33)	7 (2–17)	<0.05
Anti–CCP2 (U/mL)	97 (9–275)	43 (5–189)	<0.001
RF IgM (IU/mL)	38 (11–96)	22 (6–66)	<0.0001
RF IgA (IU/mL)	25 (10–61)	17 (8–47)	0.0001
MMP–3 (ng/mL)	90 (40–177)	45 (24–91)	<0.0001
Anti–*P. gingivalis* whole extract (AU)	238 (148–377)	274 (173–557)	<0.01
Anti–*P. gingivalis* LPS (AU)	86 (67–146)	97 (77–152)	NS
Anti–*P. intermedia* whole extract (AU)	390 (131–1558)	436 (246–853)	<0.05

Values are indicated as number of patients (%) or median (1st and 3rd quartiles). DAS28: Disease Activity Score 28; ESR: Erythrocyte sedimentation rate; CRP: C-reactive protein; Anti-CCP2: anti-cyclic citrullinated peptides 2nd generation; RF: rheumatoid factor; MMP-3: Matrix metalloproteinase-3; LPS: lipopolysaccharide; U: unit; IU: international units; AU: arbitrary units, NS: non-significant.

3.2. Immunity Against Oral Pathogens is Related to Established RA

Anti-*P. gingivalis* whole extract antibodies were more frequently positive in established RA patients (97.5%) than in healthy blood donors (5%) with higher concentrations of anti-*P. gingivalis* antibody in established RA patients (238 (148–377) AU) than in healthy blood donors (43 (24–79) AU; Figure 1A; $p < 0.001$). Similar results were observed for anti-*P. gingivalis* LPS specific antibody (data not shown). Analogous pattern was also observed for anti-*P. intermedia* whole extract antibodies with more positive in established RA patients (84.8%) than in healthy blood donors (17.8%; Figure 1A; $p < 0.001$). Anti-*P. intermedia* antibody concentrations were also higher in established RA patients (390 (131–1558) AU) than in healthy blood donors (96 (67–179) AU; Figure 1A; $p < 0.001$). Thus immunity against oral pathogens was higher in established RA patients than in healthy blood donors reinforcing association between RA and PD. Furthermore, the two ways for anti-*P. gingivalis* antibody determination strongly correlated together (Figure 1B; $p < 0.0001$) and also correlated with anti-*P. intermedia* antibody concentrations (Figure 1C; $p < 0.0001$). Since we observed a correlation between immunity against these two bacteria from the oral cavity, we investigated the specificity of our assay. For this purpose, we tested the same plasma for anti-LPS fraction of *E. coli*, another commensal bacterium of the gut. Only one patient has serum with anti-*E. coli* antibody without anti-*P. gingivalis* antibody. At the opposite, many patients had anti-*P. gingivalis* antibody without anti-*E. coli* antibody, demonstrating the absence of crossreaction between these two antibodies (Figure 1D). As *P. gingivalis* whole extract may contain citrullinated proteins, we then investigated a putative crossreactivity between anti-CCP2 and anti-*P. gingivalis* antibodies. Presence of citrullinated proteins was not observed in the whole *P. gingivalis* extract by using the monoclonal antibody to detect anti-CCP2 (data not shown).

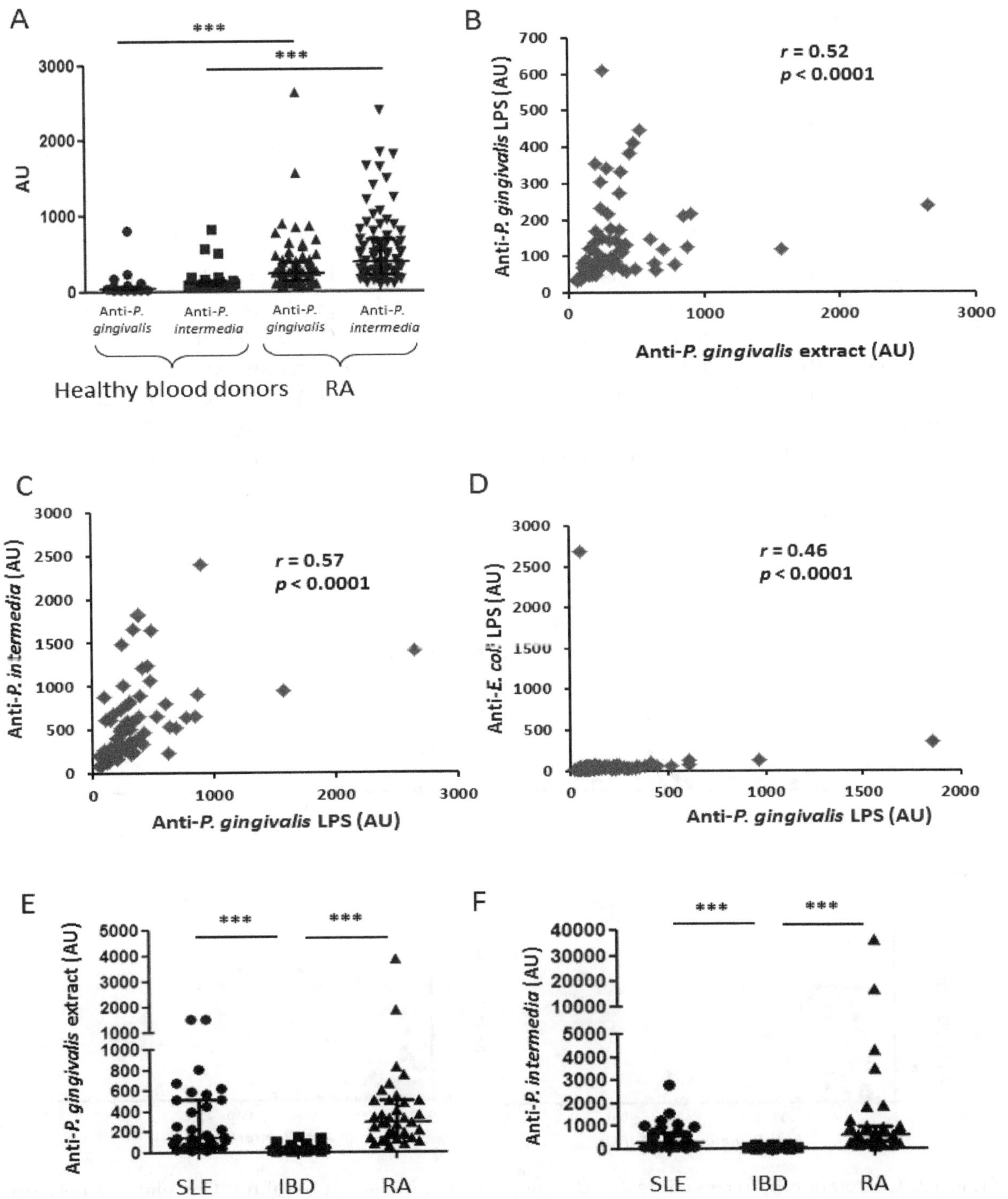

Figure 1. Evaluation of the measure of anti-*P. gingivalis* whole extract and LPS specific antibodies by ELISA. Anti-*P. gingivalis* and anti-*P. intermedia* (**A**) whole extract antibodies were measured in healthy blood donors and RA patients. Correlations between both anti-*P. gingivalis* LPS and whole extract (two ways to assess the same germ; (**B**); anti-*P. intermedia* and anti-*P. gingivalis* whole extract (assessment of two oral germs; (**C**) in RA patients. No correlation between anti-*P. gingivalis* and anti-*E. coli* LPS antibodies in RA patients (assessment of one oral germ and on commensal gut germ; (**D**). Anti-*P. gingivalis* (**E**) and anti-*P. intermedia* (**F**) whole extract antibodies were measured in SLE., IBD., and RA patients. From the bottom up, the bars indicate the interquartile range and the median. AU: arbitrary units; *r*: Spearman correlation coefficient; LPS: lipopolysaccharide; RA: rheumatoid arthritis; SLE: systemic lupus erythematosus; IBD: inflammatory bowel disease; ***: $p < 0.001$.

3.3. *Anti-P. gingivalis and anti-P. Intermedia Antibodies and RA Specificity*

To assess the specificity of these antibodies to, R.A., we then assessed them in IBD and SLE., two other inflammatory auto-immune diseases. Anti-*P. gingivalis* and anti-*P. intermedia* antibody concentrations were lower in IBD and SLE patients and established RA patients (Figure 1E,F; $p < 0.001$ for *P. gingivalis* and *P. intermedia* in RA and SLE vs. IBD).Thus high antibody concentrations against oral pathogens were specific for RA or SLE diseases involving joint.

3.4. *Differential Implication of P. Gingivalis and P. Intermedia Antibodies in Immune Response in RA Patients*

Since high antibody concentrations against *P. gingivalis* and *P. intermedia* were observed in RA patients, association of these antibodies with clinical and biological RA parameters was investigated. RF IgA concentrations were correlated with DAS28 at baseline (Figure 2A; $p < 0.01$). Furthermore, anti-CCP2 concentrations correlated with both anti-*P gingivalis* (whole extract and LPS) antibody concentrations (Figure 2B,C; $p < 0.001$ and $p < 0.01$; respectively), without correlation with IgM RF concentrations. Interestingly, anti-*P intermedia* antibody concentrations correlated with IgM RF concentrations (Figure 2D; $p < 0.05$), but not with anti-CCP2 concentrations. Since only anti-*P gingivalis* concentrations correlated with anti-CCP2 concentrations, these data reinforced the association between *P. gingivalis* and citrullination in RA.

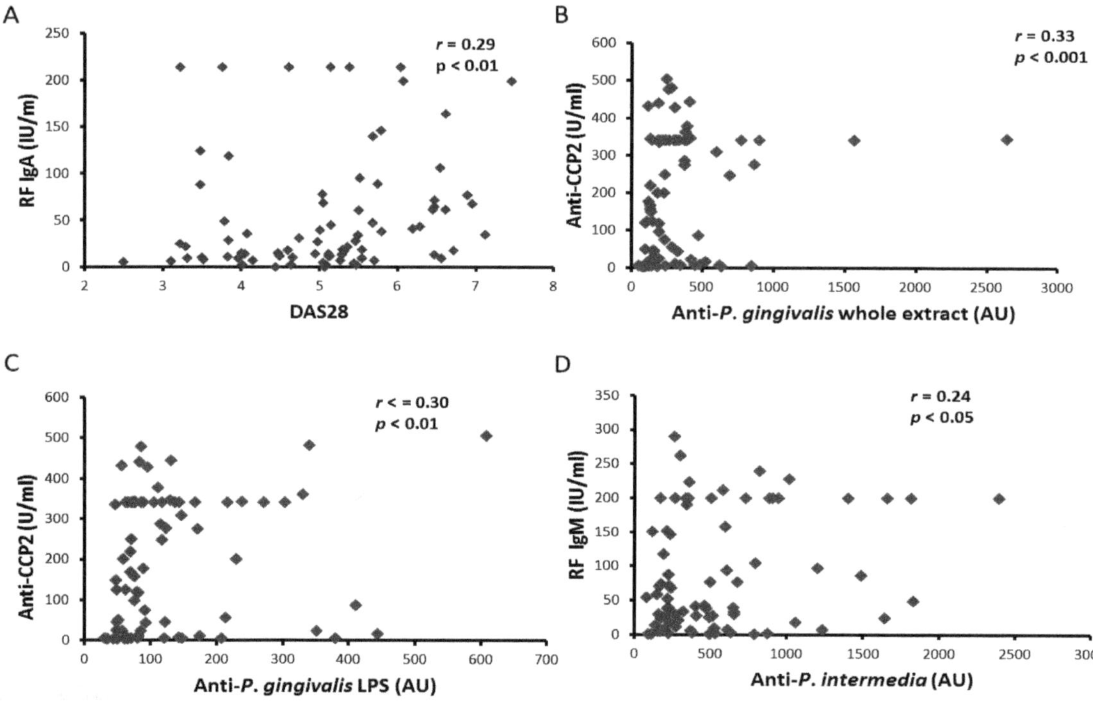

Figure 2. Correlation between clinical and biological parameters at baseline. Correlations between RF IgA and DAS28 (**A**); anti-CCP2 and anti-*P. gingivalis* whole extract antibodies (**B**); anti-CCP2 and anti-*P. gingivalis* LPS specific antibodies (**C**); and RF IgG and anti-*P. intermedia* antibodies (**D**). RF: rheumatoid factors; IU: international units; DAS28: disease activity score 28; AU: arbitrary units; anti-CCP2: anti-cyclic citrullinated petides 2nd generation; *r*: Spearman correlation coefficient; LPS: lipopolysaccharide; U: Unit; IU: International unit; NS: non-significant.

3.5. *Clinical Response to Infliximab Therapy and Joint or Periodontal Destructions*

As expected, DAS28 and inflammation markers (CRP and ESR) strongly decreased at 6 months of infliximab treatment (Table 1). DAS28 improvement was similar in RA patients with or without severe PD (1.9 (0.7–3.0) vs. 1.7 (0.5–2.5); not significant) and according to the joint damage status. Interestingly, anti-CCP2 concentrations decreased significantly during infliximab therapy (Figure 3A;

$p < 0.001$) as IgM RF concentrations (Figure 3B; $p < 0.001$). As expected, all RA parameters decreased during infliximab therapy.

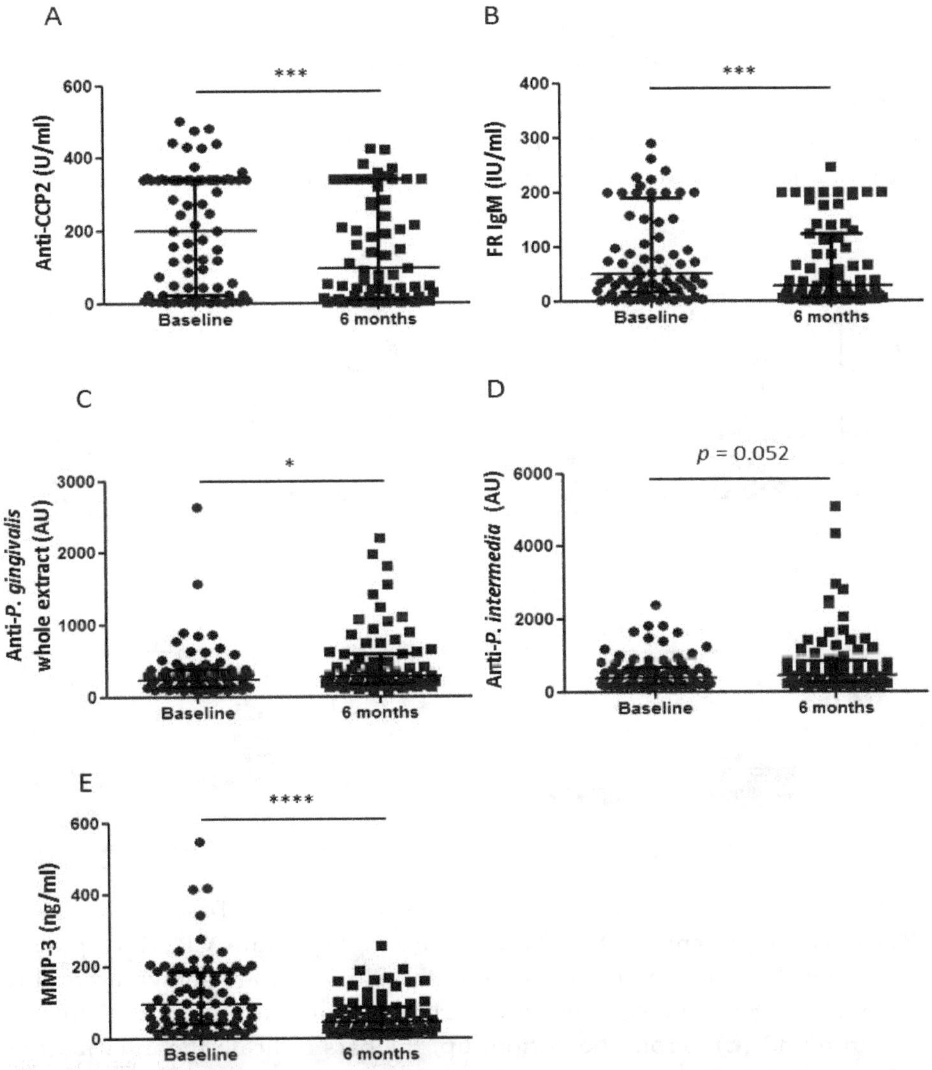

Figure 3. Effect of infliximab treatment on biological markers. Anti-CCP2 (**A**), RF IgM (**B**), anti-*P. gingivalis* antibodies (**C**), anti-*P. intermedia* antibodies (**D**), and MMP3 (**E**) were evaluated at baseline and after 6 months of infliximab therapy. Dots represent results for each patient, with values at baseline in round and at 6 months of infliximab therapy in square. From the bottom up, the bars indicate the interquartile range and the median. Anti-CCP2: anti-cyclic citrullinated petides 2nd generation; RF: rheumatoid factor; MMP-3: metalloproteinase 3; AU: arbitrary units; IU: International units; *: $p < 0.05$; ***: $p < 0.001$; ****: $p < 0.0001$.

3.6. Dissociated Effect of Infliximab Therapy on PD Biological Markers

Anti-*P. gingivalis* whole extract antibody concentrations slightly increased at 6 months of infliximab therapy (Figure 3C; $p < 0.05$) with the same trend for anti-*P. intermedia* antibody concentrations (Figure 3D; $p = 0.052$). During infliximab therapy, MMP-3 concentrations strongly decreased from 90 (14–259) ng/mL to 45 (10–160) ng/mL (Figure 3E; $p < 0.0001$). Thus, infliximab therapy induced a strong reduction of MMP-3, but slightly increased concentrations of antibodies against *P. gingivalis* and *P. intermedia*.

3.7. Biological Markers and Prediction of Clinical Response

Among biomarkers assessed in this study, baseline MMP-3 concentrations were higher in patients with a good response to infliximab (111 (49–187) ng/mL) compared to non-responders (57 (29–110) ng/mL; $p < 0.05$; Figure 4A). However, neither baseline anti-CCP2 concentrations (Figure 4B; NS) nor anti-*P. gingivalis* and anti-*P. intermedia* antibody concentrations (data not shown) were not associated with clinical response to infliximab. Furthermore, reduction of MMP-3 during infliximab therapy was higher in responders than in non-responders patients (Figure 4C; $p < 0.05$). Only a trend was observed for higher reduction of anti-CCP2 in responders compared to non-responders to infliximab (Figure 4D; $p = 0.09$).

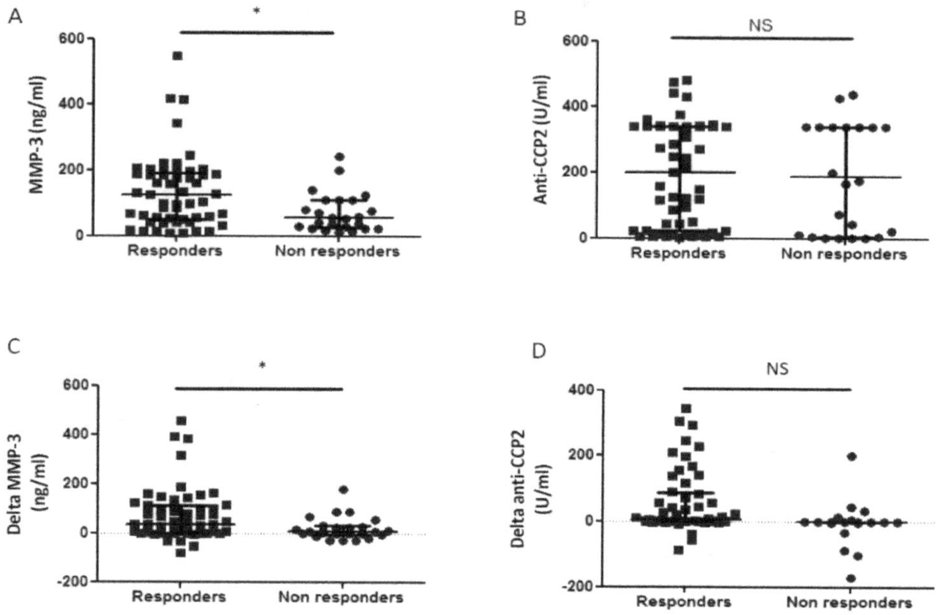

Figure 4. Predictive factors for clinical response to infliximab therapy. Baseline values of MMP-3 (**A**) and anti-CCP2 (**B**) were represented. Delta MMP-3 (**C**) and delta anti-CCP2 (**D**) represent difference of MMP-3 and ACPA (baseline value minus 6 month value) and are shown according to clinical response to infliximab. Dots represent results for each patient, with responders in square (■) and non-responders in round (●). From the bottom up, the bars indicate the interquartile range and the median. Response to infliximab treatment was defined by an improvement > 1.2 of DAS28 at 6 months. MMP-3: matrix metalloproteinase-3; anti-CCP2: anti-cyclic citrullinated petides 2nd generation; *: $p < 0.05$; NS: non significant.

4. Discussion

We confirmed a higher prevalence of PD in established RA patients (64.5%) than in the general population (30–40%) [30], as previously reported in early RA [31]. PD is related to many anaerobic periodontal pathogens including *P. intermedia*, *P. melaninogenica*, or *T. forsythia*. Antibodies against these periodontal pathogens were also more frequently detected in the serum from RA patients than controls [32]. We first confirmed higher concentrations of antibodies against *P. gingivalis* and *P. intermedia* in established RA than in healthy blood donors [32] or in two other inflammatory diseases (SLE and IBD). This is in link with a recent review considering high *P. gingivalis* antibody as a biomarker of RA [33]. Serology determination is the easiest way to assess presence of *P. gingivalis* and indirectly presence of severe PD. Gingival presence of *P. gingivalis* detected by polymerase chain reaction is strongly correlated with concentrations of anti-*P. gingivalis* antibody [13,14]. Previous studies have explored antibodies against *P. gingivalis* in RA patients by using either LPS or whole extract [12]. Here, we observed a correlation between these two assessments (LPS and bacterial extract) of antibodies against *P. gingivalis*, suggesting that LPS should be the easiest way to assess anti-*P. gingivalis*. Furthermore, antibody concentrations against *P. gingivalis* and *P. intermedia* correlated together, which was not surprising since both are involved in PD pathogenesis [34]. Despite the quite high r value for the correlation between antibodies against *P. gingivalis* LPS and against *E. coli*, we still believe that each antibody is specific due to absence of high level of antibodies for both pathogens. Our assay to detect antibodies against *P. gingivalis* LPS or *E. coli* LPS without crossreaction. This was not surprising since LPS from *P. gingivalis* has a specific structure compared to other bacteria with the ability to activate TLR2 and TLR4 [35], whereas LPS from *E. coli* activates mainly TLR4 [35].

Anti-*P. gingivalis* antibody concentrations correlated with anti-CCP2 concentrations without correlation with RF concentrations [15]. We did not expected crossreacticvity between *P. gingivalis* and anti-CCP2 due to LPS structure containing only sugars and lipids and absence of detection of citrullinated proteins in *P. gingivalis* extracts by using the monoclonal detection antibody from anti-CCP2 assay. Contrary to anti-*P. gingivalis* antibodies, anti-*P. intermedia* antibodies were not correlated with anti-CCP2, but with RF IgM concentrations, as previously described in a human [36] or in a rat model [5]. This suggested different mechanisms of action between these two bacteria in immune response induction. Assessment of several oral bacteria is required to have a discriminate role for each pathogen. For instance, recent data suggested high anti-*P. intermedia* antibodies in clinical remission RA patients with persistent PD US activity [23]. On the other hand, *Aggregatibacter actinomycetemcomitans* (*A. actinomycetemcomitans*), a periodontal pathogen associated with PD severity, has been suspected to be the culprit of the association of RA and PD [37] without confirmation since. Taken all together, our data support the specific implication of *P. gingivalis* compared to *P. intermedia* in RA pathogenesis with induction of anti-CCP2 in response to gingival citrullinated proteins, as suggested by a recent rodent model [5].

MMP-3 is a biomarker of both destruction in RA [38] and in PD [39]. So, we confirmed the reduction of inflammatory markers (ESR., CRP) and MMP-3 over infliximab treatment, as previously described with infliximab [40] or other TNF blocker [41].

Despite the growing interest for *P. gingivalis* in, R.A., this was the first observation that anti-*P. gingivalis* and *P. intermedia* antibodies were increasing over time during infliximab therapy. Only a recent study observed a stability of anti-*P. gingivalis* antibody concentrations in 50 early RA patients mainly treated with methotrexate [42]. As previously reported with methotrexate therapy [42], no patient developed seroconversion for *P. gingivalis* or *P. intermedia* with combination of infliximab and methotrexate. Despite the growing interest for *P. gingivalis* pre-existing immunity in RA patients, this was the first observation that serum anti-*P. gingivalis* antibodies were increasing over time during infliximab therapy or bDAMRDS. It is not surprinsing that bDMARD promotes infections including gingival infection. Our results are in line with previous report with infliximab showing increasing of gingival inflammation during infliximab therapy [25]. However, this increasing of gingival inflammation was not observed with rituximab or tocilizumab, two other bDMARDs targeting B cell and IL-6, respectively [27,28]. On the contrary, some studies investigated the effect of periodontal therapy on RA activity. A recent metaanalysis suggested a small effect of periodontal therapy (full-mouth scaling and root planning) on RA disease activity [43]. Reduction of ACPA during infliximab therapy was also already described [44]. Despite increased of anti-*P. gingivalis* antibody concentrations during infliximab therapy, a trend for a reduction of anti-CCP2 during infliximab therapy was observed in our study. This kind of dissociation response was also observed after non-surgical therapy for periodontal disease with a decreased of anti-*P. gingivalis* levels without effect on anti-CCP2 levels [29]. This dissociated response to infliximab of anti-*P. gingivalis* and anti-CCP2 concentrations reinforced role of *P. gingivalis* only in anti-CCP2 induction.

Prediction of TNF response remains a huge challenge and to date no biomarkers can be used in daily practice [21]. Here, we observed that high baseline MMP-3 concentrations were associated with a good clinical response. This emphasizes the role of MMP-3 for RA management strategy [20]. However, baseline MMP-3 concentrations were similar in 47 good responders vs. 29 non-responders according to response assessed earlier than in our study at 14 weeks [45]. Further studies are needed before to consider MMP-3 as a validate biomarker to predict clinical response in the daily practice [21].

Our study also has some weakness. PD assessment was only performed at baseline on panoramic X-rays without clinical assessment. Clinical PD assessment was not planned in this study. However, clinical severe PD was already extremely reported [2] with a dissociated effect of infliximab therapy. In fact, infliximab treatment worsens the gingival inflammation, but decreases the gingival destruction of bone [25]. Panoramic X-rays was not repeated due to low variation of bone loss.

5. Conclusions

Concentrations of anti-*P. gingivalis* antibody, a biomarker of PD severity correlated with anti-CCP2 concentrations in one hand and anti-*P. intermedia* antibody concentrations in another hand. Besides, anti-*P. intermedia* antibody concentrations correlated only with RF concentrations suggesting different immunologic response induced by both oral bacteria. Whereas MMP-3 is strongly decreased by infliximab therapy, serology against oral pathogen slightly increased. Furthermore, MMP-3, another biomarker of PD and RA severity, is a predictive biomarker of response to infliximab therapy. Our data reinforce interest of PD in RA pathogenesis and RA therapeutic management. They also confirm the possible involvement of *P. gingivalis* in RA physiopathology due to the correlation with ACPA.

Author Contributions: Conceptualization, M.R.-G., S.P. and H.M.; Data curation, P.M., P.G., P.F., X.R., T.T. and H.M.; Formal analysis, M.R.-G., P.F., S.P. and H.M.; Investigation, M.R.-G., P.M., P.G., P.F., X.R., T.T., S.P. and H.M.; Methodology, M.R.-G., V.B.-B., P.F., S.P. and H.M.; Project administration, P.M., P.G., T.T. and H.M.; Resources, V.B.-B., X.R., S.P. and H.M.; Supervision, H.M.; Validation, M.R.G. and H.M.; Writing-original draft, M.R.-G. and S.P.; Writing-review and editing, M.R.-G. and H.M.

Acknowledgments: This work was funded by Aide à la Recherche médicale de proximité (AIRE) and Aide à la Recherche Médicale Ondaine et Environs.

References

1. Aletaha, D.; Neogi, T.; Silman, A.J.; Funovits, J.; Felson, D.T.; Bingham, C.O.; Birnbaum, N.S.; Burmester, G.R.; Bykerk, V.P.; Cohen, M.D.; et al. 2010 rheumatoid arthritis classification criteria: An American College of Rheumatology/European League Against Rheumatism collaborative initiative. *Ann. Rheum. Dis.* **2010**, *69*, 1580–1588. [CrossRef] [PubMed]
2. Fuggle, N.R.; Smith, T.O.; Kaul, A.; Sofat, N. Hand to Mouth: A Systematic Review and Meta-Analysis of the Association between Rheumatoid Arthritis and Periodontitis. *Front. Immunol.* **2016**, *7*, 80. [CrossRef]
3. Marotte, H.; Farge, P.; Gaudin, P.; Alexandre, C.; Mougin, B.; Miossec, P. The association between periodontal disease and joint destruction in rheumatoid arthritis extends the link between the HLA-DR shared epitope and severity of bone destruction. *Ann. Rheum. Dis.* **2006**, *65*, 905–909. [CrossRef] [PubMed]
4. Rosenstein, E.D.; Greenwald, R.A.; Kushner, L.J.; Weissmann, G. Hypothesis: The humoral immune response to oral bacteria provides a stimulus for the development of rheumatoid arthritis. *Inflammation* **2004**, *28*, 311–318. [CrossRef] [PubMed]
5. Courbon, G.; Rinaudo-Gaujous, M.; Blasco-Baque, V.; Auger, I.; Caire, R.; Mijola, L.; Vico, L.; Paul, S.; Marotte, H. Porphyromonas gingivalis experimentally induces periodontis and an anti-CCP2-associated arthritis in the rat. *Ann. Rheum. Dis.* **2019**, *78*, 594–599. [CrossRef]
6. Zhang, X.; Zhang, D.; Jia, H.; Feng, Q.; Wang, D.; Liang, D.; Wu, X.; Li, J.; Tang, L.; Li, Y.; et al. The oral and gut microbiomes are perturbed in rheumatoid arthritis and partly normalized after treatment. *Nat. Med.* **2015**, *21*, 895–905. [CrossRef] [PubMed]
7. György, B.; Tóth, E.; Tarcsa, E.; Falus, A.; Buzás, E.I. Citrullination: A posttranslational modification in health and disease. *Int. J. Biochem. Cell Biol.* **2006**, *38*, 1662–1677. [CrossRef]
8. Klareskog, L.; Rönnelid, J.; Lundberg, K.; Padyukov, L.; Alfredsson, L. Immunity to citrullinated proteins in rheumatoid arthritis. *Annu. Rev. Immunol.* **2008**, *26*, 651–675. [CrossRef] [PubMed]

9. Nielen, M.M.J.; Van Schaardenburg, D.; Reesink, H.W.; Van De Stadt, R.J.; Van Der Horst-Bruinsma, I.E.; De Koning, M.H.M.T.; Habibuw, M.R.; Vandenbroucke, J.P.; Dijkmans, B.A.C.; Van Der Horst-Bruinsma, I.E. Specific autoantibodies precede the symptoms of rheumatoid arthritis: A study of serial measurements in blood donors. *Arthritis Rheum.* **2004**, *50*, 380–386. [CrossRef] [PubMed]
10. Lundberg, K.; Wegner, N.; Yucel-Lindberg, T.; Venables, P.J. Periodontitis in RA-the citrullinated enolase connection. *Nat. Rev. Rheumatol.* **2010**, *6*, 727–730. [CrossRef]
11. Mangat, P.; Wegner, N.; Venables, P.J.; Potempa, J. Bacterial and human peptidylarginine deiminases: Targets for inhibiting the autoimmune response in rheumatoid arthritis? *Arthritis Res. Ther.* **2010**, *12*, 209. [CrossRef] [PubMed]
12. Wegner, N.; Wait, R.; Sroka, A.; Eick, S.; Nguyen, K.-A.; Lundberg, K.; Kinloch, A.; Culshaw, S.; Potempa, J.; Venables, P.J.; et al. Peptidylarginine deiminase from Porphyromonas gingivalis citrullinates human fibrinogen and α-enolase: Implications for autoimmunity in rheumatoid arthritis. *Arthritis Rheum.* **2010**, *62*, 2662–2672. [CrossRef] [PubMed]
13. Seror, R.; Le Gall-David, S.; Bonnaure-Mallet, M.; Schaeverbeke, T.; Cantagrel, A.; Minet, J.; Gottenberg, J.-E.; Chanson, P.; Ravaud, P.; Mariette, X. Association of Anti-*Porphyromonas gingivalis* Antibody Titers with Nonsmoking Status in Early Rheumatoid Arthritis: Results from the Prospective French Cohort of Patients with Early Rheumatoid Arthritis: Anti-*Porphyromonas Gingivalis* Antibody and Early RA. *Arthritis Rheumatol.* **2015**, *67*, 1729–1737. [CrossRef] [PubMed]
14. Mikuls, T.R.; Payne, J.B.; Yu, F.; Thiele, G.M.; Reynolds, R.J.; Cannon, G.W.; Markt, J.; McGowan, D.; Kerr, G.S.; Redman, R.S.; et al. Periodontitis and Porphyromonas gingivalis in Patients with Rheumatoid Arthritis. *Arthritis Rheumatol.* **2014**, *66*, 1090–1100. [CrossRef] [PubMed]
15. Mikuls, T.R.; Payne, J.B.; Reinhardt, R.A.; Thielea, G.M.; Maziarz, E.; Cannell, A.C.; Holers, V.M.; Kuhnc, K.A.; O'Dell, J.R. Antibody responses to Porphyromonas gingivalis (P. gingivalis) in subjects with rheumatoid arthritis and periodontitis. *Int. Immunopharmacol.* **2009**, *9*, 38–42. [CrossRef]
16. Okada, Y.; Nagase, H.; Harris, E.D. A metalloproteinase from human rheumatoid synovial fibroblasts that digests connective tissue matrix components. Purification and characterization. *J. Biol. Chem.* **1986**, *261*, 14245–14255.
17. Toyman, U.; Tüter, G.; Kurtiş, B.; Kıvrak, E.; Bozkurt, Ş.; Yücel, A.A.; Serdar, M. Evaluation of gingival crevicular fluid levels of tissue plasminogen activator, plasminogen activator inhibitor 2, matrix metalloproteinase-3 and interleukin 1-β in patients with different periodontal diseases. *J. Periodontal Res.* **2015**, *50*, 44–51. [CrossRef]
18. Zhao, Y.; Jin, Y.; Ren, Y.; Song, L.M.; Li, J.; Lin, X.P. Expression of matrix metalloproteinase-3 in patients with rheumatoid arthritis and its correlation with chronic periodontitis and rheumatoid arthritis. *Zhonghua Kou Qiang Yi Xue Za Zhi* **2019**, *54*, 164–169.
19. da Silva, M.K.; de Carvalho, A.C.G.; Alves, E.H.P.; da Silva, F.R.P.; Pessoa, L.D.S.; Vasconcelos, D.F.P. Genetic Factors and the Risk of Periodontitis Development: Findings from a Systematic Review Composed of 13 Studies of Meta-Analysis with 71,531 Participants. *Int. J. Dent.* **2017**, *2017*, 1914073. [CrossRef]
20. Urata, Y.; Uesato, R.; Tanaka, D.; Nakamura, Y.; Motomura, S. Treating to target matrix metalloproteinase 3 normalisation together with disease activity score below 2.6 yields better effects than each alone in rheumatoid arthritis patients: T-4 Study. *Ann. Rheum. Dis.* **2012**, *71*, 534–540. [CrossRef]
21. Marotte, H.; Miossec, P. Biomarkers for prediction of TNFalpha blockers response in rheumatoid arthritis. *Jt. Bone Spine* **2010**, *77*, 297–305. [CrossRef] [PubMed]
22. Savioli, C.; Ribeiro, A.C.M.; Fabri, G.M.C.; Calich, A.L.; Carvalho, J.; Silva, C.A.; Viana, V.S.; Bonfá, E.; Siqueira, J.T.T. Persistent periodontal disease hampers anti-tumor necrosis factor treatment response in rheumatoid arthritis. *J. Clin. Rheumatol.* **2012**, *18*, 180–184. [CrossRef] [PubMed]
23. Kimura, Y.; Yoshida, S.; Takeuchi, T.; Yoshikawa, A.; Hiramatsu, Y.; Ishida, T.; Makino, S.; Takasugi, Y.; Hanafusa, T. Periodontal pathogens participate in synovitis in patients with rheumatoid arthritis in clinical remission: A retrospective case–control study. *Rheumatology* **2015**. [CrossRef] [PubMed]
24. Marotte, H. Tooth-brushing: An impact on rheumatoid arthritis. *Jt. Bone Spine* **2016**, *83*, 619–621. [CrossRef]
25. Pers, J.-O.; Saraux, A.; Pierre, R.; Youinou, P. Anti-TNF-alpha immunotherapy is associated with increased gingival inflammation without clinical attachment loss in subjects with rheumatoid arthritis. *J. Periodontol.* **2008**, *79*, 1645–1651. [CrossRef] [PubMed]

26. Rodríguez-Lozano, B.; González-Febles, J.; Garnier-Rodríguez, J.L.; Dadlani, S.; Bustabad-Reyes, S.; Sanz, M.; Sánchez-Alonso, F.; Sánchez-Piedra, C.; González-Dávila, E.; Díaz-González, F. Association between severity of periodontitis and clinical activity in rheumatoid arthritis patients: A case-control study. *Arthritis Res. Ther.* **2019**, *21*, 27. [CrossRef]
27. Coat, J.; Demoersman, J.; Beuzit, S.; Cornec, D.; Devauchelle-Pensec, V.; Saraux, A.; Pers, J.-O.; Devauchelle-Pensec, V. Anti-B lymphocyte immunotherapy is associated with improvement of periodontal status in subjects with rheumatoid arthritis. *J. Clin. Periodontol.* **2015**, *42*, 817–823. [CrossRef] [PubMed]
28. Kobayashi, T.; Okada, M.; Ito, S.; Kobayashi, D.; Ishida, K.; Kojima, A.; Narita, I.; Murasawa, A.; Yoshie, H. Assessment of interleukin-6 receptor inhibition therapy on periodontal condition in patients with rheumatoid arthritis and chronic periodontitis. *J. Periodontol.* **2014**, *85*, 57–67. [CrossRef] [PubMed]
29. Okada, M.; Kobayashi, T.; Ito, S.; Yokoyama, T.; Abe, A.; Murasawa, A.; Yoshie, H. Periodontal Treatment Decreases Levels of Antibodies to Porphyromonas gingivalis and Citrulline in Patients with Rheumatoid Arthritis and Periodontitis. *J. Periodontol.* **2013**, *84*, e74–e84. [CrossRef] [PubMed]
30. Burt, B. Research, Science and Therapy Committee of the American Academy of Periodontology. Position paper: Epidemiology of periodontal diseases. *J. Periodontol.* **2005**, *76*, 1406–1419. [CrossRef] [PubMed]
31. Scher, J.U.; Ubeda, C.; Equinda, M.; Khanin, R.; Buischi, Y.; Viale, A.; Lipuma, L.; Attur, M.; Pillinger, M.H.; Weissmann, G.; et al. Periodontal disease and the oral microbiota in new-onset rheumatoid arthritis. *Arthritis Rheum.* **2012**, *64*, 3083–3094. [CrossRef]
32. Ogrendik, M.; Kokino, S.; Ozdemir, F.; Bird, P.S.; Hamlet, S. Serum antibodies to oral anaerobic bacteria in patients with rheumatoid arthritis. *MedGenMed* **2005**, *7*, 2. [PubMed]
33. Bender, P.; Bürgin, W.B.; Sculean, A.; Eick, S. Serum antibody levels against Porphyromonas gingivalis in patients with and without rheumatoid arthritis—A systematic review and meta-analysis. *Clin. Oral Investig.* **2017**, *21*, 33–42. [CrossRef]
34. Cheng, Z.; Meade, J.; Mankia, K.; Emery, P.; Devine, D.A. Periodontal disease and periodontal bacteria as triggers for rheumatoid arthritis. *Best Pr. Res. Clin. Rheumatol.* **2017**, *31*, 19–30. [CrossRef] [PubMed]
35. Netea, M.G.; van Deuren, M.; Kullberg, B.J.; Cavaillon, J.M.; Van der Meer, J.W. Does the shape of lipid A determine the interaction of LPS with Toll-like receptors? *Trends Immunol.* **2002**, *23*, 135–139. [CrossRef]
36. Goh, C.E.; Kopp, J.; Papapanou, P.N.; Molitor, J.A.; Demmer, R.T. Association Between Serum Antibodies to Periodontal Bacteria and Rheumatoid Factor in the Third National Health and Nutrition Examination Survey: Periodontal Bacteria Antibodies and Rheumatoid Factor. *Arthritis Rheumatol.* **2016**, *68*, 2384–2393. [CrossRef]
37. Konig, M.F.; Abusleme, L.; Reinholdt, J.; Palmer, R.J.; Teles, R.P.; Sampson, K.; Rosen, A.; Nigrovic, P.A.; Sokolove, J.; Giles, J.T.; et al. Aggregatibacter actinomycetemcomitans-induced hypercitrullination links periodontal infection to autoimmunity in rheumatoid arthritis. *Sci. Transl. Med.* **2016**, *8*, 369ra176. [CrossRef]
38. Omura, K.; Takahashi, M.; Omura, T.; Miyamoto, S.; Kushida, K.; Sano, Y.; Nagano, A. Changes in the concentration of plasma matrix metalloproteinases (MMPs) and tissue inhibitor of metalloproteinases-1 (TIMP-1) after total joint replacement in patients with arthritis. *Clin. Rheumatol.* **2002**, *21*, 488–492. [CrossRef] [PubMed]
39. Reddy, N.R.; Roopa, D.; Babu, D.S.M.; Kumar, P.M.; Raju, C.M.; Kumar, N.S.; Reddy, N.; Raju, C.; Kumar, P.; Reddy, N.R.; et al. Estimation of matrix metalloproteinase-3 levels in gingival crevicular fluid in periodontal disease, health and after scaling and root planing. *J. Indian Soc. Periodontol.* **2012**, *16*, 549–552. [CrossRef]
40. Ban, A.; Inaba, M.; Furumitsu, Y.; Okamoto, K.; Yukioka, K.; Goto, H.; Nishizawa, Y. Time-course of health status in patients with rheumatoid arthritis during the first year of treatment with infliximab. *Biomed. Pharmacother.* **2010**, *64*, 107–112. [CrossRef]
41. Kawashiri, S.-Y.; Kawakami, A.; Ueki, Y.; Imazato, T.; Iwamoto, N.; Fujikawa, K.; Aramaki, T.; Tamai, M.; Nakamura, H.; Origuchi, T.; et al. Decrement of serum cartilage oligomeric matrix protein (COMP) in rheumatoid arthritis (RA) patients achieving remission after 6 months of etanercept treatment: Comparison with CRP., IgM-RF., MMP-3 and anti-CCP Ab. *Jt. Bone Spine* **2010**, *77*, 418–420. [CrossRef] [PubMed]
42. Arvikar, S.L.; Collier, D.S.; Fisher, M.C.; Unizony, S.; Cohen, G.L.; McHugh, G.; Kawai, T.; Strle, K.; Steere, A.C. Clinical correlations with Porphyromonas gingivalis antibody responses in patients with early rheumatoid arthritis. *Arthritis Res. Ther.* **2013**, *15*, R109. [CrossRef]

43. Kaur, S.; Bright, R.; Proudman, S.M.; Bartold, P.M. Does periodontal treatment influence clinical and biochemical measures for rheumatoid arthritis? A systematic review and meta-analysis. *Semin. Arthritis Rheum.* **2014**, *44*, 113–122. [CrossRef] [PubMed]
44. Bobbio-Pallavicini, F.; Alpini, C.; Caporali, R.; Avalle, S.; Bugatti, S.; Montecucco, C. Autoantibody profile in rheumatoid arthritis during long-term infliximab treatment. *Arthritis Res. Ther.* **2004**, *6*, R264–R272. [CrossRef] [PubMed]
45. Lequerré, T.; Jouen, F.; Brazier, M.; Clayssens, S.; Klemmer, N.; Ménard, J.-F.; Mejjad, O.; Daragon, A.; Tron, F.; Le Loët, X.; et al. Autoantibodies, metalloproteinases and bone markers in rheumatoid arthritis patients are unable to predict their responses to infliximab. *Rheumatology* **2007**, *46*, 446–453. [CrossRef] [PubMed]

9

Prevalence and Fracture Risk of Osteoporosis in Patients with Rheumatoid Arthritis: A Multicenter Comparative Study of the FRAX and WHO Criteria

Sang Tae Choi [1,†], Seong-Ryul Kwon [2,†], Ju-Yang Jung [3], Hyoun-Ah Kim [3], Sung-Soo Kim [4], Sang Hyon Kim [5], Ji-Min Kim [5], Ji-Ho Park [1] and Chang-Hee Suh [3,*]

1 Division of Rheumatology, Department of Internal Medicine, Chung-Ang University College of Medicine, Seoul 06973, Korea; beconst@cau.ac.kr (S.T.C.); pjh853@hanmail.net (J.-H.P.)

2 Division of Rheumatology, Department of Internal Medicine, Inha University College of Medicine, Incheon 22332, Korea; rhksr@inha.ac.kr

3 Department of Rheumatology, Ajou University School of Medicine, Suwon 16499, Korea; serinne20@hanmail.net (J.-Y.J.); nakhada@naver.com (H.-A.K.)

4 Division of Rheumatology, Department of Internal Medicine, Ulsan University College of Medicine, Gangneung Asan Hospital, Gangneung 25440, Korea; drkiss@ulsan.ac.kr

5 Division of Rheumatology, Department of Internal Medicine, Keimyung University College of Medicine, Daegu 41931, Korea; mdkim9111@hanmail.net (S.H.K.); okjimin@hanmail.net (J.-M.K.)

* Correspondence: chsuh@ajou.ac.kr

† Sang Tae Choi and Seong-Ryul Kwon contributed equally to this work.

Abstract: (1) Background: We evaluated the prevalence and fracture risk of osteoporosis in patients with rheumatoid arthritis (RA), and compared the fracture risk assessment tool (FRAX) criteria and bone mineral density (BMD) criteria established by the World Health Organization (WHO). (2) Methods: This retrospective cross-sectional study, which included 479 RA patients in 5 hospitals, was conducted between January 2012 and December 2016. The FRAX criteria for high-risk osteoporotic fractures were calculated including and excluding the BMD values, respectively. The definition of high risk for fracture by FRAX criteria and BMD criteria by WHO was 10-year probability of $\geq$ 20% for major osteoporotic fracture or $\geq$ 3% for hip fracture, and T score ≤ -2.5 or Z score ≤ -2.0, respectively. (3) Results: The mean age was 61.7 $\pm$ 11.9 years. The study included 426 female patients (88.9%), 353 (82.9%) of whom were postmenopausal. Osteoporotic fractures were detected in 81 (16.9%) patients. The numbers of candidates for pharmacological intervention using the FRAX criteria with and without BMD and the WHO criteria were 226 (47.2%), 292 (61%), and 160 (33.4%), respectively. Only 69.2%–77% of the patients in the high-risk group using the FRAX criteria were receiving osteoporosis treatments. The following were significant using the WHO criteria: female (OR 3.55, 95% CI 1.46–8.63), age (OR 1.1, 95% CI 1.08–1.13), and BMI (OR 0.8, 95% CI 0.75–0.87). Glucocorticoid dose (OR 1.09, 95% CI 1.01–1.17), age (OR 1.09, 95% CI 1.06–1.12), and disease duration (OR 1.01, 95% CI 1–1.01) were independent risk factors for fracture. (4) Conclusions: The proportion of RA patients with a high risk of osteoporotic fractures was 33.4%–61%. Only 69.2%–77% of candidate patients were receiving osteoporotic treatments while applying FRAX criteria. Independent risk factors for osteoporotic fractures in RA patients were age, the dose of glucocorticoid, and disease duration.

Keywords: osteoporosis; fracture; fracture risk assessment tool; rheumatoid arthritis

1. Introduction

Osteoporosis is one of the most well-known complications in patients with rheumatoid arthritis (RA). RA is a disease that presents a state of chronic inflammation that is known to cause an increase in osteoclastic differentiation and an inhibition of osteogenesis [1]. Furthermore, the treatment with glucocorticoids then increases the imbalance which already existed due to the disease. Moreover, this association may be due to a lack of mobility and frequent occurrences of RA during menopause as well as systemic inflammation of RA and the use of corticosteroids [1–3]. The prevalence of osteoporosis in patients with RA was reported to be approximately twice as high as in the general population [4]. The frequency of osteoporosis in patients with RA has been reported to be 6.3% to 36.3% in the hip, and 12.3% to 38.9% in the spine [4–6]. Compared with controls, the fracture risk in patients with RA also increased for the hip (relative risk (RR): 2) and spine (RR: 2.4) [7]. Moreover, hip and vertebral osteoporotic fractures are known to be associated with an immediate and long-term (up to 20 years) increased risk of mortality [8]. Excess mortality during the first year after a hip fracture ranged from 8.4% to 36%, and the risk of mortality following hip fracture was estimated to be more than 2 times higher than that of the general population [9]. Therefore, it is very important to accurately assess the risk of osteoporotic fractures in RA patients.

The fracture risk assessment tool (FRAX) criteria and the bone mineral density (BMD) criteria established by the World Health Organization (WHO) are widely used for the risk assessment of osteoporotic fractures. The WHO criteria, using BMD measured by dual-energy X-ray absorptiometry (DXA), are the most widely used in the diagnosis of osteoporosis [10]. The management guidelines for the prevention and treatment of osteoporosis, developed by an expert committee of the National Osteoporosis Foundation (NOF), are also based on BMDs [11]. In 2008, a WHO task force introduced the FRAX tool to evaluate the 10-year probability for hip and major osteoporotic fractures [12]. The FRAX model contains various risk factors for osteoporotic fractures including country, age, sex, weight, height, smoking, previous fracture, family history of fracture, glucocorticoid treatment, alcohol intake, and BMD, if available [13]. In particular, RA is the only disease risk factor in the FRAX model, even though the input for RA is just a dichotomous variable.

In clinical settings, physicians determine the proper medications to prevent osteoporotic fractures based on these criteria [11,14]. However, when assessing the risk of osteoporotic fractures in patients with RA, the relevance and benefits among the three assessment methods (WHO osteoporosis criteria and FRAX criteria with BMD and without BMD) have not been clearly studied. Therefore, in this multicenter study, we aimed to evaluate the incidence among a high-risk group for osteoporotic fracture and to identify the risk factors of osteoporotic fractures in patients with RA by comparing these criteria. We also examined the extent of treatments for osteoporosis among patients in need of osteoporosis treatment.

2. Experimental Section

2.1. Study Population

In this retrospective cross-sectional study, we assessed 479 Korean patients with RA in 5 university hospitals between January 2012 and December 2016. All recruited patients were over the age of 18 and satisfied the 1987 American College of Rheumatology (ACR) criteria or the 2010 ACR/European League Against Rheumatism (EULAR) criteria for RA [15,16]. Recorded data using a medical chart review included age, sex, body mass index (BMI), menopausal status, hormone supplement therapy in postmenopausal women, fracture history, history of parental hip fracture, daily alcohol intake, smoking status, autoantibody status, erythrocyte sediment rate (ESR), C-reactive protein (CRP), and the presence of secondary osteoporosis. The standard of BMI was 25 kg/m^2 using validated BMI categorization for the Korean population [17]. Therapeutic medication lists for the treatment of RA including current glucocorticoid use, cumulative glucocorticoid dose, and conventional and biological disease-modifying anti-rheumatic drugs, as well as pharmacological intervention for osteoporosis, such as bisphosphonate, selective estrogen receptor modulators (SERM), vitamin D and calcium, were also obtained. The study was approved by the Institutional Review Board (IRB) of each Hospital (C2015163 (1621), 2015-09-026, AJIRB-MED-MDB-15-285, 3-32100191-AB-N-01, and DSMC2015-12-017-007). Informed consent was waived by the IRB.

2.2. Evaluation of Osteoporosis by BMD Criteria

Candidates for pharmacological interventions to prevent osteoporosis were assessed using the WHO osteoporosis criteria [10]. All BMD measurements were done using the same technique. The BMD of the lumbar vertebrae (L1–L4) and both hips were measured using DXA (GE Lunar, Madison, WI, USA). *t*- and *z*-scores were calculated with the referent BMD of 5 hospitals. According to the WHO criterion, patients with osteoporosis and osteopenia were defined having a value of the *t*-score that was -2.5 or less, and from -2.5 to -1, respectively, for postmenopausal women or men $\geq$50 years old. For the evaluation of premenopausal women or men <50 years old, *z*-scores ≤ -2 were considered as osteoporosis.

2.3. Osteoporotic Fracture Risk Evaluation by FRAX

The 10-year probability of major osteoporotic and hip fractures was calculated by the FRAX tool, based on medical chart reviews and questionnaires. The FRAX criteria for high risk of osteoporotic fracture were defined as a 10-year probability of $\geq$20% for major osteoporotic fracture or $\geq$3% for hip fracture. We calculated two kinds of FRAX values using the Korean model (http://www.shef.ac.uk/FRAX/tool.aspx?country=25); FRAX with BMD was calculated including the femur neck BMD (g/cm^2) value.

2.4. Risk Factors for Fracture

Information regarding previous fractures was obtained through patient self-reporting questionnaires during routine clinic visits and spinal x-ray evaluations. Potential factors associated with osteoporotic fractures were collected by patient interviews, physical examinations, and laboratory tests. Patient baseline characteristics, including clinical variables, RA medications, and osteoporosis-related factors, were investigated at enrollment. The dose of glucocorticoid was calculated on the basis of prednisolone. Glucocorticoid use was grouped as $\geq$5 mg/day prednisolone equivalent and <5 mg/day prednisolone-equivalent. Candidates for pharmacological interventions preventing osteoporotic fracture were identified using the WHO osteoporosis or the FRAX criteria. We evaluated osteoporotic medications, such as bisphosphonate and SERM, to obtain the ratio of high-risk patients currently undergoing osteoporosis treatments.

2.5. Statistical Analysis

All measurements were expressed as means $\pm$ SD. Values that were not normally distributed were represented as medians (IQR). A Student's *t*-test was used for the comparison of mean values. A Pearson's χ^2 test was used to compare the differences between categorical variables for analyzing correlations. Multiple linear analysis, including glucocorticoid dose, age, sex, BMI, smoking, and disease duration, was used to identify factors affecting the FRAX values and BMD scores. Glucocorticoid dose, age, BMI and disease duration were continuous variables in this model. A multivariable logistic regression analysis using glucocorticoid dose, age, sex, BMI, and disease duration was performed to obtain the respective odds ratios, and all the variables except sex were continuous variables in this model. In all analyses, a p value of <0.05 was considered statistically significant. All statistical analyses were conducted using the SPSS version 20 (IBM Corp, Armonk, NY, USA).

3. Results

3.1. Baseline Characteristics of the Study Participants

The baseline characteristics of the participants are summarized in Table 1. The data of baseline characteristics in Table 1 were based on the time of BMD test, except for rheumatoid factor and anti-citrullinated protein antibody. The average age of the 479 subjects was 61.5 ± 11.5 years. Study participants included 426 female patients (88.9%) with 353 (82.9%) being postmenopausal. The median disease duration was 53 (33–72) months. The median ESR and CRP levels were 15 (7–29) mm/h and 0.18 (0.05–0.79) mg/L, respectively. The proportion of patients who were using glucocorticoids was 92.3% (442/479), and the median dose was 2.5 mg/day prednisolone-equivalent. The number of patients with biological disease-modifying anti-rheumatic drug (DMARD) use was 56 (11.7%); 13 (2.7%) etanercept, 10 (2.1%) infliximab, 9 (2.9%) adalimumab, 3 (0.6%) golimumab, 11 (2.3%) tocilizumab, 6 (1.3%) abatacept, 2 (0.4%) rituximab, and 2 (0.4%) tofacitinib. A total of 262 (54.7%) patients were receiving osteoporosis treatments: 189 (39.5%) patients were treated with bisphosphonate, and 98 (20.5%) were using SERM. Among all the participants, 81 (16.9%) patients (7 male and 74 postmenopausal females; mean age of 69.5 ± 9.3 years) had fractures, all of which were vertebral.

Table 1. Baseline characteristics of the study participants.

Variables	RA Patients (N = 479)
Age (year)	61.8 ± 11.5
Sex (female)	426 (88.9%)
Menopause	353 (82.9%)
Weight (kg)	55.4 (49.2–62.8)
Height (cm)	155.3 (150.1–160)
BMI (kg/m^2)	23.1 (20.9–25)
Smoking	33 (6.9%)
Alcohol	41 (8.6%)
Disease duration (month)	53 (33–72)
1987 ACR criteria	377 (78.7%)
2010 ACR/EULAR criteria	418 (87.2%)
RF titer (IU/mL)	67.2 (24–165.2)
ACPA titer (U/mL)	78 (0.4–179.1)
RF positive	380 (79.3%)
ACPA positive	295 (61.6%)
ESR (mm/h)	15 (7–29)
CRP (mg/L)	0.18 (0.05–0.79)
Medications	
Glucocorticoid	442 (92.3%)
Prednisolone-equivalent dose (mg/day)	2.5 (1.25–5)
NSAID	341 (71.2%)
Biologics	56 (11.7%)
Vitamin D	228 (47.6%)
Calcium	195 (40.7%)
Proton pump inhibitor	123 (25.7%)
Treatment for osteoporosis	262 (54.7%)
Bisphosphonate	189 (39.5%)
SERM	98 (20.5%)
Vertebral fracture	81 (16.9%)
Age (year)	69.5 ± 9.3
Male	7 (8.6%)
Postmenopausal woman	74 (91.4%)

BMI, body mass index; ACR, American college of rheumatology; EULAR, European League Against Rheumatism; RF, rheumatoid factor; ACPA, anti-citrullinated protein antibody; ESR, erythrocyte sedimentation rate; CRP, C-reactive protein; NSAID, non-steroidal anti-inflammatory drug; SERM, selective estrogen receptor modulator. Values were represented as mean ± standard deviation. Values that were not normally distributed are represented as medians (IQR).

Table 2. Candidates for pharmacological treatment using the FRAX criteria with and without BMD and the WHO osteoporosis criteria in patients with rheumatoid arthritis.

Patient Groups	FRAX with BMD	FRAX without BMD	Osteoporosis of the WHO	*p* Value [1]	*p* Value [2]	*p* Value [3]
Overall ($n = 479$)	226 (47.2%)	292 (61%)	160 (33.4%)	<0.001	<0.001	<0.001
Men ($n = 53$)	17 (32.1%)	27 (50.9%)	10 (18.9%)	0.006	0.070	<0.001
Women ($n = 426$)	209 (49.1%)	265 (62.2%)	150 (35.2%)	<0.001	<0.001	<0.001
Premenopausal ($n = 56$)	3 (5.4%)	2 (3.6%)	1 (1.8%)	0.659	0.322	0.568
Postmenopausal ($n = 370$)	206 (55.7%)	263 (71.1%)	149 (40.3%)	<0.001	<0.001	<0.001

FRAX, fracture risk assessment tool; BMD, bone mineral density; WHO, World Health Organization. [1] FRAX with BMD vs. FRAX without BMD. [2] FRAX with BMD vs. osteoporosis. [3] FRAX without BMD vs. osteoporosis.

3.2. Distribution of Candidates for Pharmacological Intervention Using the FRAX and the WHO Osteoporosis Criteria

The number of patients with osteoporosis according to the WHO criteria was 160 (33.4%), and the number of candidates for pharmacological intervention using the FRAX criteria with and without BMD was 226 (47.2%) and 292 (61%), respectively. There were significant differences among these three groups (Table 2). When men, women, and postmenopausal women were analyzed separately, the number of candidates for pharmacological intervention was the highest for the FRAX criteria without BMD, followed by the FRAX criteria with BMD, and finally, the WHO osteoporosis criteria (Table 2). The numbers of candidates for pharmacological intervention of women were higher than those of men using the FRAX criteria with BMD ($p = 0.014$) and when using the WHO osteoporosis criteria ($p = 0.011$); however, there were no significant differences when using the FRAX criteria without BMD ($p = 0.077$). The proportion of patients with a BMD < -1.0 was 216/226 (95.6%) among those eligible for FRAX criteria with BMD, and 265/292 (90.8%) for FRAX without BMD.

3.3. Proportion of Patients Receiving Osteoporosis Treatment in the High-Risk Group According to the FRAX Criteria and the WHO Osteoporosis Criteria

Table 3 shows the proportion of the patients currently receiving osteoporosis treatments (bisphosphonate or SERM) in the high-risk group, based on the FRAX criteria with or without BMD and the WHO osteoporosis criteria. Of the patients in the high-risk group using the FRAX criteria with BMD, only 77% were receiving osteoporosis treatments, which was similar to the percentages in sex and menopause subgroup analyses (men, 64.7%; women, 78%; postmenopausal women, 78.6%). The proportion of patients undergoing osteoporosis treatment among the high-risk group using the FRAX criteria without BMD was similar (overall, 69.2%; men, 55.6%; woman, 70.6%; postmenopausal women, 71.1%, respectively). However, when applying the WHO osteoporosis criteria, more than 90% of patients were receiving osteoporosis treatments in all patient groups or subgroups (overall, 91.3%; men, 90%; woman, 91.3%; postmenopausal women, 91.3%).

Table 3. Current osteoporosis treatments in high-risk groups according to the FRAX criteria and the WHO osteoporosis criteria.

Patient Groups	FRAX with BMD	FRAX without BMD	WHO Osteoporosis
Overall	174/226 (77%)	202/292 (69.2%)	146/160 (91.3%)
Men	11/17 (64.7%)	15/27 (55.6%)	9/10 (90%)
Women	163/209 (78%)	187/265 (70.6%)	137/150 (91.3%)
Premenopausal	0/3 (0%)	0/2 (0%)	1/1 (100%)
Postmenopausal	163/206 (78.6%)	187/263 (71.1%)	136/149 (91.3%)

FRAX, fracture risk assessment tool; BMD, bone mineral density; WHO, World Health Organization.

3.4. Fracure Risk for the FRAX Criteria, the WHO Osteoporosis Criteria and Fractures

Table 4 shows which dichotomous factors were related to the FRAX criteria with BMD and without BMD, the WHO criteria, and incidence of fractures. Patients with high fracture risk by FRAX with BMD were more likely to be female, especially postmenopausal women (female, $p = 0.019$; menopause, $p < 0.001$), with alcohol use, glucocorticoid use, and proton pump inhibitor use ($p = 0.042$, $p = 0.007$, $p = 0.018$, and $p < 0.001$, respectively), and also with lower BMI (<25 kg/m^2) ($p = 0.042$). Patients with high fracture risk by FRAX without BMD had lower BMI and longer disease duration, and were more likely to be menopausal women, alcohol users, glucocorticoid users and proton pump users than patients who were not at high risk by FRAX without BMD ($p = 0.004$, $p = 0.007$, $p < 0.001$, $p = 0.005$, $p < 0.001$, and $p < 0.001$, respectively).

The results of frequency comparison for WHO osteoporosis criteria were similar to those for the FRAX criteria with BMD except for glucocorticoid use (female, $p = 0.017$; menopause, $p < 0.001$;

BMI < 25 kg/m^2, $p < 0.001$; alcohol use, $p = 0.002$; proton pump inhibitor use, $p = 0.008$). Biologic use, seropositivity, and ESR elevation did not show any significant difference for all the criteria.

The number of patients meeting the FRAX criteria with BMD was significantly higher in the higher dose with ≥5 mg/day prednisolone group in contrast to the lower dose with < 5mg/day prednisolone group (76/127; 59.8% vs. 136/307; 44.3%, $p = 0.003$).

Multiple linear analyses were implemented to identify factors affecting the FRAX criteria and BMD scores (Table 5). The 10-year probability percentage for hip fractures and that for major osteoporotic fractures in the FRAX with BMD, the 10-year probability percentage for major osteoporotic fractures in the FRAX without BMD, and total hip BMD scores, were significantly associated with glucocorticoid dose, age, female sex, BMI, and disease duration. However, the 10-year probability percentage for hip fractures in the FRAX without BMD was only associated with age and BMI.

Multivariable logistic regression analyses were performed to identify the fracture risk for the FRAX criteria and the WHO osteoporosis criteria, and fractures in patients with RA (Table 6). Glucocorticoid dose (odds ratio (OR) 1.15, 95% confidence interval (CI) 1.03–1.28, $p = 0.016$), age (OR 1.17, CI 1.13–1.2, $p < 0.001$), female sex (OR 4.22, CI 1.8–9.9, $p = 0.001$), and BMI (OR 0.92, CI 0.85–0.99, $p = 0.002$) were independent fracture risk for the FRAX criteria with BMD. Age (OR 1.65, CI 1.47–1.84, $p < 0.001$), female sex (OR 8.23, CI 2.27–29.88, $p = 0.001$), and BMI (OR 0.6, CI 0.5–0.72, $p < 0.001$) were associated with the FRAX criteria without BMD. Likewise, age (OR 1.1, CI 1.08–1.14, $p < 0.001$), female sex (OR 3.55, CI 1.46–8.63, $p = 0.005$), and BMI (OR 0.8, CI 0.75–0.87, $p < 0.001$) were associated fracture risk for the WHO criteria. Furthermore, independent risk factors for fracture are glucocorticoid dose (OR 1.09, 95% CI 1.01–1.17, $p = 0.02$), age (OR 1.09, 95% CI 1.06–1.12, $p < 0.001$) and disease duration (OR 1.01, 95% CI 1–1.01, $p = 0.002$).

Table 4. Comparison of the frequencies for the high-risk of osteoporotic fractures according to FRAX criteria and WHO osteoporosis criteria.

Variables	FRAX Criteria with BMD (%, *p* Value)	FRAX Criteria without BMD (%, *p* value)	WHO Criteria (%, *p* Value)	Fracture (%, *p* Value)
Sex (female)	48.6%, 0.019	62.2%, 0.077	35.2%, 0.017	17.6%, 0.457
Menopause	57.2%, <0.001	71.1%, <0.001	41.9%, <0.001	21%, <0.001
BMI < 25 kg/m^2	50%, 0.042	64.9%, 0.004	39%, <0.001	17.3%, 0.868
Disease duration > 2 years	48.9%, 0.098	63.7%, 0.007	35.1%, 0.081	18.6%, 0.063
Seropositivity	46.5%, 0.970	61.4%, 0.170	35.3%, 0.118	17.5%, 0.129
ESR elevation	52.5%, 0.052	65.4%, 0.100	37.4%, 0.196	16.9%, 0.950
Smoking	30.3%, 0.092	45.5%, 0.109	21.2%, 0.209	18.2%, 0.855
Alcohol use	24.4%, 0.007	36.6%, 0.005	9.8%, 0.002	10.3%, 0.239
Glucocorticoid use	49%, 0.018	63.8%, <0.001	33.9%, 0.532	17.3%, 0.81
Biologics use	46%, 0.785	60%, 0.378	40%, 0.137	20.8%, 0.574
PPI use	62.6%, <0.001	77.2%, <0.001	43.1%, 0.008	19%, 0.524

FRAX, fracture risk assessment tool; BMD, bone mineral density; WHO, World Health Organization; BMI, body mass index; ESR, erythrocyte sedimentation rate; PPI, proton pump inhibitor.

Table 5. Multiple linear risk analyses using the FRAX criteria and the WHO osteoporosis criteria.

	Variable	β	*p* Value	Adjusted R^2
FRAX with BMD % 10-year probability for hip fracture	Constant	−13.464		0.309
	Glucocorticoid dose	0.418	<0.001	
	Age	0.254	<0.001	
	Female	3.63	<0.001	
	BMI	−0.271	0.001	
	Smoking	2.912	0.012	
	Disease duration	0.01	0.114	
FRAX with BMD % 10-year probability for major osteoporotic fracture	Constant	−24.341		0.407
	Glucocorticoid dose	0.599	<0.001	
	Age	0.386	<0.001	
	Female	7.203	<0.001	
	BMI	−0.163	0.097	
	Smoking	2.289	0.109	
	Disease duration	0.025	0.001	
FRAX without BMD % 10-year probability for hip fracture	Constant	−8.455		0.326
	Glucocorticoid dose	0.179	0.219	
	Age	0.475	<0.001	
	Female	0.515	0.75	
	BMI	−0.641	<0.001	
	Smoking	−0.399	0.832	
	Disease duration	0.004	0.722	
FRAX without BMD % 10-year probability for major osteoporotic fracture	Constant	−26.833		0.630
	Glucocorticoid dose	0.36	<0.001	
	Age	0.547	<0.001	
	Female	7.863	<0.001	
	BMI	−0.411	<0.001	
	Smoking	1.85	0.122	
	Disease duration	0.025	<0.001	

Table 5. *Cont.*

	Variable	β	*p* Value	Adjusted R^2
BMD score mean L-spine	Constant	0.705		0.322
	Glucocorticoid dose	−0.037	0.054	
	Age	−0.055	<0.001	
	Female	−0.485	0.024	
	BMI	0.097	<0.001	
	Smoking	−0.102	0.638	
	Disease duration	0.004	0.001	
BMD score total hip	Constant	1.444		0.444
	Glucocorticoid dose	−0.054	0.001	
	Age	−0.047	<0.001	
	Female	−1.072	<0.001	
	BMI	0.111	<0.001	
	Smoking	0.018	0.926	
	Disease duration	−0.004	<0.001	

FRAX, fracture risk assessment tool; BMD, bone mineral density; WHO, World Health Organization; BMI, body mass index.

Table 6. Multivariable logistic regression analyses for high-risk of fracture of FRAX criteria and WHO osteoporosis criteria, and fractures in patients with rheumatoid arthritis.

	FRAX with BMD Criteria		FRAX without BMD Criteria		WHO Criteria		Fracture	
	OR (95% CI)	*p* Value	OR (95% CI)	*p* Value	OR (95% CI)	*p* Value	OR (95% CI)	*p* Value
Constant	0		0		0.09		0	
Glucocorticoid dose (mg)	1.15 (1.03, 1.28)	0.016	1.03 (0.94, 1.12)	0.537	1.05 (0.98, 1.14)	0.187	1.09 (1.01, 1.17)	0.02
Age (year)	1.17 (1.13, 1.2)	<0.001	1.65 (1.47, 1.84)	<0.001	1.1 (1.08, 1.13)	<0.001	1.09 (1.06, 1.12)	<0.001
Female	4.22 (1.8, 9.9)	0.001	8.23 (2.27, 29.88)	0.001	3.55 (1.46, 8.63)	0.005	1.81 (0.58, 4.01)	0.395
BMI (kg/m^2)	0.92 (0.85, 0.99)	0.02	0.6 (0.5, 0.72)	<0.001	0.8 (0.75, 0.87)	<0.001	1.02 (0.95, 1.11)	0.471
Disease duration (month)	1 (1, 1.01)	0.189	1.01 (1, 1.02)	0.121	1 (1, 1.01)	0.093	1.01 (1, 1.01)	0.002

FRAX, fracture risk assessment tool; BMD, bone mineral density; WHO, World Health Organization; OR, Odds Ratio; 95% CI, 95% confidence intervals; BMI, body mass index.

4. Discussion

In this study, we compared both the WHO and the FRAX criteria to estimate the risk of osteoporotic fractures and to determine candidates for pharmacological treatments. As a result, 33.4% of patients were eligible for the WHO osteoporosis criteria, 47.2% for the FRAX criteria with BMD, and 61% for the FRAX criteria without BMD, with statistically significant differences in each high-risk group for osteoporotic fractures (Table 2). When we performed subgroup analyses separated by men, women, and postmenopausal women, all except premenopausal women showed a similar tendency.

We found that there was a significant difference between the WHO criteria and the FRAX criteria with or without BMD, as well as between the FRAX criteria with BMD and those without BMD, which is different from the previous assertion that there is a high degree of agreement [12,18]. A significant difference in the number of high-risk groups for osteoporotic fractures according to the criteria applied is a serious problem, since both the FRAX and WHO criteria are widely used in clinical practice, and drugs used to prevent osteoporotic fractures have several side effects [11,12,14]. Therefore, it is very important to determine which of the three criteria should be used. To accomplish this, we had to determine the objective standard in order to evaluate all three criteria; however, it was not easy to set standards to which everyone could agree. Ultimately, the goal of osteoporosis treatment is to prevent fractures, so in order to select the best criteria, it may be advantageous to compare the incidences of actual fractures in each criterion. Unfortunately, our study was only a retrospective cross-sectional study, and patients with actual fracture histories were confined to compression fractures of the spine, thereby limiting the prevalence of actual fractures used to evaluate the best criteria.

Recently, a study comparing the FRAX without BMD and BMD alone was published [19]. In that study, the FRAX probability of a major osteoporotic fracture in 50-year-old women was approximately two-fold higher than that for women of the same age, but with an average BMD. The authors concluded that intervention thresholds based on BMD alone do not optimally target women at higher fracture risk than age-matched individuals without clinical risk factors [19]. However, the FRAX with BMD was not evaluated in that study, and there is no comparative study in RA patients. As shown in our study, the WHO criteria may have less actual risk reflected in high-risk disease such as RA [7]. Conversely, the FRAX value may be artificially elevated because RA itself is regarded as one of the major risk factors in FRAX calculations [12].

Table 3 shows that the number of patients actually receiving pharmacological treatments for osteoporosis (bisphosphonate or SERM) was only 69.2%–77% based on the FRAX with or without BMD. Interestingly, more than 90% of patients were receiving medication for osteoporosis when the WHO criteria were applied. This is probably due to the fact that insurance, covering the treatment of osteoporosis in Korea, is based on the WHO criteria.

Osteoporotic fracture, especially hip fracture, can increase mortality rate, so there are attempts to further expand the definition of osteoporosis. For example, while osteoporosis has traditionally been diagnosed based on *t*-score of less than -2.5, osteoporosis can be clinically diagnosed if there is a low-trauma fracture in the absence of other metabolic bone disease, independent of the BMD (*t*-score) value [14]. However, there is no clear evidence that the WHO criteria reflect osteoporotic fractures better than the FRAX criteria. Considering that the FRAX criteria are calculated with BMD values and various clinical aspects of osteoporosis patients, the importance of FRAX criteria in predicting the risk of osteoporotic fracture is increasingly emphasized [19,20], making the decision to treat osteoporosis merely on the basis of WHO osteoporosis criteria problematic. Furthermore, as shown in Table 2, the number of candidates for pharmacological intervention based on the WHO osteoporosis criteria is less than those based on the FRAX criteria; therefore, candidates in need of pharmacological treatment might be missed or their numbers underestimated when applying the WHO criteria. Alternately, we may also consider the new criteria suggested by the National Bone Health Alliance, that osteoporosis may be diagnosed in patients with osteopenia and increased fracture risk using FRAX country-specific thresholds [21]. This is a kind of compromise between FRAX criteria and WHO criteria. In our study, however, almost all patients who met the FRAX criteria had a BMD of -1.0 or less (FRAX criteria with

BMD, 95.6%; FRAX criteria without BMD, 90.8%). This result implies that applying the above criteria gives almost the same result as applying the FRAX criteria at least in patients with RA.

Therefore, further study is needed on how to apply the FRAX and WHO criteria in diagnosing and treating osteoporosis, or how to combine these two criteria. In addition, since FRAX criteria with BMD and without BMD may be different, as we have seen in our study, which of these tools is better must be clarified in the future research. Ultimately, osteoporosis treatment should aim for precision medicine. In order to do this, it is necessary to evaluate and approve the risk factors of individual patients. In particular, considering that there is a high risk of osteoporosis in RA patients and that the risk of osteoporotic fracture may be overestimated by FRAX tool in RA patients, more prospective studies involving large populations are required to clarify which assessment tool can precisely estimate osteoporotic fractures in patients with RA.

Nevertheless, it is clear that more than half of postmenopausal women with RA are included in the high-risk group for osteoporotic fractures. The numbers of the high-risk group for osteoporotic fractures in RA patients with postmenopausal woman were higher than those in total RA patients, regardless of which criteria were applied (WHO criteria, 40.3% vs. 33.4%; FRAX criteria with BMD, 55.7% vs. 47.2%; FRAX without BMD, 71.1% vs. 61%, respectively) (Table 2).

The independent risk factors for pharmacological treatments to prevent osteoporotic fractures were female sex, menopause, alcohol use, glucocorticoid use, and proton pump inhibitor use (Table 4). In multiple linear analyses, female sex, older age, lower BMI, longer disease duration, and glucocorticoid dose were associated with a higher probability of osteoporotic fractures (Table 5). In multivariable logistic regression analyses, the OR of female sex was 3.55 and those of age and BMI were 1.1 and 0.8, respectively for the WHO osteoporosis criteria (Table 6). These findings agreed with previous studies [11]. Although smoking has been known to be a major risk factor in many studies [11,22], it was not a statistically significance factor in our study, which was probably due to the fact that the majority of patients enrolled in our study were postmenopausal women with a smoking rate of only 6.9%. Our results showed that the use of biologics, seropositivity, and the levels of acute phase reactants were not associated with an increased risk of osteoporotic fractures. Regarding the use of glucocorticoids, the number of patients meeting the FRAX criteria with BMD was higher in the higher dose with ≥ 5 mg/day prednisolone group. The OR of prednisolone dose was 1.15 in the FRAX criteria with BMD and 1.09 for fractures. These results suggest that no use of glucocorticoid is important in RA patients for the prevention of osteoporotic fractures, and if used, glucocorticoid use should be at a dosage of <5 mg/day.

There are some limitations to this study. The first is that it was conducted not on *all* RA patients, but on RA patients who had a BMD. There may be many patients who had been tested for BMD, given that BMD is not a routine evaluation in RA patients, which could cause a selection bias in this study. The prevalence of the high-risk group of osteoporotic fractures in patients with RA was 33.4%–61.0% in this study, which was higher than the prevalence of osteoporosis in the general population of the United States and Korea [23,24]. However, these results may be overestimated considering selection bias. There are some studies dealing with the incidence and risk factors of osteoporotic fractures in patients with RA [25–27]. In a study conducted using the WHO criteria for RA postmenopausal patients, 46.8% of the patients were considered to have osteoporosis (t-score ≤ -2.5) [25]. However, in another study using the FRAX criteria for RA patients, in which the population of this study was similar to our study population, only 17.4% of the patients were reported to meet the FRAX criteria for pharmacological interventions [27]. Therefore, a large prospective study of all RA patients is needed to more accurately evaluate the prevalence of the high-risk group of osteoporotic fractures in patients with RA.

Another limitation is that only bisphosphonate and SERM were evaluated as treatments for osteoporosis. Recently, new drugs such as teriparatide and denosumab are being used to treat osteoporosis [11,28,29], but there is no data evaluating these drugs in this study. Nevertheless, this study has important implications, in that bisphosphonate and SERM are still widely used as primary drugs in the treatment of osteoporosis [11,14]. Another limitation is that 88.9% of patients enrolled in this study were female. The final limitation is that our study did not measure vitamin D levels. Lower levels of vitamin D, which are known in addition to regulating bone homeostasis, regulate the differentiation and activities of immune cells [30]. So, vitamin D deficiency can stimulate inflammatory status influencing disease status other than increasing bone erosion. Moreover, mutation and polymorphism in vitamin D metabolism genes are associated with serum 25(OH)D levels [30]. Therefore, these factors might have been associated with the results of our study.

5. Conclusions

The proportion of RA patients with a high risk of osteoporotic fractures was 33.4% for WHO criteria, 47.2% for FRAX criteria with BMD, and 61.0% for FRAX without BMD. Only 69.2%–77% of candidate patients were receiving osteoporotic treatments when applying the FRAX criteria, in contrast to 91.3% when applying the WHO criteria. Older age, higher doses of glucocorticoid, and longer disease duration were independent risk factors for osteoporotic fractures in patients with RA.

Author Contributions: Study design, S.T.C. and C.-H.S.; data collection, S.T.C., S.-R.K., J.-Y.J., H.-A.K., S.H.K., S.-S.K., J.-M.K. and C.-H.S.; statistical analysis, S.T.C., S.-R.K., and J.-H.P.; writing-original draft preparation, S.T.C.; writing-review and editing, S.-R.K. and C.-H.S. All authors approved the final version.

Acknowledgments: This research was supported by a grant from Basic Science Research Program through the National Research Foundation of Korea (NRF) funded by the Ministry of Education, Republic of Korea (2018R1D1A1B07049248) and a grant from the Korea Health Technology R&D Project through the Korea Health Industry Development Institute (KHIDI), funded by the Ministry of Health & Welfare, Republic of Korea (HI16C0992).

References

1. Kleyer, A.; Schett, G. Arthritis and bone loss: A hen and egg story. *Curr. Opin. Rheumatol.* **2014**, *26*, 80–84. [CrossRef] [PubMed]
2. Orstavik, R.E.; Haugeberg, G.; Mowinckel, P.; Hoiseth, A.; Uhlig, T.; Falch, J.A.; Halse, J.I.; McCloskey, E.; Kvien, T.K. Vertebral deformities in rheumatoid arthritis: A comparison with population-based controls. *Arch. Intern. Med.* **2004**, *164*, 420–425. [CrossRef] [PubMed]
3. Durward, G.; Non Pugh, C.; Ogunremi, L.; Wills, R.; Cottee, M.; Patel, S. Detection of risk of falling and hip fracture in women referred for bone densitometry. *Lancet* **1999**, *354*, 220–221. [CrossRef]
4. Haugeberg, G.; Uhlig, T.; Falch, J.A.; Halse, J.I.; Kvien, T.K. Bone mineral density and frequency of osteoporosis in female patients with rheumatoid arthritis: Results from 394 patients in the Oslo County Rheumatoid Arthritis register. *Arthritis Rheum.* **2000**, *43*, 522–530. [CrossRef]
5. Sinigaglia, L.; Nervetti, A.; Mela, Q.; Bianchi, G.; Del Puente, A.; Di Munno, O.; Frediani, B.; Cantatore, F.; Pellerito, R.; Bartolone, S.; et al. A multicenter cross sectional study on bone mineral density in rheumatoid arthritis. Italian Study Group on Bone Mass in Rheumatoid Arthritis. *J. Rheumatol.* **2000**, *27*, 2582–2589. [PubMed]
6. Guler-Yuksel, M.; Bijsterbosch, J.; Goekoop-Ruiterman, Y.P.; de Vries-Bouwstra, J.K.; Ronday, H.K.; Peeters, A.J.; de Jonge-Bok, J.M.; Breedveld, F.C.; Dijkmans, B.A.; Allaart, C.F.; et al. Bone mineral density in patients with recently diagnosed, active rheumatoid arthritis. *Ann. Rheum. Dis.* **2007**, *66*, 1508–1512. [CrossRef]
7. van Staa, T.P.; Geusens, P.; Bijlsma, J.W.; Leufkens, H.G.; Cooper, C. Clinical assessment of the long-term risk of fracture in patients with rheumatoid arthritis. *Arthritis Rheum.* **2006**, *54*, 3104–3112. [CrossRef]
8. Sattui, S.E.; Saag, K.G. Fracture mortality: Associations with epidemiology and osteoporosis treatment. *Nat. Rev. Endocrinol.* **2014**, *10*, 592–602. [CrossRef]
9. Abrahamsen, B.; van Staa, T.; Ariely, R.; Olson, M.; Cooper, C. Excess mortality following hip fracture: A systematic epidemiological review. *Osteoporos. Int.* **2009**, *20*, 1633–1650. [CrossRef]
10. Report of a WHO Study Group. Assessment of fracture risk and its application to screening for postmenopausal osteoporosis. *World Health Organ. Tech. Rep. Ser.* **1994**, *843*, 1–129.

11. Cosman, F.; de Beur, S.J.; LeBoff, M.S.; Lewiecki, E.M.; Tanner, B.; Randall, S.; Lindsay, R. Clinician's guide to prevention and treatment of osteoporosis. *Osteoporos. Int.* **2014**, *25*, 2359–2381. [CrossRef] [PubMed]
12. Kanis, J.A.; Johnell, O.; Oden, A.; Johansson, H.; McCloskey, E. FRAX and the assessment of fracture probability in men and women from the UK. *Osteoporos. Int.* **2008**, *19*, 385–397. [CrossRef] [PubMed]
13. World Health Organization. Fracture Risk Assessment Tool (FRAX). Available online: http://www.shef.ac.uk/FRAX (accessed on 5 December 2016).
14. Camacho, P.M.; Petak, S.M.; Binkley, N.; Clarke, B.L.; Harris, S.T.; Hurley, D.L.; Kleerekoper, M.; Lewiecki, E.M.; Miller, P.D.; Narula, H.S.; et al. American association of clinical endocrinologists and American college of endocrinology clinical practice guidelines for the diagnosis and treatment of postmenopausal osteoporosis—2016. *Endocr. Pract.* **2016**, *22*, 1–42. [CrossRef] [PubMed]
15. Arnett, F.C.; Edworthy, S.M.; Bloch, D.A.; McShane, D.J.; Fries, J.F.; Cooper, N.S.; Healey, L.A.; Kaplan, S.R.; Liang, M.H.; Luthra, H.S.; et al. The American Rheumatism Association 1987 revised criteria for the classification of rheumatoid arthritis. *Arthritis Rheum.* **1988**, *31*, 315–324. [CrossRef] [PubMed]
16. Aletaha, D.; Neogi, T.; Silman, A.J.; Funovits, J.; Felson, D.T.; Bingham, C.O., 3rd; Birnbaum, N.S.; Burmester, G.R.; Bykerk, V.P.; Cohen, M.D.; Combe, B.; et al. 2010 rheumatoid arthritis classification criteria: An American college of rheumatology/european league against rheumatism collaborative initiative. *Ann. Rheum. Dis.* **2010**, *69*, 1580–1588. [CrossRef] [PubMed]
17. Korean Statistical Information Service. Available online: http://kosis.kr/eng/ (accessed on 14 November 2018).
18. Gadam, R.K.; Schlauch, K.; Izuora, K.E. Frax prediction without BMD for assessment of osteoporotic fracture risk. *Endocr. Pract.* **2013**, *19*, 780–784. [CrossRef] [PubMed]
19. Johansson, H.; Azizieh, F.; Al Ali, N.; Alessa, T.; Harvey, N.C.; McCloskey, E.; Kanis, J.A. FRAX- vs. T-score-based intervention thresholds for osteoporosis. *Osteoporos. Int.* **2017**, *28*, 3099–3105. [CrossRef]
20. Kanis, J.A.; Harvey, N.C.; Cooper, C.; Johansson, H.; Oden, A.; McCloskey, E.V. A systematic review of intervention thresholds based on FRAX: A report prepared for the National Osteoporosis Guideline Group and the International Osteoporosis Foundation. *Arch. Osteoporos.* **2016**, *11*, 25. [CrossRef]
21. Siris, E.S.; Adler, R.; Bilezikian, J.; Bolognese, M.; Dawson-Hughes, B.; Favus, M.J.; Harris, S.T.; Jan de Beur, S.M.; Khosla, S.; Lane, N.E.; et al. The clinical diagnosis of osteoporosis: A position statement from the National Bone Health Alliance Working Group. *Osteoporos. Int.* **2014**, *25*, 1439–1443. [CrossRef]
22. Yoon, V.; Maalouf, N.M.; Sakhaee, K. The effects of smoking on bone metabolism. *Osteoporos. Int.* **2012**, *23*, 2081–2092. [CrossRef]
23. Looker, A.C.; Melton, L.J., 3rd; Harris, T.B.; Borrud, L.G.; Shepherd, J.A. Prevalence and trends in low femur bone density among older US adults: NHANES 2005–2006 compared with NHANES III. *J. Bone Miner. Res.* **2010**, *25*, 64–71. [CrossRef] [PubMed]
24. Ha, Y. Epidemiology of osteoporosis in Korea. *J. Korean Med. Assoc.* **2016**, *59*, 836–841. [CrossRef]
25. Lee, J.H.; Sung, Y.K.; Choi, C.B.; Cho, S.K.; Bang, S.Y.; Choe, J.Y.; Hong, S.J.; Jun, J.B.; Kim, T.H.; Lee, J.; et al. The frequency of and risk factors for osteoporosis in Korean patients with rheumatoid arthritis. *BMC Musculoskelet. Disord.* **2016**, *17*, 98. [CrossRef] [PubMed]
26. Kim, D.; Cho, S.K.; Choi, C.B.; Jun, J.B.; Kim, T.H.; Lee, H.S.; Lee, J.; Lee, S.S.; Yoo, D.H.; Yoo, W.H.; et al. Incidence and risk factors of fractures in patients with rheumatoid arthritis: An Asian prospective cohort study. *Rheumatol. Int.* **2016**, *36*, 1205–1214. [CrossRef] [PubMed]
27. Lee, J.H.; Suh, Y.S.; Koh, J.H.; Jung, S.M.; Lee, J.J.; Kwok, S.K.; Ju, J.H.; Park, K.S.; Park, S.H. The risk of osteoporotic fractures according to the FRAX model in Korean patients with rheumatoid arthritis. *J. Korean Med. Sci.* **2014**, *29*, 1082–1089. [CrossRef] [PubMed]
28. Neer, R.M.; Arnaud, C.D.; Zanchetta, J.R.; Prince, R.; Gaich, G.A.; Reginster, J.Y.; Hodsman, A.B.; Eriksen, E.F.; Ish-Shalom, S.; Genant, H.K.; et al. Effect of parathyroid hormone (1–34) on fractures and bone mineral density in postmenopausal women with osteoporosis. *N. Engl. J. Med.* **2001**, *344*, 1434–1441. [CrossRef] [PubMed]

29. Cummings, S.R.; San Martin, J.; McClung, M.R.; Siris, E.S.; Eastell, R.; Reid, I.R.; Delmas, P.; Zoog, H.B.; Austin, M.; Wang, A.; et al. Denosumab for prevention of fractures in postmenopausal women with osteoporosis. *N. Engl. J. Med.* **2009**, *361*, 756–765. [CrossRef]
30. Bellavia, D.; Costa, V.; De Luca, A.; Maglio, M.; Pagani, S.; Fini, M.; Giavaresi, G. Vitamin D Level Between Calcium-Phosphorus Homeostasis and Immune System: New Perspective in Osteoporosis. *Curr. Osteoporos. Rep.* **2016**. [CrossRef]

10

Methotrexate Restores CD73 Expression on Th1.17 in Rheumatoid Arthritis and Psoriatic Arthritis Patients and may Contribute to its Anti-Inflammatory Effect through Ado Production

Marion Bossennec [1,2], Céline Rodriguez [1,2], Margaux Hubert [1,2], Anthony Di-Roio [1,2], Christelle Machon [3,4], Jérôme Guitton [4,5], Priscilla Battiston-Montagne [1,6], Mathilde Couturier [7], Hubert Marotte [8,9], Christophe Caux [1,2], Fabienne Coury [7,10,†] and Christine Ménétrier-Caux [1,2,*,†]

1. Immunology Department, University of Lyon, Claude Bernard Lyon 1 University, INSERM 1052, CNRS 5286, Cancer Research Center of Lyon (CRCL), Centre Léon Bérard, 69008 Lyon, France; marion.bossennec@gmail.com (M.B.); celine.rodriguez@lyon.unicancer.fr (C.R.); margaux.hubert@lyon.unicancer.fr (M.H.); anthony.diroio@lyon.unicancer.fr (A.D.-R.); priscillia.battiston-montagne@lyon.unicancer.fr (P.B.-M.); christophe.caux@lyon.unicancer.fr (C.C.)
2. Team "Therapeutic Targeting of the Tumor Cells and Their Immune Stroma", INSERM U1052, CRCL, 69008 Lyon, France
3. Analytical Chemistry Department, ISPB Faculty of Pharmacy, University of Lyon, Claude Bernard Lyon 1 University, 69008 Lyon, France; christelle.machon@chu-lyon.fr
4. Biochemistry and Toxicology Laboratory, Lyon Sud Hospital, 69310 Pierre-Bénite, France; jerome.guitton@univ-lyon1.fr
5. Toxicology Department, ISPB Faculty of Pharmacy, University of Lyon, Claude Bernard Lyon 1 University, 69008 Lyon, France
6. Cytometry Platform, CRCL, 69008 Lyon, France
7. Rheumatology Department, Lyon Sud Hospital, 69310 Pierre-Bénite, France; docteurcouturierrhumato@gmail.com (M.C.); fabienne.coury-lucas@chu-lyon.fr (F.C.)
8. Rheumatology Department, CHU Saint-Etienne, 42100 Saint-Etienne, France; hubert.marotte@chu-st-etienne.fr
9. INSERM U1059, Jean Monnet University, 42100 Saint-Etienne, France
10. INSERM, UMR 1033, Claude Bernard Lyon 1 University, 69008 Lyon, France

* Correspondence: christine.caux@lyon.unicancer.fr

† Co-last authorship.

Abstract: Objectives: Th1.17 are highly polyfunctional, potentially harmful $CD4^+$ effector T cells (Teff) through IFN-γ and IL-17A coproduction. Th1.17 take part in the pathophysiology of rheumatoid arthritis (RA) and psoriatic arthritis (PsA), in which their hyper activation results in part from defects in negative regulation mechanisms. We recently demonstrated that the ecto-nucleotidase CD73 delineates a Th1.17-enriched Teff population and acts as an endogenous regulatory mechanism. Because Methotrexate (MTX), used as first line treatment of RA and PsA, increases extracellular concentrations of AMP and immunosuppressive adenosine, we investigated the modulation of CD73 by MTX treatment on Teff in RA/PsA patients. Methods: In a prospective cohort of 26 RA and 15 PsA patients before or under MTX treatment, we evaluated CD73 expression on blood Teff subsets, their cytokine production and AMPase functions. Results: We showed a decreased CD73 expression on Th1.17 and Th1 in untreated patients compared to healthy donors that was partly restored under MTX. This decrease in untreated patients leads to a halved Ado production by Th1.17 cells. $CD73^+$ Teff remained functional under MTX treatment, but their CD73 re-expression may contribute to control their activation. Conclusion: Our study unveils uncovered mode of action of MTX on Teff subsets modulation and in the adenosine-dependent termination of inflammation in RA and PsA.

Keywords: Th1.17; IL-17A; IFN-γ, CD73; adenosine; rheumatoid arthritis; psoriatic arthritis; methotrexate; regulation

1. Introduction

Rheumatoid Arthritis (RA) and Psoriatic Arthritis (PsA) are chronic inflammatory disorders characterized by tenderness and swelling of the joints. If not treated, both can lead to bone erosion, resulting in joint destruction due to osteoclasts activation. RA is an autoimmune systemic disease characterized by the presence of anti-citrullinated protein antibodies (ACPA) and rheumatoid factor (RF) [1]. PsA is usually associated with the skin condition psoriasis (Pso) [2]. In both cases, study of the immune infiltrate of inflamed joints has shed light on particularly deleterious memory $CD4^+$ T helper lymphocytes (Th): Th17 and Th1.17 [3–5]. These cells, found enriched at the inflamed site, secrete high amounts of the pro-inflammatory cytokine IL-17A, responsible for many features of both RA and PsA. IL-17A indeed contributes to the recruitment of pro-inflammatory monocytes and neutrophils at the site of inflammation, and promotes the transformation of the fibroblast-like synoviocytes present in the synovial lining toward a pro-inflammatory phenotype [6–8]. In the presence of IL-17A, these cells secrete IL-6 and TNF [9] and high levels of RANKL, which in turn stimulate osteoclast differentiation [10]. Therefore, IL-17A is implicated in the positive feedback loop at the roots of the chronic inflammation and bone destruction observed in joints. Moreover, in RA and PsA, T cells display reduced sensitivity to the diverse immune suppressive functions exerted by regulatory T cells (Treg) [11]. Treg are involved in the modulation of extracellular purine derivatives levels, through their membrane expression of the ecto-enzyme CD39, which degrades pro-inflammatory extracellular ATP into AMP. AMP can, in turn, be degraded into immunosuppressive adenosine (Ado) by the ecto-nucleotidase CD73. We recently demonstrated that in human, Treg express CD39, but no CD73; therefore, third-party CD73 expressing cells are required for the degradation of AMP into Ado [12]. CD73 is in particular expressed by a fraction of non-regulatory $CD4^+$ memory T cells (Teff) strongly enriched in Th1.17 and Th17 [12]. We showed that CD73 expression by Teff renders them selectively sensitive to Ado through their cooperation with $CD39^+$ Treg for extracellular ATP degradation. In the context of chronic inflammation, modulation of expression of these ecto-enzymes on Teff, and thus of Ado production, may regulate T cell activation.

RA and PsA treatment options are mainly composed of an arsenal of disease modifying anti rheumatic drugs (DMARDs), among which Methotrexate (MTX) is still largely used due to its efficiency, low toxicity and cost effectiveness [13,14]. Its mode of action at low doses (5–20 mg/week) for RA and PsA treatment remains incompletely understood. Apart from its role as anti-folate agent, other mechanisms have been proposed to explain clinical improvement upon MTX treatment (reviewed in [13]). Robust evidence suggests that MTX acts through the potentiation of Ado signaling. Indeed, MTX inhibits the 5-Aminoimidazole-4-carboxamide ribonucleotide (AICAR) transformylase enzyme (ATIC) [13–15] resulting in increase in both intracellular AICAR levels and extracellular AMP and Ado release. However, the majority of extracellular Ado is in fact generated from extracellular transport of ATP and AMP degraded by CD39/CD73 that are required for MTX-induced immune suppression in mouse models [16]. Extracellular Ado inhibits T cell activation and proliferation in a paracrine manner, through the engagement of its A2A and A2B receptors which expression is upregulated on activated Teff [12,17,18], and through the amplification of Treg expressing A2AR [19].

In this study, we evaluated the presence and distribution of $CD73^+$ Teff among Th populations in the blood of untreated RA and PsA patients. We also assessed the functionality of these cells in patients in comparison to healthy donors' blood. We demonstrated that loss of CD73 membrane expression in untreated patients resulted in a lowered Ado production, potentially contributing to impaired control of the inflammation. Under MTX treatment, CD73 was partially recovered on Teff, which was associated with a restored capacity to degrade AMP into Ado.

Therefore, CD73 expression level on Teff may represent a therapeutic target worth considering in the treatment of RA by restoring and stabilizing it through an immunosuppressive feedback loop enabling Ado production.

2. Experimental Section

2.1. Patients

Patients aged ≥ 18 years, naive of biologics, with RA fulfilling the American College of Rheumatology and European League Against Rheumatism 2009 criteria [20] or with PsA fulfilling the Classification of PsA (CASPAR) criteria [21] were enrolled in the LADORIC study (NCT03953378) after written informed consent, in accordance with the Declaration of Helsinki. The approval of the ethics committee was not required in accordance with our institution's policy. Clinical and biological information was collected prospectively (Table 1).

Table 1. Characteristics of RA and PsA patients enrolled in the study.

	RA Patients $n = 26$	**PsA Patients** $n = 15$	**Healthy Controls** $n = 12$
Gender ratio (f/m, n)	19/7	9/6	8/4
Age (years)	56 (22–82)	53 (31–79)	49 (25–69)
DAS28 Untreated MTX-treated	4.6 (1.6–6.4) 3.4 (1.8–7.2)	-	
CRP (mg/mL) Untreated MTX-treated	17.9 (0.6–60) 5.2 (0.5–29)	16.4 (2.6–88) 4.3 (1.3–10)	
Mean MTX treatment duration (months)	9.3 (3–22)	6 (3–22)	-
MTX doses (mg/week)	(15–20)	(15–20)	-
RF detection (yes/no, n)	22/4	Not detected	-
ACPA detection (yes/no, n)	24/2	Not detected	-

Data presented as (range). RA. Rheumatoid Arthritis; PsA: Psoriatic Arthritis; DAS28: 28 joints activity score; RF: Rheumatoid Factor; ACPA: antibodies against cyclic citrullinated peptides. Two RA patients under MTX treatment also received cortancyl (7.5 mg).

Severity of the disease was assessed using the Disease Activity Score in 28 joints (DAS28-CRP) [22] for RA and CRP for PsA at baseline visit and 3 or 6 months after MTX treatment onset. DAS28-CRP ≥ 3.2 in untreated RA patients and CRP ≥ 6 mg/mL in untreated PsA patients were set as thresholds for active disease. Samples of venous blood and, when available, synovial fluid (SF) were collected for each patient before the onset of MTX (untreated patients) or during the course of MTX treatment (MTX-treated patients). Blood samples from age- and sex-matched anonymous healthy donors (HD) were obtained from the Etablissement Français du Sang.

2.2. Peripheral Blood Mononuclear Cells (PBMC) and Synovial Fluid Mononuclear Cells (SFMC) Isolation

Blood samples were centrifuged on a Ficoll (Eurobio, Les Ullis, France) density gradient to purify PBMC. SF samples were diluted in HBSS (Life Technologies, Cailloux sur Fontaines, France) containing 10 mM EDTA (Sigma, Saint Quentin-Fallavier, France), and processed as blood samples to isolate SFMC.

2.3. Flow Cytometry Analyses

Multi-parametric Flow Cytometry (FC) staining were performed on PBMC or SFMC from RA and PsA patients using different panels described in Table S1 (Panels A and B) to assess CD73 expression on total memory T cells and within Th subsets. When specified, proliferation was assessed using an anti-human anti-Ki67 antibody (Ki-67, Biolegend, Saint-Cyr-l'Ecole, CA, France). For FoxP3 intracellular staining to characterize Treg, cells were treated using the FoxP3 Fixation and Permeabilization kit (Life Technologies), according to manufacturer instructions. Samples were analyzed on a LSR-Fortessa (BD Biosciences, Pont de Claix, France) with conserved settings throughout the entire study. Data were analyzed using FlowJo Software (Tree Star v10.4, Franklin Lakes, NJ, USA).

2.4. Analysis of Cytokines Production Capacity after Reactivation

PBMC were activated with PMA and Ionomycin (Sigma-Aldrich) as previously described [12] and intracellular cytokines (IL-17A, TNF-α, IFN-γ, IL-22) produced by $CD73^{+}$ and $CD73^{neg}$ Teff were analyzed using the specific panel described in Table S1 (Panel C). Stainings were analyzed on a LSR-Fortessa and Teff polyfunctionality was evaluated using the Boolean method (FlowJo software) and then processed using Pestle and SPICE v5.3 softwares, National Institute of Allergy and Infectious Diseases, Bethesda, MD, USA.

2.5. $CD73^{+}$ Teff Sorting and In Vitro Activation to Asses CD73 Dynamic Expression

Memory $CD4^{+}$ T cells were purified from HD PBMCs using MagniSortTM Human $CD4^{+}$ Memory T Cell Enrichment Kit (LifeTechnologies). $CD73^{+}CD4^{+}$ Teff ($CD4^{+}CD45RA^{neg}CD127^{+}CD25^{neg}CD39^{neg}$ $CD73^{+}$) and $CD73^{neg}CD4^{+}$ Teff ($CD4^{+}CD45RA^{neg}CD127^{+}CD25^{neg}$ $CD39^{neg}CD73^{neg}$) were sorted from purified memory $CD4^{+}$ T cells by multi-parametric FC (FACSAria III, BD Biosciences) using antibodies against CD25 (2A3, BD-Biosciences), CD45RA (2H4LDH11LDB9, Beckman-Coulter, Brea, CA, USA), as well as CD127 (eBioRDR5), CD39 (eBioA1) and CD73 (AD2) (all from e-Bioscience), alongside a viability marker (DAPI).

Sorted populations were stained with CellTrace Violet (CTV) (20 μM, LifeTechnologies) proliferation markers before incubation with Expand beads (LifeTechnologies) (ratio 1:4) in 96-round-bottomed-well plates in 200 μL of complete RPMI medium for 4 days at 37 °C under 5% CO_2.

After 4 days' proliferation, part of the cells was stained for viability and CD73 expression with anti-human anti-CD73 and cells were fixed with 2% Formaldehyde solution (Sigma) and stored at 4 °C. The rest of the cells were washed and removed from Expand beads using a magnet. They were then incubated for a 2-day period without TCR signal in 200 μL of complete RPMI medium containing IL-2 (50 UI, Chiron). Cells were then stained for viability and CD73 expression as well. All time points were analyzed concomitantly by FC for viability, proliferation and CD73 expression (LSR Fortessa, BD Biosciences).

2.6. Th1.17, Th1 and Th17 Sorting for In Vitro AMP Degradation Assay

Memory $CD4^{+}$ Teffs were purified using MojoSort Human $CD4^{+}$ Memory T Cell Isolation Kit (Biolegend). Th1, Th17 and Th1.17 cells were sorted from purified memory $CD4^{+}$ T cells by multi-parametric FC (FACSAria III, BD Biosciences) based on chemokine receptors expression [23] (Figure S1) using the combination of antibodies described in Table S1 (Panel D).

The capacity of 5×10^4 cells of each Th subpopulation of HD, RA untreated or MTX-treated patients to degrade AMP was analyzed after 2 h incubation at 37 °C under 5% CO_2 with labeled AMP ($AMP_{13C,15N}$, 37.5 μM, Sigma-Aldrich) in 200 μL of serum-free RPMI medium supplemented with antibiotics and L-glutamine (Life Technologies). As a control, cells were pre-incubated with a CD73 chemical inhibitor (APCP, 50 μM, Sigma) for 30 min before adding $AMP_{13C,15N}$ to assess CD73-specific degradation.

2.7. Nucleotides and Nucleosides Quantification by Liquid Chromatography Coupled with Tandem Mass Spectrometry (LC-MS/MS)

Cell supernatants were harvested, boiled at 65 °C for 5 s and frozen at −20 °C. $AMP_{13C,15N}$ and $Ado_{13C,15N}$ were quantified in 50 µL of supernatant, after solid phase extraction, using a LC-MS/MS method as described [12,24]. Concentrations of nucleotides in the supernatants were calculated using calibration curves of the corresponding labeled nucleotides (AMP_{15N} and Ado_{13C}). AMP_{13C} and Ado_{15N} were used as internal standards. We also verified that APCP did not interfere with AMP and Ado quantification.

2.8. Statistical Analysis

Data formatting and statistical tests were performed using Prism software (Graphpad Inc., San Diego, CA, USA). Kruskal-Wallis test, Mann-Whitney test and ANOVA2 were used when comparing unpaired data according to the parameters considered. Wilcoxon test and ANOVA2 with paired values were performed to analyze patients' data follow up. We evaluated correlation between biological parameters and activity of the disease (DAS28-CRP) using Spearman correlation tests.

3. Results

3.1. Activated Th1.17 from Peripheral Blood of Untreated RA and PsA Patients Express Low Levels of CD73

Total memory $CD4^+$ and $CD8^+$ T cells frequencies were not modified in peripheral blood of untreated RA and PsA patients compared to HD (Figure S2A), neither were frequencies of Th subpopulations based on their CCR6 and CXCR3 expression [23] (Figure 1A). Treg frequency was unaltered in untreated RA and PsA patients' blood (Figure 1B). However, in RA patients, Treg displayed a higher frequency of CD39 expression compared to HD and PsA patients, although the mean fluorescence intensity (MFI) of CD39 was not different (Figure 1C). Interestingly, we found a significantly lower CD73 expression on total Teff population from RA and PsA patients compared to HD (Figure 1D). Since we established that, in HD, CD73 is enriched in Th1.17 and Th17 phenotype [12], we stratified our analysis on Th subpopulations based on CXCR3 and CCR6 expression that allows to distinguish Th subsets with different cytokine pattern (Figure S1). CD73 expression was significantly decreased on Th1.17 (by 1.5 and 1.4 fold on RA and PsA patients respectively) and Th1 (by 1.9 fold on both RA and PsA patients) (Figure 1E).

Using CD39 [25,26], we demonstrated a significantly increased activation of blood-associated Th1.17 and Th17 in RA and PsA patients compared to HD ones (Figure 1F). In parallel, we observed that in vitro TCR stimulation was sufficient to decrease CD73 expression in sorted $CD73^+$ Teff from HD (Figure S2B). Taken together, these results indicate that loss of CD73 expression on Th1.17 associated to high CD39 expression in untreated RA and PsA patients' blood could reflect the activated state of this population. The access to paired samples of PBMC and SFMC for RA and PsA patients before treatment enabled us to show that the decrease of CD73 expression and CD39 up-regulation on total Teff was even more dramatic at the site of inflammation both in RA (Figure 1G) and in PsA (Figure S2C). In addition, proliferating cells (identified as $Ki67^+$ cells) were included within $CD39^+CD73^{neg}$ Teff in RA (Figure 1H and Figure S2E) and PsA (Figure S2D,F) SF, further highlighting the absence of CD73 expression by proliferating Teff.

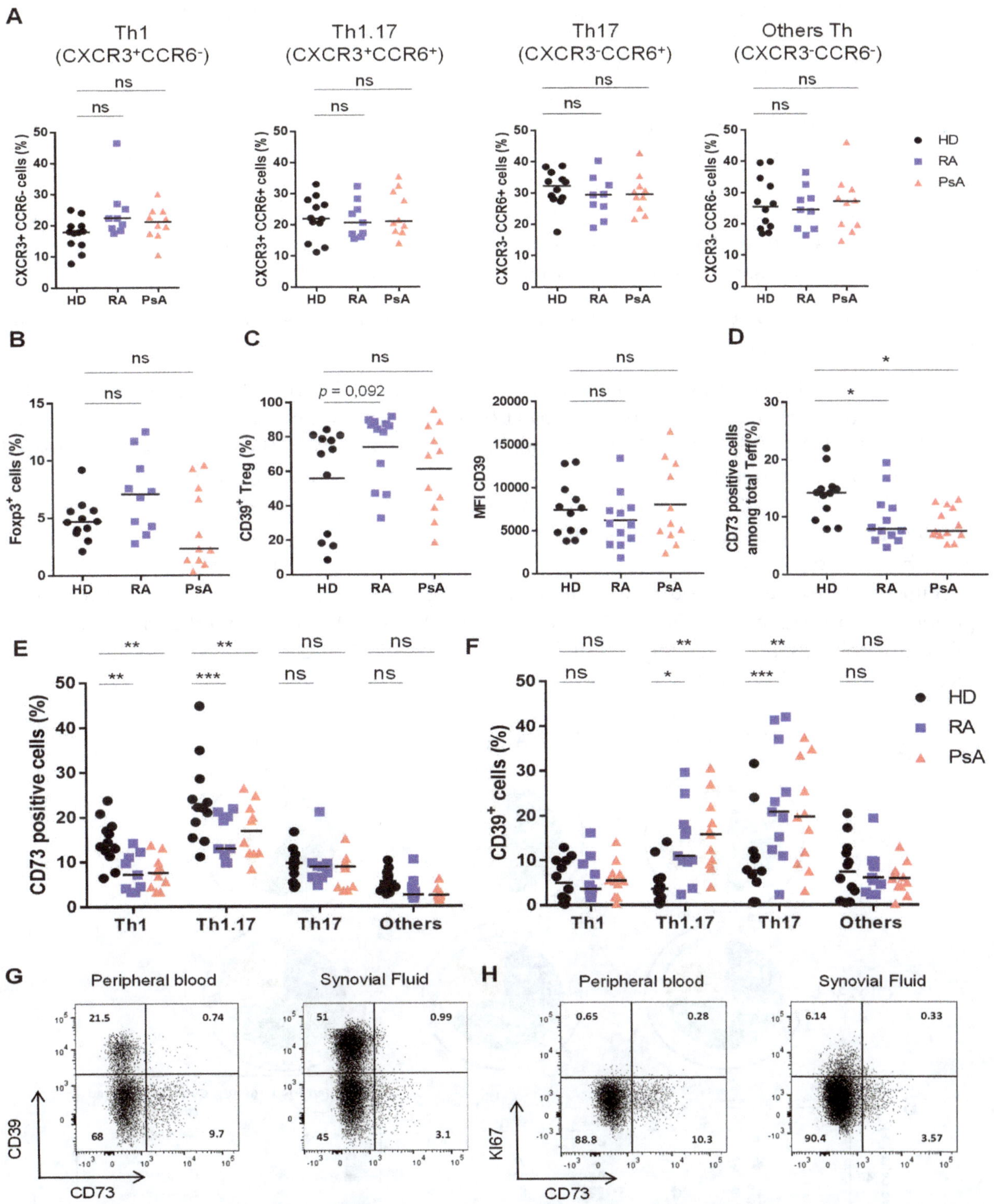

Figure 1. Unchanged Th populations but impaired CD73 expression on Th1 and Th1.17 from RA and PsA patients. (**A**). Th subsets frequencies based on phenotypic analysis (CXCR3/CCR6 staining) among memory CD4+ T cells. (**B**). Frequencies of FoxP3+ Treg among memory CD4+ T cells. (**C**). Frequencies (left) and MFI (right) of CD39+ Treg among memory CD4+ T cells. (**D**). CD73 expression on total Teff. (**E**). CD73 expression by Th subsets. (**F**). CD39 expression by Th subsets. (from A to F: analyses performed on peripheral blood). (**G**,**H**). Flow cytometry plots on total Teff in peripheral blood and SF of an untreated RA patient showing CD73/CD39 (**G**) and CD73/Ki67 (**H**) staining. (**A**–**D**): Kruskal-Wallis test, (**E**,**F**): ANOVA-2. * $p < 0.05$, ** $p < 0.001$, *** $p < 0.0001$.

In untreated RA patients, percentage of CD39$^+$ Treg positively correlated ($r = 0.68$, $p = 0.03$) with the severity of the disease evaluated through DAS28-CRP score. In contrast, no correlation was noticed for CD39 percentage on Th1, Th1.17 and Th17 subsets (not shown). No correlation with the severity of the disease was noticed for global CD73 expression on Teff nor global Th1, Th1.17 and Th17 proportions in blood. Moreover, the proportion of CD73 expressed by Th1 and Th1.17 populations did not correlate with disease severity despite they were strongly reduced in untreated RA patients compared to HD. In contrast expression of CD73 on Th17 and IL-17A production by CD73$^+$ Teff tend to inversely correlate with disease severity ($r = -0.65$, $p = 0.06$ and $r = -0.63$, $p = 0.07$, respectively) (Figure S3). For PsA untreated patients no correlation was observed probably because either the heterogeneity of the disease or too small cohort size to achieve robust correlations.

3.2. Untreated RA and PsA Patients' Blood Teff are Polyfunctional but Express Lower Levels of CD73 among IFN-γ/IL-17A Expressing Cells

We previously showed that CD73 marks polyfunctional Teff in blood but also in healthy (tonsil, colon) and tumor (breast and ovarian) tissues [12]. In our setting, no striking modifications of the polyfunctionality (IFN-γ, IL-17A, and TNF-α) of CD73$^+$ and CD73^{neg} Teff was noticed in untreated RA and PsA patients compared to HD (Figure 2A) and global levels of each cytokine were unchanged (Figure S4A). Of note, CD73$^+$ Teff, which were higher single IL-22 producers in HD [12] were an even more important source of IL-22 in PsA (9.1 ± 2.6% versus 4.2 ± 1.3% of CD73$^+$ Teff) (Figure S4B). In line with phenotypic analyses (Figure 1E), the IFN-γ/IL-17A coproducing cells, corresponding to Th1.17 (Figure S1), expressed significantly less CD73 (Figure 2B). Finally, Teff from untreated RA and PsA patients according to their DAS28-CRP or CRP level, respectively, showed enhanced IFN-γ and IL-17A production by CD73$^+$ Teff in patients with active RA (DAS28-CRP ≥ 3.2), although not reaching statistical significance (Figure 2C).

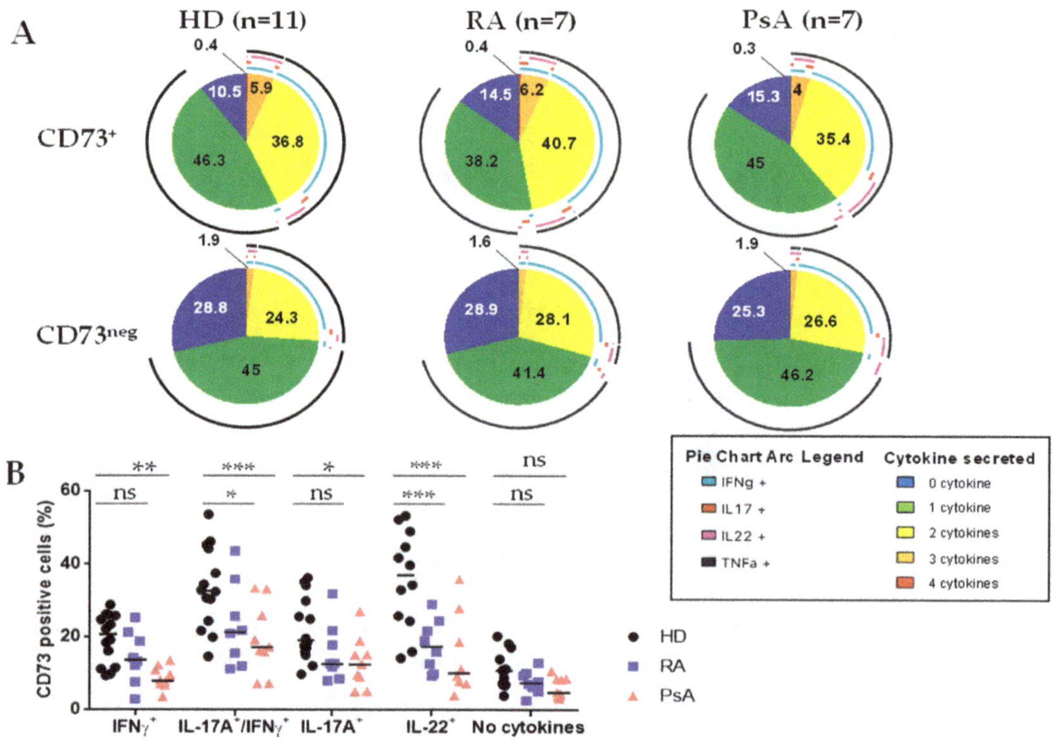

Figure 2. *Cont.*

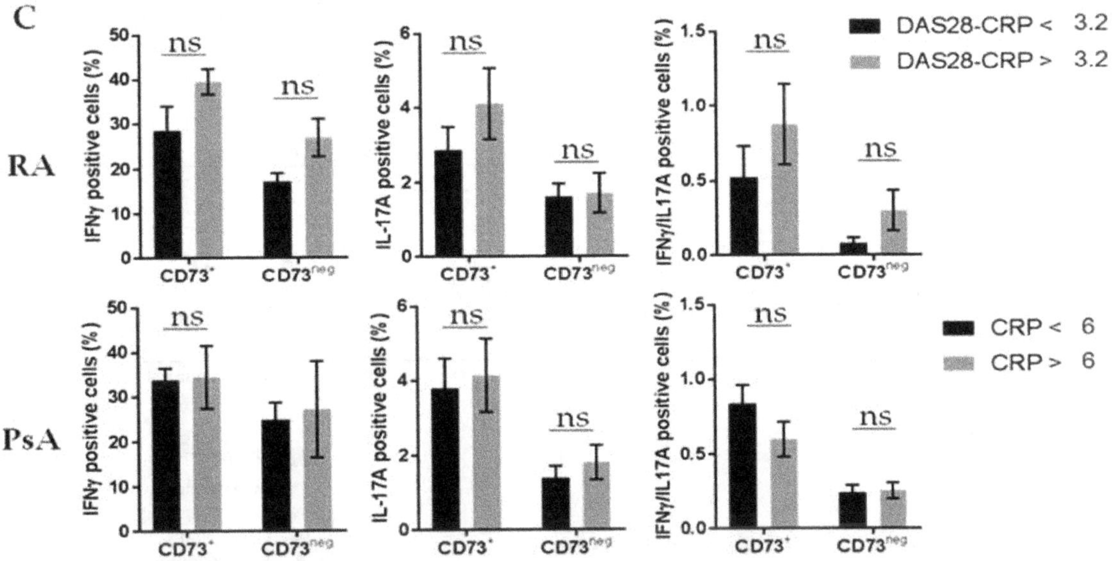

Figure 2. Polyfunctionality of Teff is not altered in RA and PsA patients but there are less CD73^{+} cells identified in IL-17A/IFN-γ secreting Teff. (**A**): SPICE® representation of the cytokines secreted by either CD73^{+} or CD73^{neg} Teff from peripheral blood of HD, or untreated RA and PsA patients. (**B**): CD73 expression on Teff according to their secretion of IFN-γ, IL-17A and IL-22 in peripheral blood of HD or untreated RA and PsA patients. (**C**): IFN-γ and IL-17A mono- or co-production by Teff according to their CD73 expression in untreated RA and PsA patients stratified on DAS28-CRP score and CRP seric level respectively. (**B**,**C**): ANOVA-2. * $p < 0.05$, ** $p < 0.001$, *** $p < 0.0001$.

3.3. Treatment of Patients with MTX Partially Restores CD73 Expression on Teff Resulting in an Enhanced Ado Production

Due to the described MTX involvement in the regulation of purine metabolism [13,26], we also analyzed the impact of MTX treatment on CD73 expression by Th subpopulations. We recently demonstrated that exogenously added Ado on CD73^{+} Teff blocked their proliferation and cytokine secretion [12]. Here, we evidenced that CD73^{+} Teff re-acquired CD73 expression after two days in resting condition (no TCR signaling), demonstrating dynamic CD73 protein expression at the surface of Teff (Figure S2B). In this context, we analyzed CD73 expression on Th subsets in MTX-treated RA and PsA patients, considering that a gain of CD73 expression could reflect drug efficiency on these populations and could contribute to its anti-inflammatory effects. MTX did not impact Th subsets frequencies compared to untreated RA and PsA patients (Figure 3A). However, CD73 expression on Teff was increased in MTX-treated RA patients compared to untreated ones while no significant variation was observed in PsA patients (Figure 3B). Interestingly, in RA patients, CD73 expression was especially increased within Th1.17 (Figure 3C) and overall CD73 expression level tended towards those observed in HD. Finally, the analysis of paired patients' blood samples (for, respectively, four and seven patients for RA and PsA) before and under MTX treatment showed significantly increased CD73 levels on Th1 and Th1.17 subsets (Figure 3D), the two populations with significantly altered CD73 expression in untreated patients compared to HD (Figure 1E). This impact of MTX was restricted to CD4^{+}CD73^{+} Teff, as we did not notice striking variations in memory CD8^{+} T cell frequencies (Figure S5A) or in Treg or CD39^{+} Treg frequencies (Figure S5B,C) even in paired samples (Figure S5D–F). Of note, CD39 levels did not seem to be modulated by MTX treatment on Teff either (Figure S5G,H).

Among HD donors' Th subsets, Th1.17 was the main subset able to degrade AMP into Ado (Figure S6), in line with its strongest expression of CD73 (Figure 1E). This generation of Ado was dependent on CD73, as demonstrated by the loss of Ado in the presence of APCP (Figure S6). In comparison the quantities of Ado generated was four-fold lower for the Th1 subset. Interestingly, we evidenced that reduced CD73 expression on Th1.17 and Th1 of untreated RA patients was associated with 50% decrease in Ado production (Figure 3E). Strikingly, upon MTX treatment, the level of Ado production was restored to HD donor levels (Figure 3E).

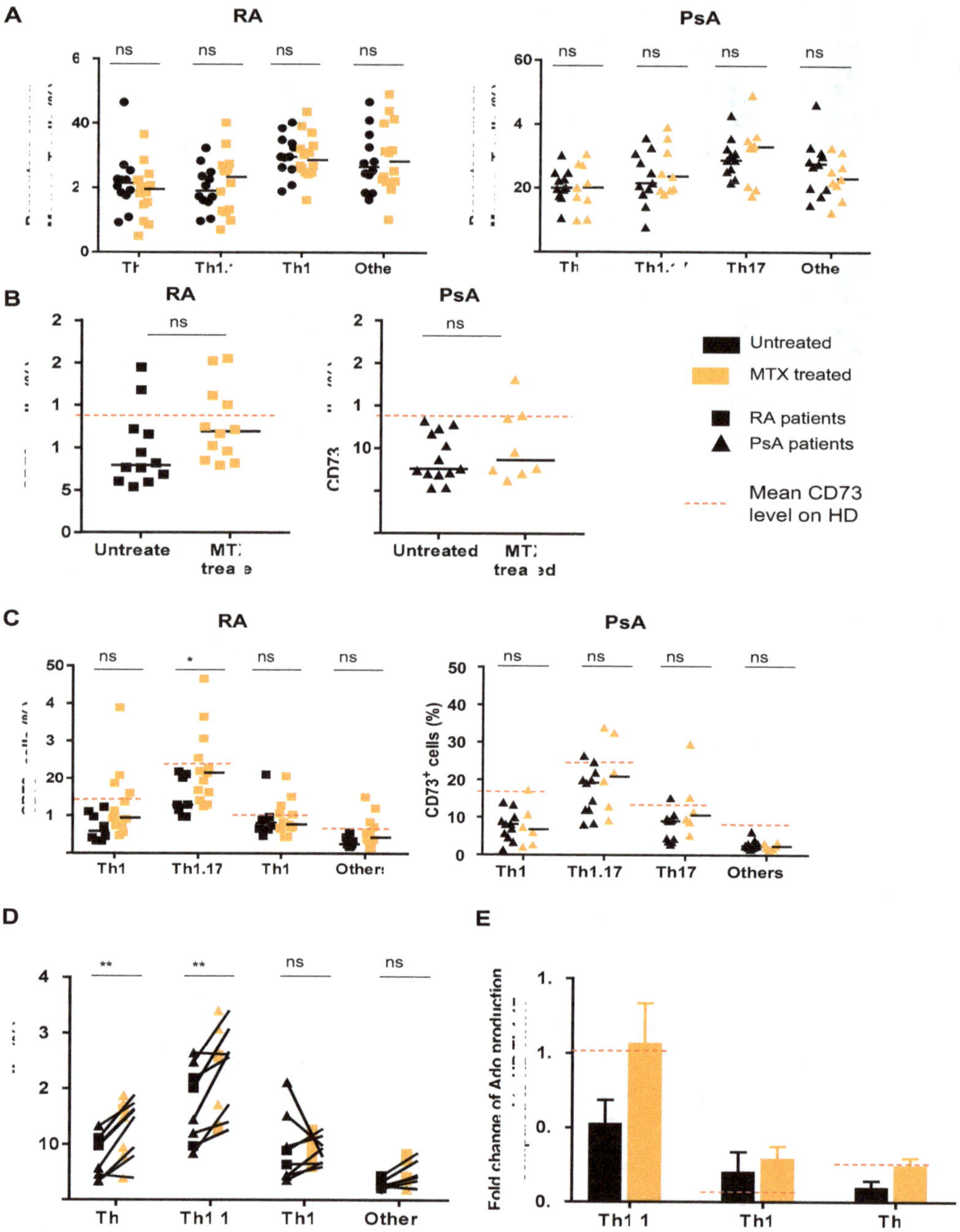

Figure 3. MTX treatment restores CD73 levels on Teff populations in RA patients but not in PsA patients. (**A**) Frequencies of Th subsets in peripheral blood of untreated versus MTX-treated RA (left) and PsA (right) patients. (**B**) CD73 percentages on total Teff in peripheral blood of untreated versus MTX treated RA (left) and PsA (right) patients. (**C**) CD73 percentages on Th subsets of untreated versus MTX-treated RA (up) and PsA (down) patients. (**D**) Paired samples showing CD73 percentages modulation in Th subsets upon MTX treatment in RA ($n = 4$) and PsA ($n = 7$) patients. (**E**) Fold change of Ado produced by sorted Th1.17, Th17 and Th1 subsets from untreated ($n = 3$) and MTX-treated RA ($n = 3$) patients. Cells were incubated for 2 h with AMP_{13C15N} isotope (37.5 µM) +/− APCP (50 µM) before Ado quantification in supernatants by LC-MS/MS. Ado production was normalized to the production by Th1.17 from HD's blood used as reference. **A** and **C**: ANOVA-2, **B**: Mann-Whitney test, **D**: ANOVA-2 with paired values. * $p < 0.05$, ** $p < 0.001$.

3.4. MTX Treatment Impacts Teff Polyfunctionality

Interestingly, we showed that CD73 expression was increased on cells coproducing IFN-γ and IL-17A, corresponding to Th1.17, from MTX-treated RA patients (Figure 4A,B). These results mirror the phenotypic analysis obtained for the Th1.17 subset (Figure 3C). In addition, we evidenced that MTX treatment significantly increased CD73 frequency among IL-22 producing cells in RA patients (Figure 4A). Of note, no major variation on global pattern of cytokines production was detected in RA patients when comparing untreated and MTX-treated samples (Figure S7A) and a rather modest increase of IL-17A$^+$ and IFN-γ^+/IL-17A$^+$ coproducing cells was observed in MTX-treated PsA patients compared to untreated ones (Figure S7B). CD73^{neg} Teff functionality was not altered by MTX neither in RA nor in PsA patients (Figure 4C,D). Surprisingly, CD73$^+$ Teff displayed increased capacity to produce IFN-γ in RA patients (Figure 4C) and to co-produce IFN-γ and IL-17A after MTX treatment in both RA (Figure 4C) and PsA patients (Figure 4D).

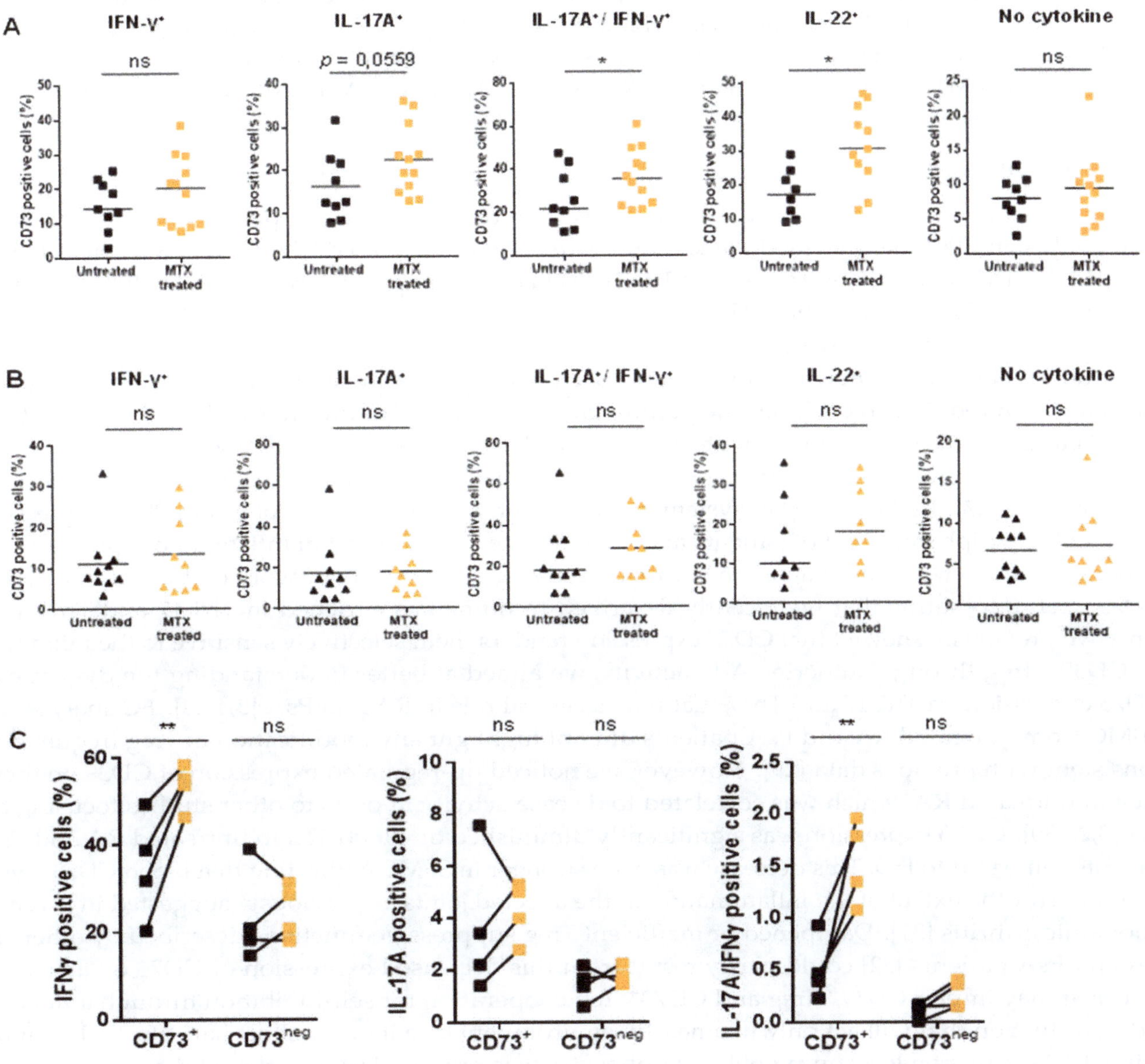

Figure 4. *Cont.*

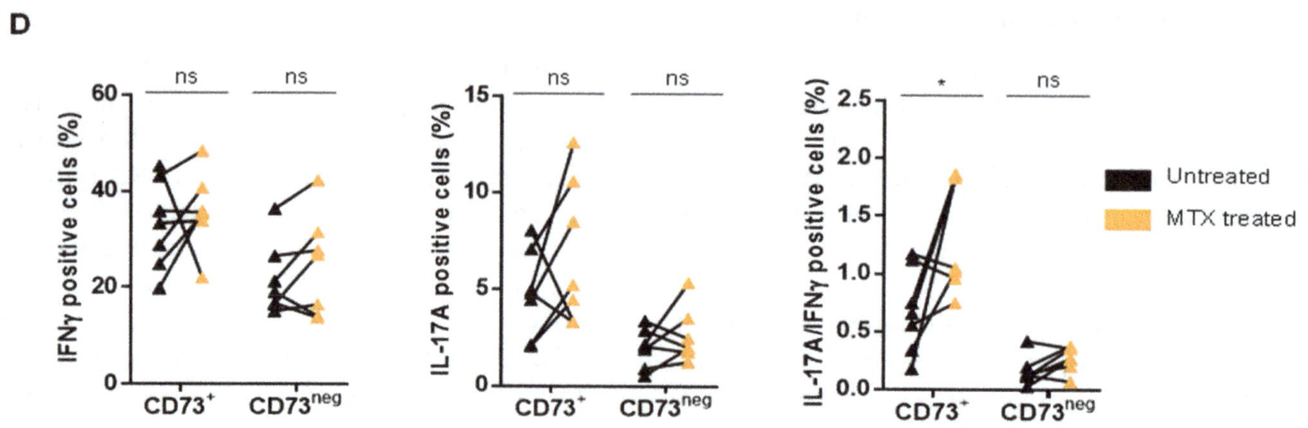

Figure 4. Impact of MTX treatment on Teff polyfunctionality. (**A**,**B**). Analysis of CD73 expression on cytokine secreting Teff mirrors phenotypic analysis in RA (**A**) and PsA (**B**) patients. (**C**,**D**). IFN-γ, IL-17A producing and IFN-γ/IL-17A co-producers in RA ($n = 4$) (**C**) and PsA ($n = 7$) (**D**) patients before initiation of MTX treatment and under MTX treatment. **A**,**B**: Mann-Whitney tests, **C**,**D**: ANOVA-2 paired samples * $p < 0.05$, ** $p < 0.001$.

4. Discussion

In this study, we demonstrated a dynamic expression of CD73 on Th populations in peripheral blood of RA and PsA patients modulated by MTX treatment. Decreased CD73 levels were detected on Th1, Th1.17, Th22 and to a lesser extent on Th17 cells in untreated patients compared to HD. The partial restoration of CD73 levels on these Th effectors upon MTX treatment reveals a novel regulatory action of this immunosuppressive drug.

The development of new therapeutic approaches for the treatment of RA and PsA is an ongoing challenge that requires to decipher the pathologic modifications of immune cells at the roots of the establishment of the chronic inflammatory state that characterizes these pathologies.

The diverse pro-inflammatory Th populations appear as good targets to breakdown the chronic inflammation [27]. In the context of systemic inflammation, the monitoring of CD39/CD73 expression levels in the peripheral blood of patients may therefore be a marker of Teff inflammatory potential, an important parameter in the evaluation of disease activity. We focused our work on the polyfunctional CD73$^+$ Teff population that we recently described in human as enriched in Th1.17 and Th17 [12]. Since we previously showed that CD73 expression renders them selectively sensitive to the inhibition by CD39$^+$ Treg through autocrine Ado activity, we aimed at better understanding the dynamic of CD73 expression on Th1.17 and Th17 that play a central role in RA and PsA [3,4,28]. FC analyses on PBMC from untreated RA and PsA patients did not highlight any modification in Treg frequencies, consistent with previous data [29]. However, we noticed up-regulated expression of CD39 on these Treg in untreated RA, which was correlated to disease activity at odds to other studies focusing on RA [3,28,30]. CD73 expression was significantly diminished on blood Teff in untreated RA and PsA patients compared to HD. This decrease was even stronger in SFMC, indicating that blood CD73 levels might mirror the extent of the inflammation in the affected joints as previously suggested in juvenile idiopathic arthritis [31]. Dampened or inefficient Treg suppressive functions described by others in RA and PsA patients [32] could partly result from this decreased expression of CD73 on activated Teff, as it may impair CD39$^+$ Treg and CD73$^+$ Teff cooperation for self-inhibition through autocrine Ado production that will act only in a nearby environment due its very short half-life. In line with this, CD73 expression level on synovial lymphocytes was proposed as a marker of disease activity in idiopathic juvenile arthritis [31] and could also be monitored in adults.

This decreased CD73 expression was particularly pronounced on Th1 and Th1.17 subsets compared to HD. Considering the strong plasticity of Th differentiation and recent data showing that Th1.17 can shift to unconventional Th1 cells when exposed to inflammatory cytokines [3,33], we suggest this decreased CD73 expression observed on Th1 might comprise activated non-classical Th1 cells phenotypically characterized by CXCR3 expression. Interestingly, this loss of CD73 expression was associated with a decreased production of Ado by Th1.17 and Th1 cells from untreated patients. Therefore, we propose that loss of CD73 expression on Teff might be a mechanism of escape to the suppression exerted by Treg, thereby enabling them with uncontrolled proliferation and secretion of pro-inflammatory cytokines. Although not reaching statistical significance, CD73 downregulation was also observed on Th17 cells that highly express CD39, suggesting an activated state. In addition, the only parameter that negatively correlated to disease activity in RA was CD73 expression by Th17 cells. This suggests that CD73 expression on Th17 cells could contribute in RA to limit the aggressiveness of the disease through the generation of Ado that could impair their own expansion but not IL-17A production as we previously demonstrated the inability of Ado to alter IL-17A secretion in contrast to other cytokines (IFN-γ, GM-CSF, IL-22, IL-10, IL-13) [12,30].

Considering the polyfunctionality of Teff in untreated patients, we did not notice significant variations compared to HD in contrast to other studies reporting higher frequency of IL-17A producing cells in peripheral blood of PsA patients [34,35]. These discrepancies may rely on the methodology used to investigate IL-17A production, and also from patients' medical history and sampling criteria. These results remain however to be confirmed in a bigger cohort of untreated RA and PsA patients. It would also be interesting to confirm that Teff from untreated patients display low or no alteration of their cytokine production in presence of exogenous AMP because of their low expression of CD73 contrary to HD [12]. In addition, we evidenced that the frequency of single IL-22 producing cells is higher in untreated PsA patients compared to HD and to untreated RA patients (Figure S4B). This is in line with the high IL-22 production by Teff previously reported in blood of PsA patients [36]. CD73 expression could not precisely investigated on Th22 cells using as specific phenotypic markers are lacking so far, but we demonstrated that single IL-22-producing cells were enriched among CD73^{+} Teff compared to CD73^{neg} counterparts, although this population was decreased in untreated patients. While IL-22 has been reported to contribute to Pso pathogenesis [37], there is, however, no clear consensus as to whether this cytokine is deleterious in PsA. In our study, we reported no variation in the proportion of single IL-22 producing cells between untreated and MTX treated PsA patients. From our point of view, it is therefore important to evaluate the CD73 status of these IL-22 secreting cells to determine if they can be regulated by Ado. A recent study on the contrary suggests a regulatory role of IL-22 in PsA patients with a reported decreased IL-22^{+} cells frequency in PsA patients compared to HD [38]. However, in this paper, treated and untreated patients have been pooled together, making the interpretation more difficult. In RA, inflammation in the SF seems mediated by IL-17A independently of IL-22 signaling [39]. Nevertheless, IL-22 can be found in high concentrations in RA patients due to its production by Th17 and Th1.17 cells that are subsets highly active in the pathology.

In our study, MTX treatment of RA and PsA patients did not induce changes on Treg frequency and CD39 MFI (Figure S5C,E,F). This contrasts with another study showing increased CD39^{+} Treg frequencies in MTX responders [40]. However, in this study, the authors suggest the direct production of Ado by Treg expressing both CD39 and CD73 which is in contradiction with observations we and others have reported [12,41]. However, high CD39^{+} Treg frequency at baseline could correlate with good MTX response, and CD39 is therefore suggested as a biomarker of the MTX response in RA [40,42]. Our analysis of untreated and MTX-treated paired samples of RA and PsA patients demonstrated a CD73 frequency in Th subsets closer to HD in MTX-treated patients. This could result from an arrest in cell proliferation due to A2AR engagement by Ado released after MTX-induced AICAR blockade [15]. We hypothesize that restoration of CD73 expression, through degradation of AMP, in turn accentuates the Ado-mediated immunosuppression initiated by MTX. The loss of CD73 expression on Teff could indeed be necessary for their proliferation and pro-inflammatory features to escape CD39^{+} Treg-mediated suppression through cooperative Ado production.

In MTX-treated PsA patients, up-regulation of CD73 on Teff appears less important than in RA patients. This could rely on the fact that PsA is a joint affection mostly developing subsequently to established Pso, that is more heterogeneous in its characterization and symptoms. The immune-biological regulation of PsA inflammation is therefore different from RA and joint inflammation in PsA might be fueled by specific immune cells active in Pso, possibly interfering with the biological effect of MTX. Indeed, auto-reactive CD8$^+$ T cells have been shown to contribute to Pso and should be considered.

We also showed an enhanced cytokine production capacity of CD73$^+$ Teff in RA patients after MTX treatment (IFN-γ, IL-17A, IL-17A/IFN-γ, IL-22). However, we can expect these cells to be less pro-inflammatory in vivo, since they express higher level of CD73, favoring Ado production. We and others have indeed previously showed that Ado strongly reduced CD73$^+$ Teff cytokine pattern except IL-17A and, to a lesser extent, IL-22 [12,30]. These data suggest a benefit of MTX treatment, which may have synergistic effect with anti-IL-17A in contrast to TNF inhibitors in PsA [43]. Similarly, in RA, although combination of MTX and anti-IL-6R such as Tocilizumab has not shown clinically relevant short-term superiority over Tocilizumab monotherapy [44], concomitant MTX treatment with Tocilizumab may have an interest in low Tocilizumab responders first under monotherapy. Indeed, we evidenced down-regulation of IL-6R on CD73$^+$ Teff compared to CD73^{neg} Teff (unpublished results), suggesting a reduced impact of anti-IL-6R on CD73$^+$ Teff. Therefore, MTX could better neutralize activated and proliferating CD73$^+$ Teff, while anti-IL-6R might target CD73^{neg} Teff; their combined action provide a better regulation of the overall hyper activated Teff population in the contexts of auto-immune disorders.

Purine metabolism and its regulation emerges as a pivotal regulator of immunity and inflammation, Modulation of this pathway in combination with MTX therefore appears as a promising target for new therapeutic strategies.

Supplementary Materials:
Figure S1: Co analysis of phenotypic and functional characteristics of Th subsets; Figure S2: Altered frequencies of CD73+ T cells in patients blood reflecting their high activation; Figure S3: Correlation between proportion of CD39+ Treg, CD73 on Th1, Th17 and Th1.17 and disease activity score (DAS28) in untreated RA patients; Figure S4: Teff from RA and PsA patients evidence the same capacities for cytokine secretion but an increase in Th22 cells is observed in peripheral blood of PsA patients; Figure S5: MTX treatment induces a slight decrease of memory CD8+ T cells frequency in PsA patients and does not modify Treg proportion and activation status in RA and PsA patients; Figure S6: Th1.17 cells are the major producers of Ado among Teff in a CD73 dependent manner; Figure S7: MTX treatment moderately increase IL-17A secretion by Teff in PsA but not in RA patients; Table S1: Panels of antibodies used for multi-parametric flow cytometry analysis throughout the study.

Author Contributions: Conceptualization: C.M.-C., C.C. and F.C.; Methodology: M.B., C.R., M.H., A.D.-R., P.B.-M. and C.M.; J.G.; Formal analysis: M.B., C.R., M.H., A.D.-R., C.M.-C. and C.C.; Investigation: M.B., C.R., M.H. and C.M.; Biological resources: F.C., H.M. and M.C.; Data curation: F.C. and H.M.; Writing—original draft preparation: M.B., C.M.-C., C.C. and F.C.; Visualization: M.B., C.R. and M.H.; Supervision: C.M.C., C.C. and F.C.; Project administration: C.M.C. and F.C.; Funding acquisition: C.M.C. and C.C.

Acknowledgments: We wish to thank the staff of the Rheumatology department at the Hôpital Lyon-Sud for providing patients samples.

References

1. Firestein, G.S. Evolving concepts of rheumatoid arthritis. *Nature* **2003**, *423*, 356–361. [CrossRef] [PubMed]
2. Gladman, D.D.; Antoni, C.; Mease, P.; Clegg, D.O.; Nash, P. Psoriatic arthritis: Epidemiology, clinical features, course, and outcome. *Ann. Rheum. Dis.* **2005**, *64*, ii14–ii17. [CrossRef] [PubMed]
3. Basdeo, S.A.; Cluxton, D.; Sulaimani, J.; Moran, B.; Canavan, M.; Orr, C.; Veale, D.J.; Fearon, U.; Fletcher, J.M. Ex-Th17 (Nonclassical Th1) Cells Are Functionally Distinct from Classical Th1 and Th17 Cells and Are Not Constrained by Regulatory T Cells. *J. Immunol.* **2017**, *198*, 2249–2259. [CrossRef] [PubMed]
4. Nistala, K.; Adams, S.; Cambrook, H.; Ursu, S.; Olivito, B.; de Jager, W.; Evans, J.G.; Cimaz, R.; Bajaj-Elliott, M.; Wedderburn, L.R. Th17 plasticity in human autoimmune arthritis is driven by the inflammatory environment. *Proc. Natl. Acad. Sci. USA* **2010**, *107*, 14751–14756. [CrossRef]

5. Raychaudhuri, S.P.; Raychaudhuri, S.K.; Genovese, M.C. IL-17 receptor and its functional significance in psoriatic arthritis. *Mol. Cell Biochem.* **2012**, *359*, 419–429. [CrossRef]
6. Burman, A.; Haworth, O.; Bradfield, P.; Parsonage, G.; Filer, A.; Thomas, A.M.; Amft, N.; Salmon, M.; Buckley, C.D. The role of leukocyte-stromal interactions in chronic inflammatory joint disease. *Jt. Bone Spine* **2005**, *72*, 10–16. [CrossRef]
7. Hot, A.; Zrioual, S.; Lenief, V.; Miossec, P. IL-17 and tumour necrosis factor α combination induces a HIF-1α-dependent invasive phenotype in synoviocytes. *Ann. Rheum. Dis.* **2012**, *71*, 1393–1401. [CrossRef]
8. Raychaudhuri, S.K.; Saxena, A.; Raychaudhuri, S.P. Role of IL-17 in the pathogenesis of psoriatic arthritis and axial spondyloarthritis. *Clin. Rheumatol.* **2015**, *34*, 1019–1023. [CrossRef]
9. van Hamburg, J.P.; Asmawidjaja, P.S.; Davelaar, N.; Mus, A.M.C.; Colin, E.M.; Hazes, J.M.W.; Dolhain, R.J.; Lubberts, E. Th17 cells, but not Th1 cells, from patients with early rheumatoid arthritis are potent inducers of matrix metalloproteinases and proinflammatory cytokines upon synovial fibroblast interaction, including autocrine interleukin-17A production. *Arthritis Rheum.* **2011**, *63*, 73–83. [CrossRef]
10. Kotake, S.; Udagawa, N.; Takahashi, N.; Matsuzaki, K.; Itoh, K.; Ishiyama, S.; Saito, S.; Inoue, K.; Kamatani, N.; Gillespie, M.T.; et al. IL-17 in synovial fluids from patients with rheumatoid arthritis is a potent stimulator of osteoclastogenesis. *J. Clin. Investig.* **1999**, *103*, 1345–1352. [CrossRef]
11. Ménétrier-Caux, C.; Curiel, T.; Faget, J.; Manuel, M.; Caux, C.; Zou, W. Targeting regulatory T cells. *Target. Oncol.* **2012**, *7*, 15–28. [CrossRef] [PubMed]
12. Gourdin, N.; Bossennec, M.; Rodriguez, C.; Vigano, S.; Machon, C.; Jandus, C.; Faget, J.; Durand, I.; Chopin, N.; Bauché, D.; et al. Autocrine Adenosine regulates tumor polyfunctional CD73+CD4+ effector T cells devoid of immune checkpoints. *Cancer Res.* **2018**, *78*, 3604–3618. [CrossRef] [PubMed]
13. Brown, P.M.; Pratt, A.G.; Isaacs, J.D. Mechanism of action of methotrexate in rheumatoid arthritis, and the search for biomarkers. *Nat. Rev. Rheumatol.* **2016**, *12*, 731–742. [CrossRef] [PubMed]
14. Taylor, P.C.; Criado, A.B.; Mongey, A.B.; Avouac, J.; Marotte, H.; Mueller, R.B. How to Get the Most from Methotrexate (MTX) Treatment for Your Rheumatoid Arthritis Patient?-MTX in the Treat-to-Target Strategy. *J. Clin. Med.* **2019**, *8*, 515. [CrossRef]
15. Montesinos, M.C.; Takedachi, M.; Thompson, L.F.; Wilder, T.F.; Fernández, P.; Cronstein, B.N. The antiinflammatory mechanism of methotrexate depends on extracellular conversion of adenine nucleotides to adenosine by ecto-5′-nucleotidase: Findings in a study of ecto-5′-nucleotidase gene-deficient mice. *Arthritis Rheum.* **2007**, *56*, 1440–1445. [CrossRef]
16. Mirabet, M.; Herrera, C.; Cordero, O.J.; Mallol, J.; Lluis, C.; Franco, R. Expression of A2B adenosine receptors in human lymphocytes: Their role in T cell activation. *J. Cell Sci.* **1999**, *112*, 491–502.
17. Zarek, P.E.; Huang, C.-T.; Lutz, E.R.; Kowalski, J.; Horton, M.R.; Linden, J.; Drake, C.G.; Powell, J.D. A2A receptor signaling promotes peripheral tolerance by inducing T-cell anergy and the generation of adaptive regulatory T cells. *Blood* **2008**, *111*, 251–259. [CrossRef]
18. Ohta, A.; Kini, R.; Ohta, A.; Subramanian, M.; Madasu, M.; Sitkovsky, M. The development and immunosuppressive functions of CD4+ CD25+ FoxP3+ regulatory T cells are under influence of the adenosine-A2A adenosine receptor pathway. *Front. Immunol.* **2012**, *3*, 190. [CrossRef]
19. Aletaha, D.; Neogi, T.; Silman, A.J.; Funovits, J.; Felson, D.T.; Bingham, C.O.; Birnbaum, N.S.; Burmester, G.R.; Bykerk, V.P.; Cohen, M.D.; et al. 2010 rheumatoid arthritis classification criteria: An American College of Rheumatology/European League Against Rheumatism collaborative initiative. *Ann. Rheum. Dis.* **2010**, *69*, 1580–1588. [CrossRef]
20. Taylor, W.; Gladman, D.; Helliwell, P.; Marchesoni, A.; Mease, P.; Mielants, H.; CASPAR Study Group. Classification criteria for psoriatic arthritis: Development of new criteria from a large international study. *Arthritis Rheum.* **2005**, *54*, 2665–2673. [CrossRef]
21. Wells, G.; Becker, J.C.; Teng, J.; Dougados, M.; Schiff, M.; Smolen, J.; Aletaha, D.; van Riel, P.L. Validation of the 28-joint Disease Activity Score (DAS28) and European League Against Rheumatism response criteria based on C-reactive protein against disease progression in patients with rheumatoid arthritis, and comparison with the DAS28 based on erythrocyte sedimentation rate. *Ann. Rheum. Dis.* **2009**, *68*, 954–960.
22. Sallusto, F.; Lanzavecchia, A. Heterogeneity of CD4+ memory T cells: Functional modules for tailored immunity. *Eur. J. Immunol.* **2009**, *39*, 2076–2082. [CrossRef] [PubMed]

23. Machon, C.; Jordheim, L.P.; Puy, J.-Y.; Lefebvre, I.; Dumontet, C.; Guitton, J. Fully validated assay for the quantification of endogenous nucleoside mono- and triphosphates using online extraction coupled with liquid chromatography-tandem mass spectrometry. *Anal. Bioanal. Chem.* **2014**, *406*, 2925–2941. [CrossRef] [PubMed]
24. Moncrieffe, H.; Nistala, K.; Kamhieh, Y.; Evans, J.; Eddaoudi, A.; Eaton, S.; Wedderburn, L.R. High Expression of the Ectonucleotidase CD39 on T Cells from the Inflamed Site Identifies Two Distinct Populations, One Regulatory and One Memory T Cell Population. *J. Immunol.* **2010**, *185*, 134–143. [CrossRef] [PubMed]
25. Zhou, Q.; Yan, J.; Putheti, P.; Wu, Y.; Sun, X.; Toxavidis, V.; Tigges, J.; Kassam, N.; Enjyoji, K.; Robson, S.C.; et al. Isolated CD39 Expression on CD4+ T Cells Denotes both Regulatory and Memory Populations. *Am. J. Transpl.* **2009**, *9*, 2303–2311. [CrossRef] [PubMed]
26. Cronstein, B.N.; Sitkovsky, M. Adenosine and adenosine receptors in the pathogenesis and treatment of rheumatic diseases. *Nat. Rev. Rheumatol.* **2017**, *13*, 41–51. [CrossRef] [PubMed]
27. Sarkar, S.; Cooney, L.A.; Fox, D.A. The role of T helper type 17 cells in inflammatory arthritis. *Clin. Exp. Immunol.* **2010**, *159*, 225–237. [CrossRef]
28. Kotake, S.; Yago, T.; Kobashigawa, T.; Nanke, Y. The Plasticity of Th17 Cells in the Pathogenesis of Rheumatoid Arthritis. *J. Clin. Med.* **2017**, *6*, 67. [CrossRef]
29. Walter, G.J.; Fleskens, V.; Frederiksen, K.S.; Rajasekhar, M.; Menon, B.; Gerwien, J.G.; Evans, H.G.; Taams, L.S. Phenotypic, Functional, and Gene Expression Profiling of Peripheral CD45RA+ and CD45RO+ CD4+CD25+CD127low Treg Cells in Patients with Chronic Rheumatoid Arthritis. *Arthritis Rheum.* **2016**, *68*, 103–116. [CrossRef]
30. Herrath, J.; Chemin, K.; Albrecht, I.; Catrina, A.I.; Malmström, V. Surface expression of CD39 identifies an enriched Treg-cell subset in the rheumatic joint, which does not suppress IL-17A secretion. *Eur. J. Immunol.* **2014**, *44*, 2979–2989. [CrossRef]
31. Botta Gordon-Smith, S.; Ursu, S.; Eaton, S.; Moncrieffe, H.; Wedderburn, L.R. Correlation of Low CD73 Expression on Synovial Lymphocytes with Reduced Adenosine Generation and Higher Disease Severity in Juvenile Idiopathic Arthritis. *Arthritis Rheum.* **2015**, *67*, 545–554. [CrossRef] [PubMed]
32. Prakken, B.; Wehrens, E.; van Wijk, F. Editorial: Quality or quantity? Unraveling the role of Treg cells in rheumatoid arthritis. *Arthritis Rheum.* **2013**, *65*, 552–554. [CrossRef] [PubMed]
33. Maggi, L.; Santarlasci, V.; Capone, M.; Rossi, M.C.; Querci, V.; Mazzoni, A.; Cimaz, R.; De Palma, R.; Liotta, F.; Maggi, E.; et al. Distinctive features of classic and nonclassic (Th17 derived) human Th1 cells. *Eur. J. Immunol.* **2012**, *42*, 3180–3188. [CrossRef] [PubMed]
34. Jandus, C.; Bioley, G.; Rivals, J.-P.; Dudler, J.; Speiser, D.; Romero, P. Increased numbers of circulating polyfunctional Th17 memory cells in patients with seronegative spondylarthritides. *Arthritis Rheum.* **2008**, *58*, 2307–2317. [CrossRef]
35. Zhang, L.; Li, Y.; Li, Y.; Qi, L.; Liu, X.; Yuan, C.; Hu, N.W.; Ma, D.X.; Li, Z.F.; Yang, Q.; et al. Increased Frequencies of Th22 Cells as well as Th17 Cells in the Peripheral Blood of Patients with Ankylosing Spondylitis and Rheumatoid Arthritis. *PLoS ONE* **2012**, *7*, e31000. [CrossRef]
36. Benham, H.; Norris, P.; Goodall, J.; Wechalekar, M.D.; FitzGerald, O.; Szentpetery, A.; Smith, M.; Thomas, R.; Gaston, H. Th17 and Th22 cells in psoriatic arthritis and psoriasis. *Arthritis Res. Ther.* **2013**, *15*, R136. [CrossRef]
37. Wolk, K.; Witte, E.; Warszawska, K.; Schulze-Tanzil, G.; Witte, K.; Philipp, S.; Kunz, S.; Döcke, W.D.; Asadullah, K.; Volk, H.D.; et al. The Th17 cytokine IL-22 induces IL-20 production in keratinocytes: A novel immunological cascade with potential relevance in psoriasis. *Eur. J. Immunol.* **2009**, *39*, 3570–3581. [CrossRef]
38. Ezeonyeji, A.; Baldwin, H.; Vukmanovic-Stejic, M.; Ehrenstein, M.R. CD4 T-Cell Dysregulation in Psoriatic Arthritis Reveals a Regulatory Role for IL-22. *Front. Immunol.* **2017**, *8*, 1403. [CrossRef]
39. van Hamburg, J.P.; Corneth, O.B.J.; Paulissen, S.M.J.; Davelaar, N.; Asmawidjaja, P.S.; Mus, A.M.; Lubberts, E. IL-17/Th17 mediated synovial inflammation is IL-22 independent. *Ann. Rheum. Dis.* **2013**, *72*, 1700–1707. [CrossRef]
40. Peres, R.S.; Liew, F.Y.; Talbot, J.; Carregaro, V.; Oliveira, R.D.; Almeida, S.L.; França, R.F.; Donate, P.B.; Pinto, L.G.; Ferreira, F.I.; et al. Low expression of CD39 on regulatory T cells as a biomarker for resistance to methotrexate therapy in rheumatoid arthritis. *Proc. Natl. Acad. Sci. USA* **2015**, *112*, 2509–2514. [CrossRef]

41. Dwyer, K.M.; Hanidziar, D.; Putheti, P.; Hill, P.A.; Pommey, S.; McRae, J.L.; Winterhalter, A.; Doherty, G.; Deaglio, S.; Koulmanda, M.; et al. Expression of CD39 by human peripheral blood CD4+CD25+ T cells denotes a regulatory memory phenotype. *Am. J. Transplant.* **2010**, *10*, 2410–2420. [CrossRef] [PubMed]
42. Gupta, V.; Katiyar, S.; Singh, A.; Misra, R.; Aggarwal, A. CD39 positive regulatory T cell frequency as a biomarker of treatment response to methotrexate in rheumatoid arthritis. *Int. J. Rheum. Dis.* **2018**, *21*, 1548–1556. [CrossRef] [PubMed]
43. Fagerli, K.M.; Lie, E.; van der Heijde, D.; Heiberg, M.S.; Lexberg, A.S.; Rødevand, E.; Kalstad, S.; Mikkelsen, K.; Kvien, T.K. The role of methotrexate co-medication in TNF-inhibitor treatment in patients with psoriatic arthritis: Results from 440 patients included in the NOR-DMARD study. *Ann. Rheum. Dis.* **2014**, *73*, 132–137. [CrossRef] [PubMed]
44. Dougados, M.; Soubrier, M.; Antunez, A.; Balint, P.; Balsa, A.; Buch, M.; Kalstad, S.; Mikkelsen, K.; Kvien, T.K. Prevalence of comorbidities in rheumatoid arthritis and evaluation of their monitoring: Results of an international, cross-sectional study (COMORA). *Ann. Rheum. Dis.* **2013**, *73*, 62–68. [CrossRef]

Achieving Pain Control in Rheumatoid Arthritis with Baricitinib or Adalimumab Plus Methotrexate: Results from the RA-BEAM Trial

Peter C. Taylor [1,*], Yvonne C. Lee [2], Roy Fleischmann [3], Tsutomu Takeuchi [4], Elizabeth L. Perkins [5], Bruno Fautrel [6], Baojin Zhu [7], Amanda K. Quebe [7], Carol L. Gaich [7], Xiang Zhang [7], Christina L. Dickson [7], Douglas E. Schlichting [7], Himanshu Patel [7], Frederick Durand [7] and Paul Emery [8]

1 Botnar Research Centre, University of Oxford, Oxford OX3 7LD, UK
2 Division of Rheumatology, Northwestern University Feinberg School of Medicine, Chicago, IL 60611, USA; yvonne.lee@northwestern.edu
3 Metroplex Clinical Research Center, University of Texas Southwestern Medical Center, Dallas, TX 75231, USA; RFleischmann@arthdocs.com
4 Division of Rheumatology, Department of Internal Medicine, Keio University, Tokyo 162-5882, Japan; tsutake@z5.keio.jp
5 Rheumatology Care Center, Birmingham, AL 35244, USA; eperkins@rheumatologycarecenter.com
6 AP-HP, Pitie-Salpetriere Hospital, Dept of Rheumatology, Sorbonne Université, Pierre Louis Institute for Epidemiology and Public Health, 705013 Paris, France; bruno.fautrel@aphp.fr
7 Eli Lilly and Company, Indianapolis, IN 46285, USA; zhu_baojin@lilly.com (B.Z.); amanda.quebe@lilly.com (A.K.Q.); gaich_carol_lynn@lilly.com (C.L.G.); zhang_xiang@lilly.com (X.Z.); dickson_christina_l@lilly.com (C.L.D.); schlichting_douglas_e@lilly.com (D.E.S.); himanshu.patel@lilly.com (H.P.); durand_frederick@lilly.com (F.D.)
8 Leeds Institute of Rheumatic and Musculoskeletal Medicine University of Leeds, Leeds LS1 3EX, UK; p.emery@leeds.ac.uk
* Correspondence: peter.taylor@kennedy.ox.ac.uk

Abstract: The purpose of the study was to assess the proportion of patients who achieve pain relief thresholds, the time needed to reach the thresholds, and the relationship between pain and inflammation among patients with rheumatoid arthritis (RA) and an inadequate response to methotrexate in RA-BEAM (NCT0170358). A randomized, double-blind trial was conducted, comparing baricitinib (N = 487), adalimumab (N = 330), and placebo (N = 488) plus methotrexate. Pain was evaluated by patient's assessment on a 0–100 mm visual analog scale (VAS). The following were assessed through a 24-week placebo-controlled period: the proportion of patients who achieved ≥30%, ≥50%, and ≥70% pain relief, the time to achieve these pain relief thresholds, remaining pain (VAS ≤ 10 mm, ≤20 mm, or ≤40 mm), and the relationship between inflammation markers and pain relief. Baricitinib-treated patients were more likely ($p < 0.05$) to achieve ≥30%, ≥50%, and ≥70% pain relief than placebo- and adalimumab-treated patients, as early as Week 1 vs. placebo and at Week 4 vs. adalimumab. A greater proportion of baricitinib-treated patients achieved ≤20 mm or ≤40 mm remaining pain vs. placebo- and adalimumab-treated patients. Baricitinib-treated patients tended to demonstrate consistent pain relief independent of levels of inflammation control. In RA patients with an inadequate response to methotrexate, baricitinib provided greater and more rapid pain relief than adalimumab and placebo. Analyses suggest the relationship between inflammation and pain may be different for baricitinib and adalimumab treatments.

Keywords: baricitinib; disease-modifying antirheumatic drugs; pain perception; outcomes research; patient perspective; rheumatoid arthritis

1. Introduction

Rapid, sustained pain control is a foremost goal for many patients with rheumatoid arthritis (RA); notably, in a survey approximately two-thirds of patients responded that pain was their treatment priority [1]. Many patients with RA who have achieved control of inflammation associated with good clinical response with RA therapy continue to report pain, including at levels described as moderate to severe [1–4]. This remaining pain may be a result of the multifactorial nature of pain associated with RA, which is not solely a result of inflammation; rather it may also be associated with structural damage, peripheral sensitization, or central amplification [2,5,6]. For other patients, despite a treat-to-target approach, the desired goal of remission cannot be attained. For these patients, ongoing pain is often a predominant symptom.

In RA-BEAM, a Phase 3 clinical trial of baricitinib, an oral, selective inhibitor of Janus kinase (JAK)1 and JAK2, baricitinib plus methotrexate (MTX) was associated with significant clinical improvements compared to patients treated with adalimumab plus MTX or placebo plus MTX. Baricitinib- and adalimumab-treated patients demonstrated similar improvement in swollen joint count (SJC), with both groups demonstrating significantly greater improvement relative to the placebo group beginning at Week 1 that was maintained through the placebo-controlled period (Week 24). For patient-reported pain, however, baricitinib-treated patients reported significantly greater improvements as early as Week 1 compared to placebo-treated patients, and as early as Week 2 when compared with adalimumab-treated patients. These statistical differences in pain relief between the active treatment arms were maintained through the duration of RA-BEAM (Week 52) [7]. This observation prompted us to explore differences in pain relief with baricitinib- and adalimumab-treated patients in RA-BEAM.

Publications of clinical trials in RA traditionally evaluate pain improvement only as central tendencies (i.e., mean change from baseline). To our knowledge, no prior reports have more fully characterized treatment effects or explored the relationship between the control of pain and inflammation with treatment. The objectives of this analysis were two-fold: first, to use the RA-BEAM data to assess the proportion of patients who achieve pain relief thresholds and the time needed to achieve these thresholds, and second, to investigate the relationship between inflammation and patient-reported pain.

2. Patients and Methods

2.1. *Trial Design*

The design and procedure of RA-BEAM have been described previously [7,8]. Briefly, RA-BEAM was a randomized, double-blind, double-dummy, placebo-controlled and active-controlled, parallel-arm, 52-week study conducted at 281 centers in 26 countries between 2012 and 2015 (ClinicalTrials.gov: NCT01710358). A total of 1305 patients on stable background MTX were randomly allocated (3:2:3) to placebo, adalimumab 40 mg, or baricitinib 4 mg. At Week 16, those patients considered non-responders received open-label rescue treatment with baricitinib 4 mg. After Week 16, patients may have received rescue treatment at investigator discretion. At Week 24, placebo-treated patients were switched to baricitinib. The study was conducted in accordance with the ethical principles of the Declaration of Helsinki and Good Clinical Practice guidelines. The study protocol was approved by each center's institutional review board or ethics committee. All patients provided written informed consent.

2.2. *Patients*

Patients were ≥18 years old with active RA (≥6/68 tender and ≥6/66 swollen joints; serum high-sensitivity C-reactive protein (CRP) ≥6 mg/L). Patients had an inadequate response to MTX and either ≥3 joint erosions (based on radiographs), or ≥1 joint erosion with seropositivity for rheumatoid factor or anti-citrullinated peptide antibodies [7].

2.3. Pain Measures

Pain was measured with the patient's assessment of pain visual analog scale (VAS), consisting of one question, "How much pain are you currently having because of your rheumatoid arthritis?" Responses range from 0 mm (no pain) to 100 mm (worst possible pain). The pain VAS was administered at every study visit.

Pain Thresholds

Our initial observation of differential pain response between baricitinib and adalimumab was based on mean change from baseline. We wanted to understand if these differences persisted when pain relief was evaluated against various thresholds of success, as is typical for other patient-reported outcomes in RA. Because there are no established, standard pain thresholds in RA, we reviewed the literature and selected two approaches. First, we applied percent change from baseline threshold recommendations from the general chronic pain literature, specifically those from the Initiative on Methods, Measurement, and Pain Assessment in Clinical Trials (IMMPACT), a multidisciplinary organization with the mission to develop consensus reviews and recommendations and to improve clinical trials of treatments for pain [9,10]. A 30% improvement threshold is described as "much improved, meaningful differences" and 50% represents "very much improved, substantial improvement" in chronic pain conditions. A 70% improvement threshold, although not defined in IMMPACT, was also evaluated because it is analogous to American College of Rheumatology response endpoints and was observed with patients in RA-BEAM. Second, while relative improvement is important, so is absolute pain; thus we evaluated thresholds of remaining pain (i.e., the absolute value of patient-reported pain) of ≤10 mm, ≤20 mm, or ≤40 mm, at Week 24. The ≤10 mm threshold reflects limited pain to no pain and is extrapolated from data by Wells et al. [11]. The ≤20 mm threshold represents a threshold when satisfaction with health is not negatively affected by pain [11,12]. The ≤40 mm threshold was derived from observed cut-off points between the pain VAS and the Patient Acceptable Symptom State (PASS) [13].

2.4. Outcomes

The proportion of patients achieving ≥30%, ≥50%, or ≥70% improvement from baseline by Week 24 was assessed, as was the median time when 50% of patients achieved these thresholds of pain relief. The proportion of patients achieving remaining pain VAS values of ≤10 mm, ≤20 mm, or ≤40 mm was assessed at Week 24. To evaluate if the differences in pain response were associated with inflammation, we assessed the relationship between levels of inflammation and pain relief at Week 24.

2.5. Statistical Analyses

All analyses were conducted with an intention-to-treat approach in which data from patients who received ≥1 dose of study drug were assessed, regardless of whether they completed the trial. Missing values were imputed with modified last observation carried forward for all analyses where applicable. Analyses were not adjusted for multiplicity.

Comparisons were made on the percent change in pain VAS from baseline to Week 24 using analysis of covariance (ANCOVA) and on the proportion of patients achieving pain relief at Week 24 between treatment arms using logistic models, adjusted for randomization factors (region, baseline joint erosion status (1–2 erosions plus seropositivity vs. ≥3 erosions)) and baseline pain VAS score. The median time needed for patients to achieve these pain relief thresholds were assessed through Week 24 using the cumulative incidence estimate with 'competing risks' which included rescue or discontinuation due to lack of efficacy before reaching the pain relief threshold. The Cox proportional hazards model with 'competing risks' (proportional sub-distribution hazards model) [14,15] was used to obtain the hazard ratio.

Remaining pain was analyzed across treatment groups with logistic regression models. Pain relief at Week 24 by CRP was evaluated using ANCOVA.

A mediation analysis with multiple mediators was conducted to evaluate the relationship between levels of inflammation and pain relief. The effects of change in inflammatory factors (CRP, erythrocyte sedimentation rate (ESR), SJC) as multiple mediators on change in pain outcome for each treatment over placebo during the 24-week period were evaluated in this analysis [16]. The total treatment effect on pain relief over placebo that can be accounted for by changes in CRP, ESR, and SJC in the mediation analysis is the 'indirect' or mediation effect, while the total treatment effect that cannot be accounted for by the 'indirect' effect is called the 'direct' effect. Observed data were used for the mediation analysis.

Statistical analyses were performed in SAS (SAS Institute; Cary, NC, USA, version 9.4). A two-sided p value < 0.05 was considered statistically significant.

3. Results

3.1. Pain Relief

As noted by Taylor et al. [7], patients had established and active RA. The mean baseline pain scores were well matched across treatment groups in this study and ranged from 60 to 62 mm with the median baseline pain of 62 mm [7]. Other baseline characteristics were well-balanced between the treatment arms [7]. A detailed description of the safety of baricitinib and adalimumab is available in the RA-BEAM publication [7]. In brief, adverse events were more frequent with baricitinib (71%) and adalimumab (68%) than with placebo (60%) through Week 24. Rates of serious adverse events through Week 24 were 5% with placebo, 5% with baricitinib, and 2% with adalimumab.

As early as Week 1, significantly greater improvement in pain relief was observed between baricitinib and placebo (25% for baricitinib vs. 4% for placebo, $p < 0.0001$). At Week 24, the mean percentage reduction in pain from baseline for baricitinib, adalimumab, and placebo, respectively, were 51%, 39%, 17% ($p = 0.001$ for baricitinib and adalimumab vs. placebo and $p = 0.030$ for baricitinib vs. adalimumab).

A greater proportion of patients treated with baricitinib or adalimumab achieved the ≥30%, ≥50%, or ≥70% pain relief thresholds compared with placebo-treated patients at Week 1 (Figure 1). Compared with adalimumab-treated patients, a greater proportion ($p < 0.05$) of baricitinib-treated patients achieved ≥30% and ≥50% pain relief as early as Week 4 and ≥70% pain relief at Week 8. Differences between baricitinib and adalimumab for ≥50% and ≥70% pain relief were maintained through Week 24 (Figure 1).

At Week 24, for the placebo-, adalimumab-, and baricitinib-treated patients, respectively, the proportion of patients who achieved ≥30% pain relief were 49%, 69%, and 74%; for ≥50% pain relief, the values were 32%, 52%, and 61%; and for ≥70% pain relief, the values were 16%, 32%, and 41%.

The median time to achieve the ≥30% pain relief threshold was 2 weeks for baricitinib- and adalimumab-treated patients and 5 weeks for those on placebo (Figure 2). For ≥50% pain relief, the median time was 4 weeks for baricitinib, 8 weeks for adalimumab, and 14 weeks for placebo (Figure 2). For ≥70% pain relief, the median time was 12 weeks for baricitinib, 20 weeks for adalimumab, and >24 weeks for placebo (Figure 2). Compared with placebo, baricitinib-treated patients were more likely to achieve ≥30%, ≥50%, or ≥70% pain relief with Hazard Ratio (HR) values of 1.7, 1.9, and 2.5, respectively ($p \leq 0.001$). Compared with adalimumab, baricitinib-treated patients were more likely to achieve ≥50% or ≥70% pain relief; the HR values for the ≥30%, ≥50%, or ≥70% pain relief thresholds, respectively, were 1.1 ($p = 0.145$), 1.2 ($p = 0.032$), and 1.3 ($p = 0.003$).

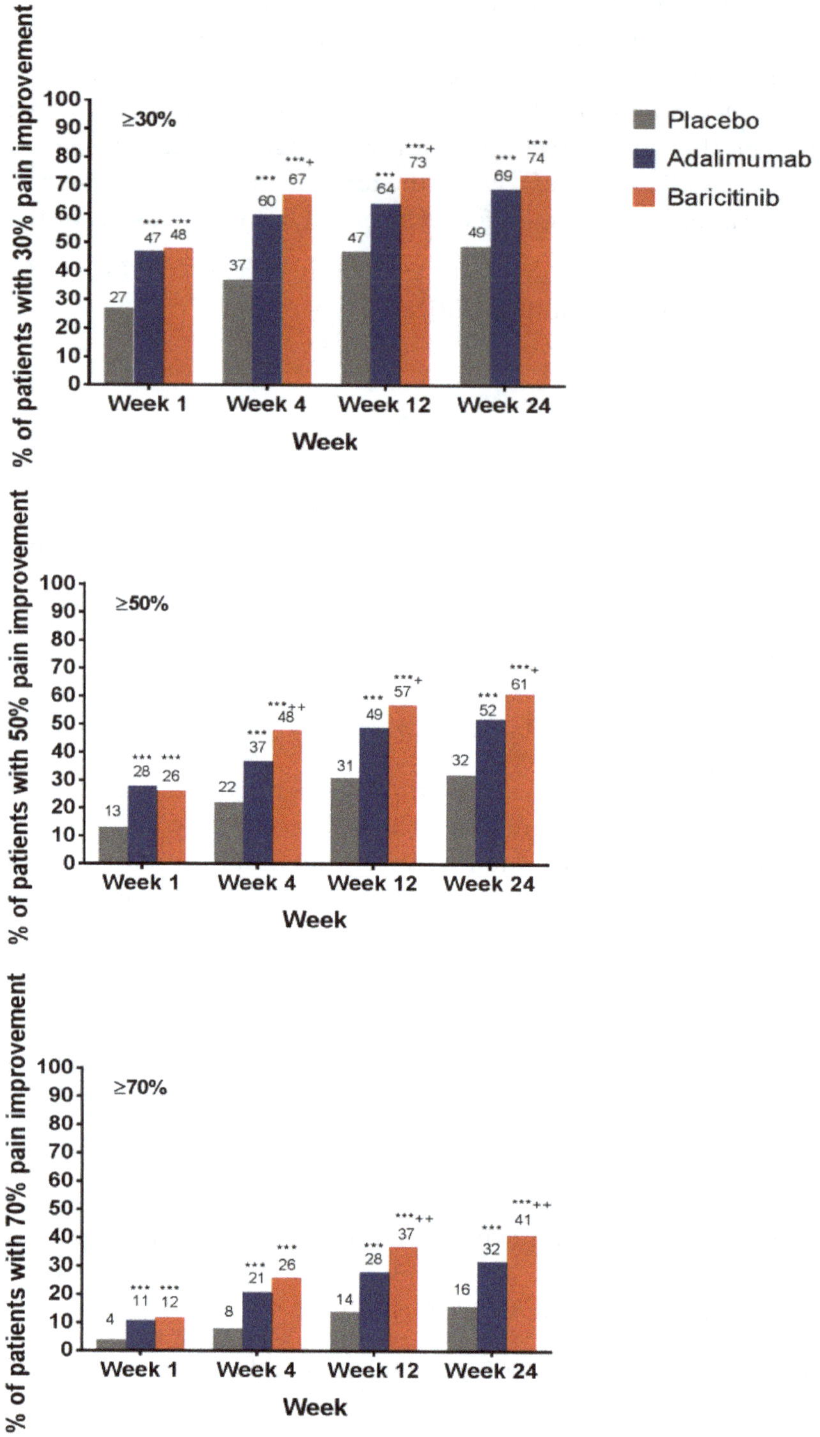

Figure 1. Percentage of patients who achieved pain relief thresholds from baseline, as measured by the pain VAS. *** $p \leq 0.001$ vs. placebo; † $p \leq 0.05$; †† $p \leq 0.01$, ††† $p \leq 0.001$ vs. adalimumab. Abbreviations: VAS = visual analog scale. Number of respondents who answered the pain question by week: placebo, $n = 481$ at Week 1 and $n = 483$ at all other weeks; adalimumab, $n = 325$ at Week 1 and $n = 327$ at all other weeks; baricitinib, $n = 482$ at all weeks.

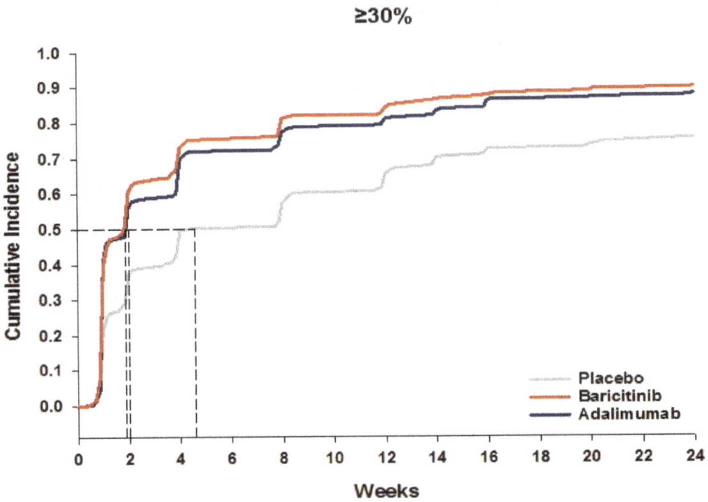

The median time (weeks) for patients to attain pain VAS improvement ≥30% was 1.9 weeks for baricitinib, 2.0 weeks for adalimumab, and 4.6 weeks for placebo. Compared with placebo, baricitinib-treated patients were more likely to achieve ≥30% pain relief with Hazard Ratio (HR) of 1.7 ($p \leq 0.001$).

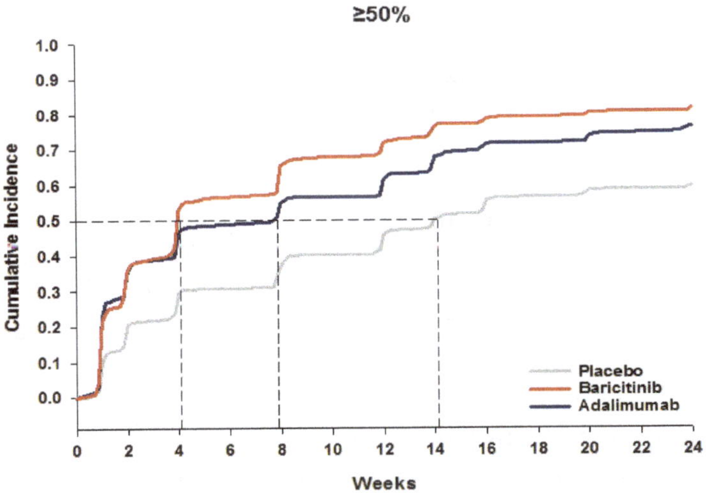

The median time (weeks) for patients to attain pain VAS improvement ≥50% was 4.0 weeks for baricitinib, 7.9 weeks for adalimumab, and 14.0 weeks for placebo. Compared with placebo, baricitinib-treated patients were more likely to achieve ≥50% pain relief with an HR of 1.9 ($p \leq 0.001$). Compared with adalimumab, baricitinib-treated patients were more likely to achieve ≥50% pain relief with an HR of 1.2 ($p = 0.032$).

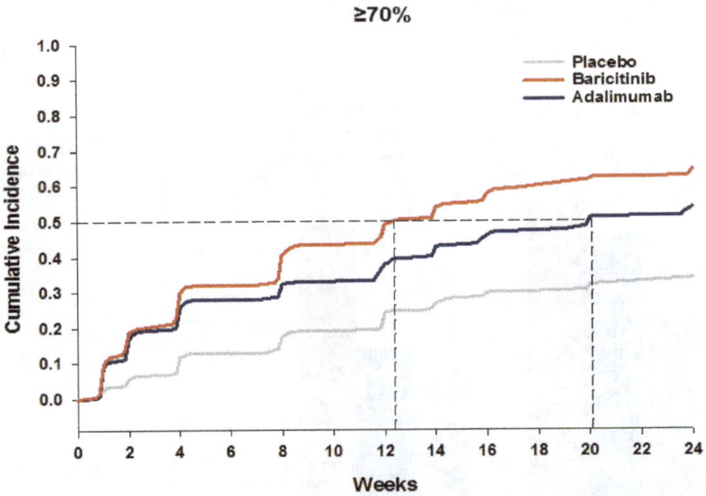

The median time (weeks) for patients to attain pain VAS improvement ≥70% was 12.4 weeks for baricitinib, 20.0 weeks for adalimumab, and >24.0 weeks for placebo. Compared with placebo, baricitinib-treated patients were more likely to achieve ≥70% pain relief with an HR of 2.5 ($p \leq 0.001$). Compared with adalimumab, baricitinib-treated patients were more likely to achieve ≥70% pain relief; the HR value was 1.3 ($p = 0.003$).

Figure 2. Time course for patients attaining pain relief thresholds.

3.2. Remaining Pain

The differences in the proportion of patients who achieved the ≤40 mm, ≤20 mm, and ≤10 mm remaining pain thresholds were significantly greater for baricitinib and adalimumab compared with placebo as early as Week 1 (Table 1). Compared with adalimumab-treated patients, a greater proportion of baricitinib-treated patients achieved the ≤40 mm threshold ($p \leq 0.001$) at Week 4, and a difference was observed between the active treatment groups at the ≤20 mm threshold by Week 12 ($p \leq 0.001$; Table 1). Differences were maintained through Week 24. The percentage of patients who achieved the ≤10 mm remaining pain threshold was greater for baricitinib compared to adalimumab, but the difference reached statistical significance only at Week 12.

Table 1. Percentage of patients who met the thresholds of remaining pain (VAS) over time by treatment groups. *** $p \leq 0.001$ vs. placebo; † $p \leq 0.05$; ††† $p \leq 0.001$ vs. adalimumab.

Threshold of Remaining Pain at Each Time Point (Week)	Placebo *n* (%)	Adalimumab *n* (%)	Baricitinib *n* (%)
≤40 mm			
1	150 (31)	132 (41) ***	208 (43) ***
4	193 (40)	169 (52) ***	298 (62) ***,†††
12	225 (46)	202 (62) ***	335 (69) ***,†
24	236 (49)	218 (66) ***	351 (73) ***,†
≤20 mm			
1	51 (11)	64 (20) ***	90 (19) ***
4	80 (17)	93 (28) ***	158 (33) ***
12	103 (21)	120 (37) ***	209 (43) ***,†
24	105 (22)	121 (37) ***	239 (49) ***,†††
≤10 mm			
1	20 (4)	32 (10) ***	40 (8) ***
4	29 (6)	49 (15) ***	88 (18) ***
12	52 (11)	63 (19) ***	124 (26) ***,†
24	56 (12)	86 (26) ***	144 (30) ***

3.3. Relationship between Inflammation and Pain Relief

At Week 24, among patients with varying levels of inflammation, as measured by CRP as an objective marker of inflammation, baricitinib-treated patients tended to demonstrate consistent pain relief regardless of the CRP levels. In contrast, patients treated with adalimumab and placebo demonstrated less pain relief at higher CRP levels (Figure 3).

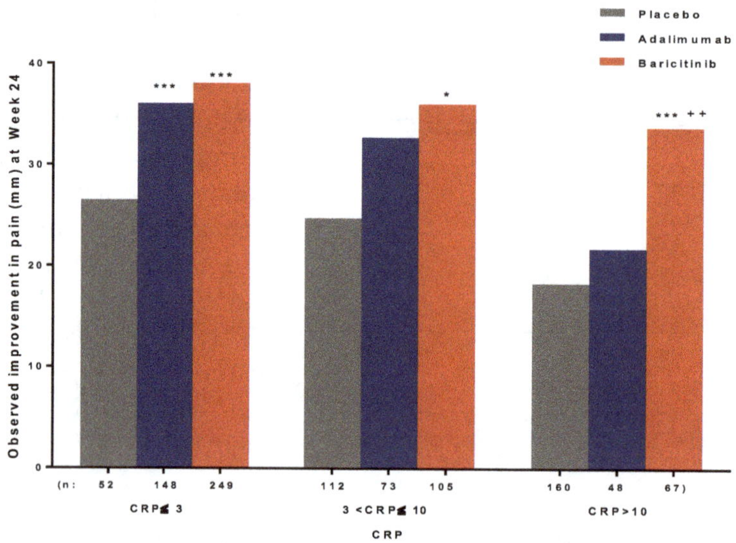

Figure 3. Pain improvement by remaining inflammation (CRP, mg/L) at Week 24. * $p \leq 0.05$, *** $p \leq 0.001$ vs. placebo; †† $p \leq 0.01$ vs. adalimumab. Abbreviations: CRP = C-reactive protein.

While the total effect of baricitinib on pain relief over placebo at Week 24 was greater than that for adalimumab, changes in inflammation accounted for approximately 40% of the pain improvement with baricitinib and 50% of pain improvement with adalimumab (Figure 4; Table S1). In this analysis, the direct effects (i.e., those not associated with these markers of inflammation) of drug on pain relief were higher for baricitinib than for adalimumab after accounting for indirect inflammatory effects (Figure 4).

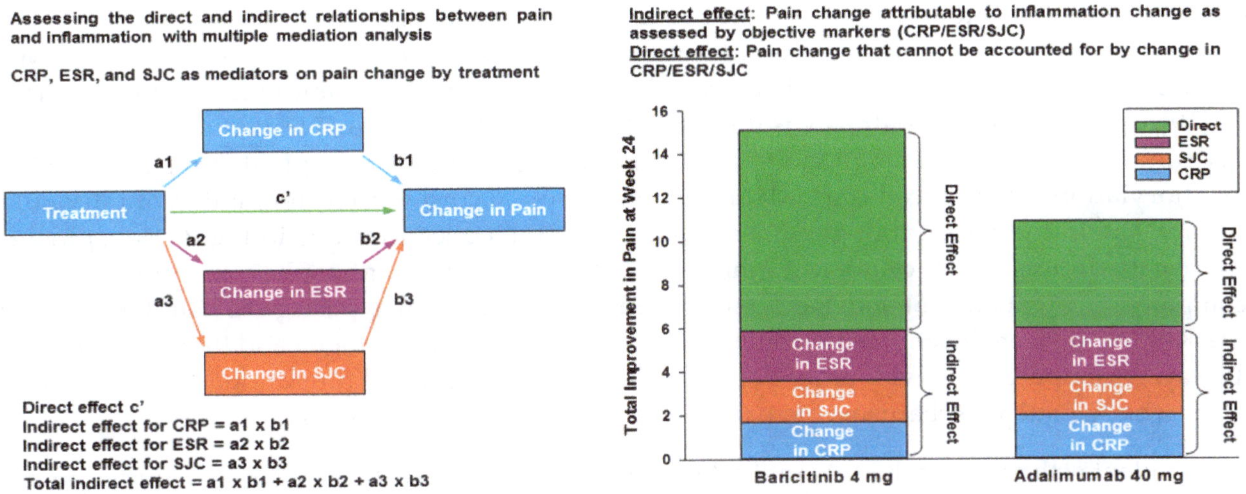

Figure 4. Relative contribution of inflammatory control to pain control.

4. Discussion

In the RA-BEAM trial, patient-reported improvements in disease activity, physical function, and pain were greater for baricitinib plus MTX than for adalimumab plus MTX within 4 weeks of starting treatment and were maintained throughout the 52-week observation period [7]. In this analysis, we further explored pain relief experienced by patients. Baricitinib demonstrated greater and more rapid achievement of clinically significant levels of pain relief than adalimumab or placebo through Week 24. Furthermore, this differential effect became more marked as the pain relief thresholds increased, with approximately 40% of the patients receiving baricitinib achieving ≥70% pain relief from baseline by Week 24.

Another striking feature of this analysis was the rapid onset of effective mean pain relief at a cohort level with baricitinib plus MTX. Here, we show that for those patients achieving ≥50% or ≥70% pain relief, baricitinib had a shorter median time to achieving these pain relief thresholds than placebo or adalimumab. Specifically, for ≥50% pain relief, the 4 weeks needed for baricitinib was approximately half that of adalimumab treated patients (8 weeks). For patients achieving ≥30% pain relief, baricitinib and adalimumab had similar median time to onset (approximately 2 weeks).

Remaining pain is commonly reported by patients with RA despite achieving satisfactory disease control by adopting the treat-to-target approach in disease management. A threshold of ≤20 mm remaining pain is considered to represent a point where health satisfaction is not adversely affected [11,12]. In our study, we found that patients treated with either baricitinib plus MTX or adalimumab plus MTX were significantly more likely to achieve ≤10 mm, ≤20 mm, and ≤40 mm thresholds for remaining pain compared to placebo plus MTX. Baricitinib separated from adalimumab by Week 4 for the ≤40 mm and by Week 8 for the ≤20 mm threshold.

To explore the relative contribution of anti-inflammatory and other mechanisms of pain relief obtained with either baricitinib or adalimumab, we explored relationships between changes in patient-reported pain and an objective marker of inflammation, namely CRP. This analysis suggests that the difference in pain relief between baricitinib and adalimumab cannot be solely accounted for by differential effects on inflammation.

While it is clear from multiple clinical studies that baricitinib has a profound anti-inflammatory effect, as would be expected of a multi-cytokine inhibitor, these observations imply that JAK1 and JAK2 inhibition also has anti-nociceptive effects that are independent of at least certain aspects of the inflammatory process [17]. A rodent model indicated that treatment with baricitinib attenuates complete Freund's adjuvant-induced joint deficits, a surrogate measure of joint pain [18]. At present, the mechanisms by which baricitinib modulates the pain experience independently of at least some generic features of inflammation is unknown. One possible mechanism could involve granulocyte-macrophage colony-stimulating factor (GM-CSF). GM-CSF is a cytokine that signals through JAK2 homodimers. In a rodent collagenase-induced instability model of osteoarthritis, pain was shown to be GM-CSF dependent, and therapeutic neutralization of GM-CSF rapidly and completely abolished arthritis pain [19]. Another possible pathway is through phosphorylation of signal transducer and activator of transcription 3 (STAT3). In rodent models of neuropathic pain following spinal nerve ligation, STAT3 phosphorylation was induced centrally in the dorsal spinal cord with upregulation of interleukin-6 (IL-6) mRNA in the dorsal root ganglia and elevated IL-6 concentrations in the dorsal spinal cord. Intrathecal administration of a JAK2 inhibitor blocked this STAT3 phosphorylation pathway with accompanying attenuation of both mechanical allodynia and thermal hyperalgesia [20]. It is known that the JAK-STAT3 system is activated through IL-6 signaling in spinal microglia and that this transduction pathway participates in development of pain associated with nerve alteration. However, it is not known whether such mechanisms have relevance to pain in established RA.

In rodent arthritis models, autoantibodies to citrullinated proteins (ACPA) are reported to induce joint pain independent of inflammation via a chemokine-dependent mechanism [21]. However, this is unlikely to account for the differences in pain relief between TNF blockade and JAK inhibition in our study as we did not observe statistically significant differences in ACPA change from baseline between baricitinib and adalimumab at Week 24.

This analysis has limitations. Specifically, the present findings represent post hoc analyses in which patients were not randomized according to their baseline pain. Pain studies may be complicated by the subjective experience of pain and the inherent limitations of a VAS as an instrument to measure pain experience. Additionally, the pain relief thresholds and remaining pain values are not yet firmly established for RA [12,13]. Further, some concomitant medication use (e.g., glucocorticoids) are controlled within a clinical trial, precluding assessment of any potential relationship between pain improvement and medication changes.

Pain relief with treatment may have clinical and holistic implications. Patients who experience pain relief are likely to report clinically significant improvements in other patient-reported outcomes, such as the Patient's Global Assessment of Disease Activity and functional disability [22,23]. More broadly, reductions in pain have been associated with improvements in daily activity and work productivity [24]. In this analysis, we have presented evidence that baricitinib rapidly provides pain relief in patients with active RA on concomitant MTX to a magnitude greater than that observed with the TNF inhibitor, adalimumab. We have expanded prior research through a new and detailed analysis of the range of magnitude and kinetics of pain relief in a head-to-head study of baricitinib versus adalimumab and by exploring the relationship between the control of pain and inflammation with treatment. We observed that the inhibition of JAK1/JAK2 or TNF similarly ameliorate inflammatory markers, but the overall pain and the non-inflammatory component are faster and more markedly improved by baricitinib. Our findings merit further investigation into the biological mechanisms underlying pain relief.

The observations from this analysis may be of importance in managing the unmet needs of adequate pain relief in RA, whether in patients attaining the treatment targets of remission or low disease activity or in those who are unable to achieve these targets with biologic anti-TNF treatment.

Author Contributions: Conceptualization: P.C.T., Y.C.L., R.F., T.T., E.L.P., B.F., B.Z., A.K.Q., C.L.G., X.Z., C.L.D., D.E.S., H.P., F.D., P.E.; methodology: P.C.T., Y.C.L., R.F., T.T., E.L.P., B.F., B.Z., A.K.Q., C.L.G., X.Z., C.L.D., D.E.S., H.P., F.D., P.E.; software, validation, formal analyses, data curation: B.Z. and X.Z.; writing—original draft preparation: P.C.T., B.Z., A.K.Q.; writing—review and editing, visualization: P.C.T., Y.C.L., R.F., T.T., E.L.P., B.F., B.Z., A.K.Q., C.L.G., X.Z., C.L.D., D.E.S., H.P., F.D., P.E.; funding acquisition: B.Z., A.K.Q.

Acknowledgments: The authors would like to thank Molly Tomlin, MS, of Eli Lilly and Company for her assistance with manuscript preparation and process support; Julie Sherman, of Eli Lilly and Company, for her assistance with the manuscript figures; and Jiaying Guo, MS, of Eli Lilly and Company, for her review of the data. P.C.T. would like to acknowledge support by the National Institute for Health Research (NIHR) Oxford Biomedical Research Centre (BRC) and by AR UK.

Conflicts of Interest: P.C.T. has received grant/research support from Celgene, Eli Lilly and Company, Galapagos, UCB and is a consultant for AbbVie, Eli Lilly and Company, Galapagos, GlaxoSmithKline, Pfizer, UCB, Biogen, Sandoz, Novartis, Gilead and Janssen. Y.C.L. has stock in Express Scripts and has received a research grant from Pfizer. R.F. has received grant/research support from AbbVie, Amgen, AstraZeneca, Bristol-Myers Squibb, Celgene, Centrexion, Genetech, GlaxoSmithKline, Janssen, Eli Lilly and Company, Merck, Pfizer, Regeneron, Roche, Sanofi, Aventis, UCB and is a consultant for AbbVie, Amgen, Bristol-Myers Squibb, Celgene, Celltrion, GSK, Janssen, Eli Lilly and Company, Novartis, Pfizer, Samsung, Sanofi-Aventis, Tahio. T.T. has received consulting support and/or speakers bureau fees from AbbVie GK, Asahi Kasei Medical KK, Astellas Pharma, AstraZeneca KK, Bristol-Myers KK, Chugai Pharma Ltd., Daiichi Sankyo Ltd., Eisai Co Ltd., Eli Lilly and Company, Janssen Pharma KK, Mitsubishi Tanabe Pharma, Nipponkayaku Ltd., Novartis Pharma KK, Pfizer Japan, Takeda Pharma Ltd., Taiho Pharmaceutical Co., Ltd., Taisho Toyama Pharmaceutical Co., Ltd., GlaxoSmithKline K.K., and UCB Japan. E.L.P. is a consultant for Novartis and Eli Lilly and Co. B.F. is a consultant for AbbVie, Biogen, BMS, Celgene, Janssen, Lilly, Medac, MSD, NORDIC Pharma, Novartis, Pfizer, Roche, Sanofi-Aventis, SOBI, UCB and has received research grants from AbbVie, MSD, Pfizer. B.Z., C.L.G., X.Z., A.K.Q., C.L.D., D.E.S., H.P., F.D.: All authors are employees and stock holders in Eli Lilly and Company. P.E. has provided expert advice for Pfizer, MSD, Abbvie, BMS, UCB, Roche, Novartis, Samsung, Sandoz, Eli Lilly and Company.

References

1. Taylor, P.C.; Manger, B.; Alvaro-Gracia, J.; Johnstone, R.; Gomez-Reino, J.; Eberhardt, E.; Wolfe, F.; Schwartzman, S.; Furfaro, N.; Kavanaugh, A. Patient perceptions concerning pain management in the treatment of rheumatoid arthritis. *J. Int. Med. Res.* **2010**, *38*, 1213–1224. [CrossRef] [PubMed]
2. Boyden, S.D.; Hossain, I.N.; Wohlfahrt, A.; Lee, Y.C. Non-inflammatory causes of pain in patients with rheumatoid arthritis. *Curr. Rheumatol. Rep.* **2016**, *18*, 30. [CrossRef] [PubMed]
3. Altawil, R.; Saevarsdottir, S.; Wedren, S.; Alfredsson, L.; Klareskog, L.; Lampa, J. Remaining Pain in Early Rheumatoid Arthritis Patients Treated with Methotrexate. *Arthritis Care Res.* **2016**, *68*, 1061–1068. [CrossRef] [PubMed]
4. Ishida, M.; Kuroiwa, Y.; Yoshida, E.; Sato, M.; Krupa, D.; Henry, N.; Ikeda, K.; Kaneko, Y. Residual symptoms and disease burden among patients with rheumatoid arthritis in remission or low disease activity: A systematic literature review. *Mod. Rheumatol.* **2018**, *28*, 789–799. [CrossRef] [PubMed]
5. Meeus, M.; Vervisch, S.; De Clerck, S.; Moorkens, G.; Hans, G.; Nijs, J. Central sensitization in patients with rheumatoid arthritis: A systematic literature review. *Semin. Arthritis Rheum.* **2012**, *41*, 556–567. [CrossRef]
6. McWilliams, D.F.; Walsh, D.A. Pain mechanisms in rheumatoid arthritis. *Clin. Exp. Rheumatol.* **2017**, *35* (Suppl. 107), 94–101.
7. Taylor, P.C.; Keystone, E.C.; van der Heijde, D.; Weinblatt, M.E.; del Carmen Morales, L.; Reyes Gonzaga, J.; Yakushin, S.; Ishii, T.; Emoto, K.; Beattie, S.; et al. Baricitinib versus placebo or adalimumab in rheumatoid arthritis. *N. Engl. J. Med.* **2017**, *376*, 652–662. [CrossRef]
8. Keystone, E.C.; Taylor, P.C.; Tanaka, Y.; Gaich, C.; DeLozier, A.M.; Dudek, A.; Zamora, J.V.; Cobos, J.A.C.; Rooney, T.; de Bono, S.; et al. Patient-reported outcomes from a phase 3 study of baricitinib versus placebo or adalimumab in rheumatoid arthritis: Secondary analyses from the RA-BEAM study. *Ann. Rheum. Dis.* **2017**, *76*, 1853–1861. [CrossRef]
9. Dworkin, R.H.; Turk, D.C.; Wyrwich, K.W.; Beaton, D.; Cleeland, C.S.; Farrar, J.T.; Haythornthwaite, J.A.; Jensen, M.P.; Kerns, R.D.; Ader, D.N.; et al. Interpreting the clinical importance of treatment outcomes in chronic pain clinical trials: IMMPACT recommendations. *J. Pain* **2008**, *9*, 105–121. [CrossRef]
10. IMMPACT: Initiative on Methods, Measurement, and Pain Assessment in Clinical Trials. Available online: http://www.immpact.org/ (accessed on 24 April 2019).

11. Wells, G.A.; Boers, M.; Shea, B.; Brooks, P.M.; Simon, L.S.; Strand, C.V.; Aletaha, D.; Anderson, J.J.; Bombardier, C.; Dougados, M.; et al. Minimal disease activity for rheumatoid arthritis: A preliminary definition. *J. Rheumatol.* **2005**, *32*, 2016–2024.
12. Wolfe, F.; Michaud, K. Assessment of pain in rheumatoid arthritis: Minimal clinically significant difference, predictors, and the effect of anti-tumor necrosis factor therapy. *J. Rheumatol.* **2007**, *34*, 1674–1683. [PubMed]
13. Tubach, F.; Ravaud, P.; Martin-Mola, E.; Awada, H.; Bellamy, N.; Bombardier, C.; Felson, D.T.; Hajjaj-Hassouni, N.; Hochberg, M.; Logeart, I.; et al. Minimum clinically important improvement and patient acceptable symptom state in pain and function in rheumatoid arthritis, ankylosing spondylitis, chronic back pain, hand osteoarthritis, and hip and knee osteoarthritis: Results from a prospective multinational study. *Arthritis Care Res.* **2012**, *64*, 1699–1707.
14. Gooley, T.A.; Leisenring, W.; Crowley, J.; Storer, B.E. Estimation of failure probabilities in the presence of competing risks: New representations of old estimators. *Stat. Med.* **1999**, *18*, 695–706. [CrossRef]
15. Fine, J.P.; Gray, R.J. A proportional hazards model for the subdistribution of a competing risk. *J. Am. Stat. Assoc.* **1999**, *94*, 496–509. [CrossRef]
16. Preacher, K.J.; Hayes, A.F. Asymptotic and resampling strategies for assessing and comparing indirect effects in multiple mediator models. *Behav. Res. Methods* **2008**, *40*, 879–891. [CrossRef] [PubMed]
17. Busch-Dienstfertig, M.; González-Rodríguez, S. IL-4, JAK-STAT signaling, and pain. *JAK-STAT* **2013**, *2*, e27638. [CrossRef] [PubMed]
18. Knopp, K.L.; Kato, A.; Wall, T.M.; McDermott, J.S.; Nisenbaum, E.S.; Adams, B.L.; Johnson, M. SAT0051 Baricitinib improves joint mobility after injury in a rodent forced-ambulation model. *Ann. Rheum. Dis.* **2019**, *78*, A1089.
19. Cook, A.D.; Pobjoy, J.; Steidl, S.; Durr, M.; Braine, E.L.; Turner, A.L.; Lacey, D.C.; Hamilton, J.A. Granulocyte-macrophage colony-stimulating factor is a key mediator in experimental osteoarthritis pain and disease development. *Arthritis Res. Ther.* **2012**, *14*, R199. [CrossRef] [PubMed]
20. Dominguez, E.; Rivat, C.; Pommier, B.; Mauborgne, A.; Pohl, M. JAK/STAT3 pathway is activated in spinal cord microglia after peripheral nerve injury and contributes to neuropathic pain development in rat. *J. Neurochem.* **2008**, *107*, 50–60. [CrossRef] [PubMed]
21. Wigerblad, G.; Bas, D.B.; Fernades-Cerqueira, C.; Krishnamurthy, A.; Nandakumar, K.S.; Rogoz, K.; Kato, J.; Sandor, K.; Su, J.; Jimenez–Andrade, J.M.; et al. Autoantibodies to citrullinated proteins induce joint pain independent of inflammation via chemokine-dependent mechanism. *Ann. Rheum. Dis.* **2016**, *74*, 730–738. [CrossRef]
22. Augustsson, J.; Neovius, M.; Cullinane-Carli, C.; Eksborg, S.; van Vollenhoven, R.F. Patients with rheumatoid arthritis treated with tumour necrosis factor antagonists increase their participation in the workforce: Potential for significant long-term indirect cost gains (data from a population-based registry). *Ann. Rheum. Dis.* **2010**, *69*, 126–131. [CrossRef] [PubMed]
23. Taylor, P.C.; Moore, A.; Vasilescu, R.; Alvir, J.; Tarallo, M. A structured literature review of the burden of illness and unmet needs in patients with rheumatoid arthritis: A current perspective. *Rheumatol. Int.* **2016**, *36*, 685–695. [CrossRef] [PubMed]
24. Michaud, K.; Pope, J.; Emery, P.; Zhu, B.; Gaich, C.; DeLozier, A.M.; Zhang, X.; Dickson, C.; Smolen, J.S. Relative impact of pain and fatigue on work productivity in patients with rheumatoid arthritis from the RA-BEAM baricitinib trial. *Rheumatol. Ther.* **2019**, in press.

12

Current Therapeutic Options in the Treatment of Rheumatoid Arthritis

Birgit M. Köhler, Janine Günther, Dorothee Kaudewitz and Hanns-Martin Lorenz *

Internal Medicine 5, Division of Rheumatology, University Hospital Heidelberg, 69120 Heidelberg, Germany
* Correspondence: Hannes.Lorenz@med.uni-heidelberg.de

Abstract: Rheumatoid arthritis (RA) is a systemic autoimmune disease characterized by chronic inflammation of the joints. Untreated RA leads to a destruction of joints through the erosion of cartilage and bone. The loss of physical function is the consequence. Early treatment is important to control disease activity and to prevent joint destruction. Nowadays, different classes of drugs with different modes of action are available to control the inflammation and to achieve remission. In this review, we want to discuss differences and similarities of these different drugs.

Keywords: Rheumatoid Arthritis; therapy; DMARD; MTX; Tumor Necrosis Factor-Alpha Inhibitors

1. Introduction

Rheumatoid Arthritis (RA) is an autoimmune disease characterized by chronic inflammation of the synovial membrane. Untreated RA can lead to progressive joint destruction, resulting in disability, poor quality of life, and increased mortality. About 1% of the population is affected, and the disease onset generally occurs between 30 years and 50 years of age, with a higher incidence in women.

The therapy is complex and includes different classes of drugs with different routes of application but also nonpharmacologic interventions. The most important are patient education followed by exercise and physical and occupational therapy. Because of an increased risk of coronary atherosclerosis, efforts should be made to reduce risk factors such as smoking, hyperlipidemia, hypertension, and obesity.

To relieve pain and swelling fast and to gain control of the inflammation, glucocorticoids (GC) are used widely in acute disease flares either orally or as intraarticular injections. Oral GC is for short-term use (up to 3–4 month) only and should be tapered to prevent side effects as soon as possible [1]. To control inflammation in the long run, Disease Modifying Anti-Rheumatic Drugs (DMARD) to spare GC are needed. Nowadays, there are a bunch of opportunities that can be challenges or chances.

The treatment of patients with RA aims to relieve pain and to control inflammation, and the final goal is to achieve remission or at least low disease activity for all patients. In this context, the European League Against Rheumatism (EULAR) has composed 10 international recommendations on how to treat patients [2]. An algorithm based on the EULAR recommendations is shown in Figure 1. In 2010, an international committee developed the treat-to-target (T2T) initiative. The centerpiece of this initiative is the shared decision-making and regular patient revaluation that targets remission or at least low disease activity (LDA) [3].

By now, there is evidence from different studies that the T2T principle is superior, and it forms part of the treatment guidelines of the European League Against Rheumatism and the American College of Rheumatology. The core principles of T2T are shown in Table 1. Even more important is that an early start of therapy is required in order to achieve optimal outcomes.

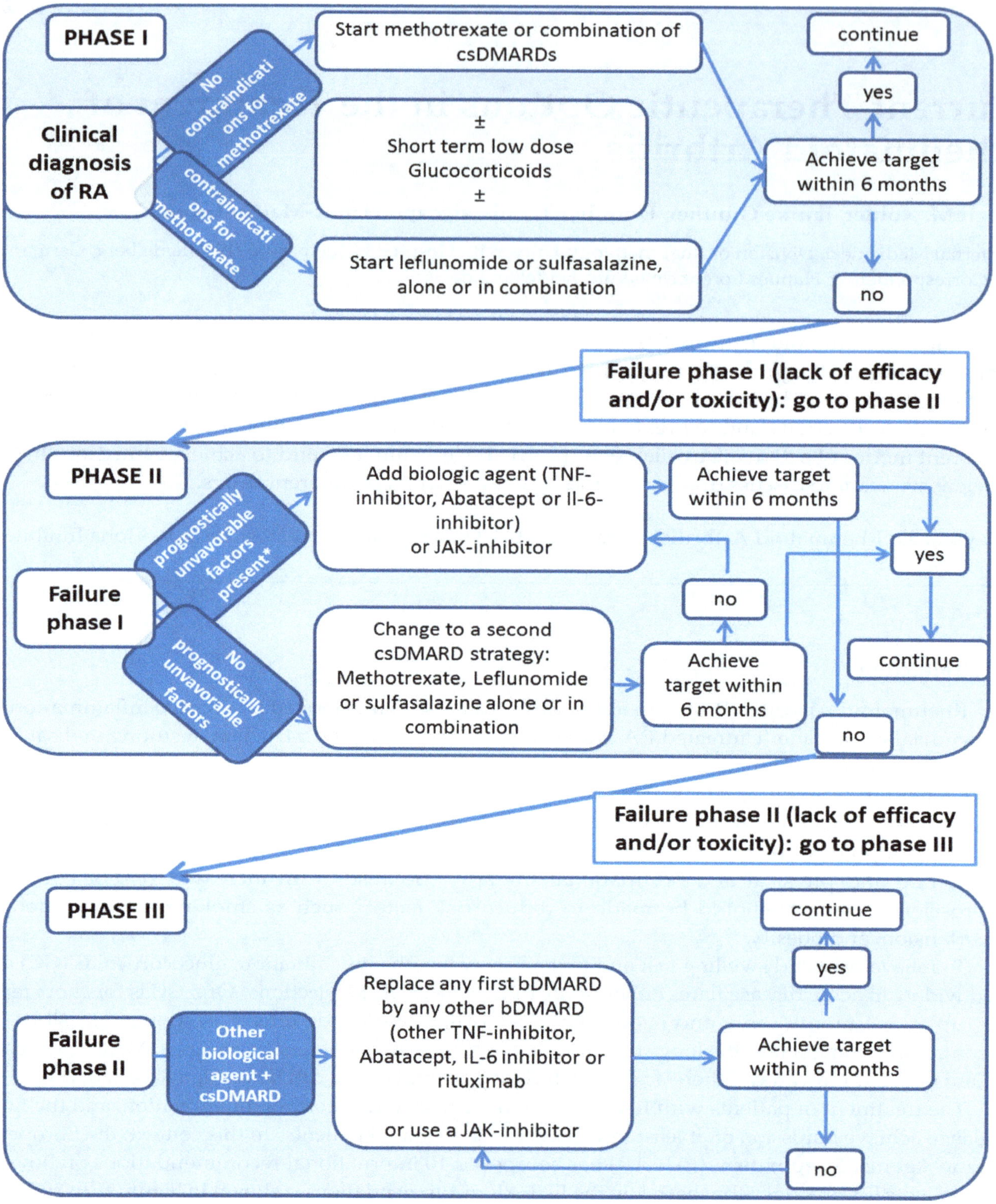

Figure 1. Algorithm adapted from the 2016 European League Against Rheumatism (EULAR) recommendationson rheumatoid arthritis (RA) management. bDMARD, biological; bsDMARD, biosimilar DMARDs; csDMARDs, conventional synthetic DMARDs; DMARDs disease modifying amtirheumatic drug; IL, Interleukin; MTX, methotrexate; TNF, tumor necrosis factor; tsDMARDs, targeted synthetic DMARDS.

Table 1. Overarching principles of the T2T strategy (modified after Smolen J.S., et al. Ann Rheum Dis 2016;75:3–15). [3].

	Overarching Principles of the T2T Strategy
1	Basis for the treatment is a shared decision making between patient and doctor
2	Major treatment goals are: maximization of quality of life, normalisation of function and participation in social and professional life
3	The elimination of inflammation is essential to achieve the treatment goals
4	Outcomes in rheumatoid arthritis are improved by implementing T2T

2. Treatment Guidelines: Conventional Synthetic DMARD (csDMARD)

As soon as the diagnosis of rheumatoid arthritis is made, a treatment with a csDMARD should be started [4].

A controlled comparison between csDMARDs for the first-line therapy does not exist; however, within this group, methotrexate should be the first choice because, for this drug, most clinical experience exists in monotherapy and as a combination partner with other DMARDs [5]. Methotrexate is usually started at a dose of 15 mg/week and can be stepwise increased up to 25 mg/week. The combination with glucocorticoids is recommended [3]. Due to the decreased bioavailability, a subcutaneous way of administration is recommended [5].

The induction of remission with a combination of conventional synthetic DMARDs at this stage is not superior to methotrexate monotherapy; however, these combinations are associated with more adverse events and a higher rate of drug discontinuation [4,6]. Patients with a higher baseline disease activity and Rheumatoid factor (RF)-positive patients have an increased risk of methotrexate (MTX) failure due to inefficacy [6].

If MTX cannot be used, e.g., due to intolerance or contraindications, leflunomide (20 mg/week) or sulfasalazine (2 g/day) should be started. In a placebo-controlled randomized controlled trial (RCT), both substances showed a similar efficacy [7].

If by week 12 after the start of MTX therapy no adequate response is achieved or no remission is reached with optimum doses after 24 weeks, the therapy should be adjusted [5]. To find the best individual treatment strategy, patients should be categorized using prognostic markers. Poor prognostic markers such as the presence of autoantibodies, early joint damage, and high disease activity are associated with rapid disease progression; therefore, a biologic DMARD or a targeted synthetic DMARD should be added at this stage [4]. In the absence of poor prognostic markers and with moderate disease activity, a second csDMARD should be added to the therapy [5].

2.1. MTX

Unlike targeted DMARDs, conventional synthetic DMARDs came into clinical practice based on empiric observations and their mechanisms of action are still incompletely understood [4].

The mode of action of high-dose methotrexate via the depletion of thymidine and purine residues and cell-cycle arrest at S1 are well-known [8]. However, this mechanism does not seem to play a major role in the clinical effect of low-dose MTX, as folate co-therapy does not result in a loss of clinical benefit. Methotrexate has pleiotropic therapeutic effects on various immune cells and mediators, resulting in an overall dampening of the inflammatory response. The main mode of action of low-dose MTX in rheumatoid arthritis is thought to be via the potentiation of adenosine signaling. Adenosine acts as a paracrine signaling agent via four distinct purinergic G-protein-coupled receptors, which in rheumatoid arthritis are overexpressed. In addition to downregulating the production of tumor necrosis factor (TNF) and NF-kB, adenosine might be one of the main mediators of the downregulation of the activation and proliferation of T-lymphocytes, creating an immunotolerant environment [8].

Side effects of MTX are usually dependent on dose, mode of application, and duration of methotrexate therapy. Unlike high-dose MTX, the side effects of low-dose MTX are rarely life-threatening and can often be relieved by substituting folate. Common side effects of low-dose MTX are hematologic abnormalities (thrombocytopenia and leucopenia), stomatitis, gastrointestinal problems (e.g., anorexia, loose stools, nausea, or stomach upset), elevation of liver enzymes, or central nervous system symptoms like fatigue or headache [9]. The substitution of folate significantly lowers the risk for side effects like hepatotoxicity (relative risk reduction of 77%) and decreases the number of serious adverse events (by 61%) [5,10]. If side effects occur, substituting folate acid regularly and gradually increasing the dose up to 5 mg daily can help to control the symptoms. Overall, fewer than 5% of patients have to stop using methotrexate because of adverse events [4].

MTX therapy can, in many cases, be safely continued perioperatively; however, a potentially decreased kidney function in this setting should be taken into account. In addition, to decrease the risk of pneumonia, the treatment should be paused if pulmonary comorbidities exist. At high doses (25 mg/week), a temporary dose reduction should be considered [11].

MTX exposure during pregnancy can induce multiple congenital deformities. Therefore, MTX therapy during pregnancy is not recommended. MTX should be withdrawn prophylactically 3 months before conception. Daily folate supplementation should be continued antenatal and throughout pregnancy. At the present stage of knowledge, it is not clear whether MTX transiently influences male fertility and sperm DNA integrity [12].

2.2. *Leflunomide*

The primary mechanism of action of leflunomide (LEF) is the reversible inhibition of the mitochondrial enzyme dihydroorotate dehydrogenase (DHODH), the rate limiting step in the de novo synthesis of pyrimidines. Activated lymphocytes expand their pyrimidine pool by approximately eightfold during proliferation. Therefore, the inhibition of DHODH prevents activated lymphocytes from moving from G1 to the S phase, hence triggering apoptosis [13]. The leflunomide effect seems to be rather lymphocyte-specific on other cells, can reuptake pyrimidines, and can thereby overcome the DHODH blockade.

The rate of discontinuation due to side effects is similar with methotrexate [14]. Potential side effects include diarrhea and nausea as well as the elevation of liver enzymes. The changes in liver function are generally reversible with dose reduction or a discontinuation of the drug, but in rare cases, hepatotoxicity can be severe. However, transaminase elevation mainly occurs if other comorbidities contributing to hepatotoxicity, e.g., concomitant non-steroidal anti-inflammatory drugs (NSAID) or MTX therapy, previous or concurrent alcohol abuse, or viral or autoimmune hepatitis, are present [15]. A small percentage of patients with RA develop hypertension when taking LEF; therefore, blood pressure monitoring is recommended during treatment [14].

The active metabolite of leflunomide is detectable in plasma until 2 years after the discontinuation of the drug; therefore, a discontinuation of leflunomide perioperatively is generally not recommended. Only at a high risk of infection or if a greater intervention is planned, a wash out with cholestyramine should be initiated as recommended [11].

Leflunomide is contraindicated during pregnancy. Safe contraception during therapy in both women and men is recommended. Before conception, leflunomide must be withdrawn and a washout should be carried out until the drug is undetectable in the blood [12].

2.3. *Sulfasalazine*

Sulfasalazine SSZ was specifically designed in 1938 for the treatment of rheumatoid arthritis. The idea behind the drug was to combine an antibacterial and an anti-inflammatory agent [16]. Sulfasalazine is effective in the treatment of rheumatoid arthritis; however, the mode of action is incompletely understood. The main pharmacological effects of SSZ include effects on the gut bacterial flora, on inflammatory cell functions, and on immunological processes [16]. Several plausible mechanisms of action have been observed in vitro, such as the inhibition of NF-kB and osteoclast formation via modulatory effects on the receptor activators of NF-kB (RANK), osteoprotegerin (OPG), and RANK-ligand. In addition, SASP can inhibit tumor necrosis factor (TNF)-alpha expression and may reduce the secretion of inflammatory cytokines such as interleukin (IL)-8 as well as may suppress B-cell function [17]. An additional mechanism that has been suggested is the increased production of adenosine at sites of inflammation similar to the mode of action of methotrexate.

Adverse reactions, including idiosyncratic (e.g., hypersensitivity-/immune-related) and dose-related effects, are common with sulfasalazine, especially gastrointestinal, central nervous system, cutaneous, and hematologic adverse effects. The withdrawal rate for adverse events is about 25%, two thirds of which are due to gastrointestinal and central nervous system toxicity. If dose-related side effects occur, treatment can be paused for a week and after a resolution of the symptoms, the treatment can be restarted at a lower dose [18]. However, if idiosyncratic effects like skin reactions, hepatitis, pneumonitis, or hematologic side effects like agranulocytosis and hemolytic anemia occur, immediate discontinuation of the drug is necessary; patients with this type of adverse effect should not be rechallenged with the drug [18].

As sulfasalazine only has a short half-life of about 4–5 h and only a minimal immunosuppressive effect, it can usually be continued perioperatively. If there is a risk of interaction or a potential additive hepatotoxic effect with medication used preoperatively, sulfasalazine can be paused on the day of the operation [11].

If treatment of rheumatoid arthritis is required during pregnancy, SSZ is an acceptable therapeutic option, as the continuation of SSZ during pregnancy is very unlikely to cause fetal harm [12,19]. To increase safety, a concomitant folate supplementation before and throughout pregnancy is advised and the dose of SSZ should not exceed 2 g per day to prevent neutropenia in the newborns. SSZ can cause reduced male fertility; however, spermatogenesis recovers at about 2–3 months after a withdrawal of the drug [12].

3. Biologic DMARDs (bDMARD)

According the EULAR guidelines, a bDMARD should be considered if remission or LDA is not achieved with the first DMARD strategy, if poor prognostic factors (i.e., high acute phase reactant levels, high swollen joint counts, or the presence of early erosions) exist, or if the patient responds inadequately to MTX and/or other csDMARD strategies.

Before starting a therapy with bDMARD, active or latent infections with hepatitis or tuberculosis must be ruled out. Patients, if possible, should be brought up to date with all immunizations before initiating therapy. Blood cell counts and liver and kidney function also need to be evaluated prior to treatment.

3.1. Tumor Necrosis Factor-Alpha Inhibitors (TNFi)

Until now, five TNFi were available. Although all anti-TNF drugs bind TNF-α, there are differences in their molecular structures, their administration regimens, and their modes of action.

The first preclinical studies using antibodies against TNF- α were performed in animal models of sepsis in 1985. About 6 years later, Keffer et al. provided the first evidence that TNF plays a role in developing arthritis [20]. In 1994, *The Lancet* published the first RCT showing that the blockade of a specific cytokine can be an effective treatment in patients with rheumatoid arthritis [21]. Since then, antibodies against TNF-alpha have gotten an important cornerstone in the treatment of RA and changed the lives of our patients.

Nowadays, we could not think of a world without antibodies against TNF-α or other cytokines. For our patients, this changed the game.

The first TNF-α-inhibitor, approved in 2000 for the therapy of RA, was the chimeric murine/human IgG1 monoclonal antibody Infliximab (IFX) that binds to both soluble and membrane-bound TNF-α [21]. The administration is intravenous every 8 weeks at a dosage between 3–5 mg/kg. Another TNF-inhibitor also approved in 2000 is Etanercept (ETN), a recombinant fusion protein compound of the soluble TNF-alpha receptor linked to the Fc portion of human IgG. ETN binds to the TNF receptor, preventing

TNF-mediated cellular responses. ETN is administered subcutaneously at a dose of 25 mg twice a week or 50 mg weekly [22,23]. The third inhibitor approved in 2003 by the European Medicines Agency (EMA) is Adalimumab (ADA) [24]. It is a recombinant human IgG1 monoclonal antibody that binds to soluble and membrane-bound TNF-α with a high affinity. It is administered by subcutaneous injection once every 2 weeks. Golimumab (GOL) is a human IgG1 monoclonal antibody neutralizing both soluble and membrane-bound TNF-α. GOL was approved in 2010 and is administered as a subcutaneous injection at an initial dose of 50 mg every 4 weeks that can be increased to 100 mg if there is no response after 4 doses (in patients with a body weight > 100 kg) [25]. Certolizumab Pegol (CZP) was approved by the EMA in 2007. CZP is a recombinant humanized Fab' fragment of a TNF antibody coupled to polyethylene glycol (PEG) that prolongs its plasma half-life to approximately 2 weeks. It has an initial loading dose of 400 mg every 2 weeks for 6 weeks, followed by 200 mg every 2 weeks [26,27].

Only certolizumab, adalimumab, and etanercept are approved as monotherapy as well as in combination with methotrexate [27–31].

Adverse effects include skin reactions characterized by itching, pain, and redness at the site of medication injection. Such injection site reactions characteristically occur during the first weeks of treatment. For intravenously administered agents, acute infusion reactions can occur with hypotension, bronchospasm, wheezing, and/or urticaria. Acute reactions may, in some cases, represent immunoglobulin-E-mediated type I reactions. The majority of acute infusion reactions that occur are anaphylactoid reactions and not immunoglobulin E mediated. These reactions can be managed by just reducing the rate of infusion [32,33].

However, delayed infusion reactions can also occur, and they are associated with skin rash, diffuse joint pains, myalgia, and fatigue and sometimes accompanied by fever. Delayed reactions may represent mild type III (immune complex-mediated) reactions [34]. It has been shown that the formation of Anti-monoclonal antibodies may lead to a greater risk of infusion reactions and also may limit the long-term efficacy of the drug. It has also been shown that the use of concomitant immunomodulators prior to starting a TNF-α-inhibitor is effective in reducing antibody production and therefore decreasing immunogenicity [32,34].

As TNF-alpha is a key player of the immune system during infections, this treatment has been associated with an increased risk of serious infections. These include bacterial infections (particularly pneumonia), herpes zoster, tuberculosis, and opportunistic infections [35]. As mentioned above, screening for latent tuberculosis infections should be performed before the initiation of TNF-alpha inhibitor therapy. If there is an indication of latent tuberculosis, a treatment for latent tuberculosis should be initiated before starting therapy with a TNF-alpha inhibitor [36]. Another side effect occurring in a few cases is neutropenia. Other cytopenias are uncommon [37]. The association between TNF-alpha inhibitors and demyelinating diseases remains uncertain. However, anti-TNF-alpha agents should generally be avoided in patients with established diseases that are associated with demyelination and should be discontinued directly in any patient with suspected demyelination [38]. Treating patients with NYHA III or IV cardiac failure is not recommended [2,39]. However, data regarding cardiac failure in patients treated with anti-TNF-alpha agents are inconclusive [40]. While Kwon et al. reported 38 patients who developed new-onset heart failure and 9 patients who experienced heart failure exacerbation after therapy [39], others report a reduced risk of cardiovascular events in patients treated with TNF-alpha inhibitors [40].

Pregnancy

Observational studies and case reports of women exposed to TNF inhibitors during pregnancy suggest that their pregnancy outcomes, including rates of preterm birth, spontaneous miscarriage, and congenital anomalies, are similar to those in women with RA who have not received a TNFi [41].

Complete immunoglobulin G (IgG) antibodies—maternal as well as therapeutic—cross placenta via active transport facilitated by the neonatal fragment crystallizable (Fc) receptor on the placenta.

IgG1 is the most effectively transported of the four subclasses of IgG (G1–G4) [42]. This is relevant to adalimumab, golimumab, and infliximab which are complete IgG1 anti-TNF. Etanercept is comprised of the Fc domain of human IgG1 fused with the extracellular ligand binding domain of human tumor necrosis factor receptor-2. Transplacental transport via the neonatal Fc receptor would theoretically be plausible. In contrast to the complete IgG1 anti-TNF antibodies certolizumab pegol differs structurally as it is a humanized PEG (polyethylene glycol)-ylated antibody Fab′ fragment lacking the IgG1 Fc portion. Without the Fc portion it should, in theory, not be transported actively across the placenta [43]. So passive diffusion would be the only option for any detectable concentrations in exposed infants. This was shown in two trials. Based on these trials the EMA has approved a label change for CZP, making it the first anti-TNF for potential use in women with chronic rheumatic disease during both pregnancy and breastfeeding [44].

TNFi may have different structures, morphology, pharmacokinetic properties, and activity, but their clinical efficiency is comparable. If drug survival and safety are similar or different is still a matter of debate.

3.2. Interleukin 1 Inhibitor

Anakinra was first approved in the US in 2001 and in Europe in March 2002. It is a recombinant human IL-1 receptor antagonist with a short half-life (4–6 h), administered subcutaneously at a dose of 100 mg once a day. It was first developed for use in RA and showed some effects in early trials. A big systematic review of the literature in 2009 showed only a moderate effectiveness [45,46]. Anakinra plays not a very great role in RA therapy; today, it is much more effective in the therapy of auto-inflammatory diseases, gout, or polyserositis [45–50].

Adverse effects include injection site reactions characterized by itching, pain, and redness at the site of medication injection and lasting days to weeks. Between one and ten percent of people have severe infections, decreased white blood cells, or decreased platelets [51].

Pregnancy

There have been no adequate studies for the safety of Anakinra in Pregnancy, although several case reports of women with adult-onset Still's disease treated through pregnancy resulted in healthy neonates [52].

4. Interleukin 6 and Interleukin 6 Receptor Inhibitors

Interleukin-6 (IL-6) was identified in 1986 as a key cytokine in the pathogenesis of RA with proinflammatory activity. It is able to enhance the production of acute-phase proteins involved in the systemic inflammation process. Tocilizumab (TCZ) is the first humanized recombinant IgG1monoclonal antibody that binds to both the soluble and membrane-bound IL-6 receptor, blocking its action and leading to the decrease of the inflammatory response cascade. Its half-life (10–13 days) allows its administration intravenously (8 mg/kg) every 4 weeks. A subcutaneous formulation of TCZ (162 mg/week) has been approved, with an efficacy and safety profile comparable to intravenous administration [52,53]. A second agent, Sarilumab is a human immunoglobulin G1 anti-interleukin-6 (IL-6) receptor monoclonal antibody that blocks IL-6 from binding to membrane-bound and soluble IL-6 receptor alpha [54].

Events of gastrointestinal (GI) perforations have been reported in Phase III clinical trials, primarily as complications of diverticulitis, including generalized purulent peritonitis, lower GI perforation, fistula, and abscess. Tocilizumab or Sarilumab should be used with caution in patients who may be at increased risk for GI perforation. Patients presenting with new-onset abdominal symptoms should be evaluated promptly for the early identification of GI perforation. It is important to keep in mind that, during IL-6 blockade, C-reactive protein or other acute phase reactants will increase slowly and less pronounced [55,56].

Other side effects are neutropenia or thrombocytopenia as well as hyperlipidemia. Also, serious infections and liver enzyme elevations were observed and can require dose adjustments or drug discontinuation [56].

4.1. Pregnancy

Based upon animal data, tocilizumab may cause fetal harm, but there are no adequate studies of its effects on human pregnancy to allow an assessment of its risk. There are a few case series available. No teratogenic effects were observed. In a case series of 50 pregnancies exposed to tocilizumab with known outcomes, 36 resulted in live births, while there were five low-birthweight infants born and one case of neonatal asphyxia [57,58].

4.2. CD80/86-CD 28 Inhibitor

Abatacept is a fusion protein constituted by an immunoglobulin fused to the extracellular domain of cytotoxic T-lymphocyte antigen 4 (CTLA-4). This is a molecule that binds with a high affinity to the CD80/86 ligand on antigen-presenting cells. Therefore, abatacept is able to block the interaction between the antigen-presenting cell's CD80/86 ligand and the CD28 ligand on the T cell [59]. This results in decreased T cell proliferation and cytokine production. Abatacept is administered intravenously once every 4 weeks or subcutaneously once a week [60,61].

Adverse effects including cases of hypersensitivity and anaphylaxis or anaphylactoid reactions have been reported with iv administration. As in other bDMARDs, serious infections (including tuberculosis and sepsis) have been reported, particularly in patients receiving concomitant immunosuppressive therapy [59].

The use of CTLA-4 Inhibitors due to its T cell inhibition affect defenses against malignancies. As compared to the general population, an increased risk of lymphoma has been noted in clinical trials; however, rheumatoid arthritis has been previously associated with an increased rate of lymphoma. Abatacept itself seems not to further increase this risk [62].

Pregnancy

Abatacept is not teratogenic in animals, but there are no adequate studies of its effects on human pregnancy to allow an assessment of its risk.

5. Anti-CD 20 Antibody

Rituximab (RTX) was initially developed for the treatment of hematologic malignancies. Since 2006, RTX is approved for the therapy of RA refractory to a combination therapy of anti-TNF-alpha, an MTX [60]. RTX is a chimeric murine-human monoclonal antibody that binds to the CD20 membrane receptor, leading to the depletion of circulating B cells. It is also able to inhibit the activation of T cells that produce proinflammatory cytokines. A cycle of RTX consists in 1000 mg by intravenous infusion, followed by a second 1000-mg intravenous infusion two weeks later. This is then repeated every 6 months. Different studies showed that particularly patients who are autoantibody-positive benefit from RTX [63,64].

According to results of different studies, patients benefit more from switching to RTX when an initial TNFi was discontinued due to inefficacy.

One of the common side effects is an infusion reaction especially during the first infusion, occurring in up to 30 to 45 percent of patients. Symptoms include headache, fever, skin rash, dyspnea, hypotension, nausea, rhinitis, pruritus, and mild angioedema [65].

Repeated courses of RTX are associated with an increasing risk of hypogammaglobinemia. A meta-analysis in 2009 found no increase in serious infections associated with the use of rituximab with or without MTX compared with MTX plus a placebo, but other studies have found that repeated courses may be associated with a higher rate of serious infections. The risk of serious infections seems to increase with age [65].

Pregnancy

There is only limited information about the use of RTX during pregnancy. Rituximab has been detected in high concentrations in umbilical cord blood. There are case reports available, but in most cases, the mother took RTX due to hematologic malignancies. Congenital anomalies were not reported. As for all babies indirectly exposed to immunosuppressant biologics during pregnancy, immunization with live vaccines should be postponed until the age of 6 months [66].

6. Targeted Synthetic DMARDS: JAK-Inhibitors

Recently, with the Janus–Kinase (JAK) Inhibitors, a new group of drugs for the treatment of rheumatoid arthritis was introduced. These targeted, synthetic DMARDS (tsDMARDS) are effective in inflammatory diseases by intracellularly blocking tyrosine kinase [67].

The JAK are cytoplasmic protein tyrosine kinases that are critical for signal transduction to the nucleus from the common gamma chain of the plasma membrane receptors for interleukin (IL)-2, -4, -7, -9, -15, and -21. JAK are receptor-associated intracellular proteins, with a tyrosine-kinase component. They are important downstream mediators of many pro-inflammatory cytokines, e.g., interferons or interleukin 6. Once a ligand binds to its receptor, the intracellular kinase is phosphorylated, which further leads to the phosphorylation and activation of the signal transducer and activator of transcription (STAT)-pathway. Accordingly, blocking these enzymes with a targeted molecule affects multiple inflammatory pathways [65,66]. How JAKs transmit signals from cytokines and thereby activates gene transcription is shown in Figure 2.

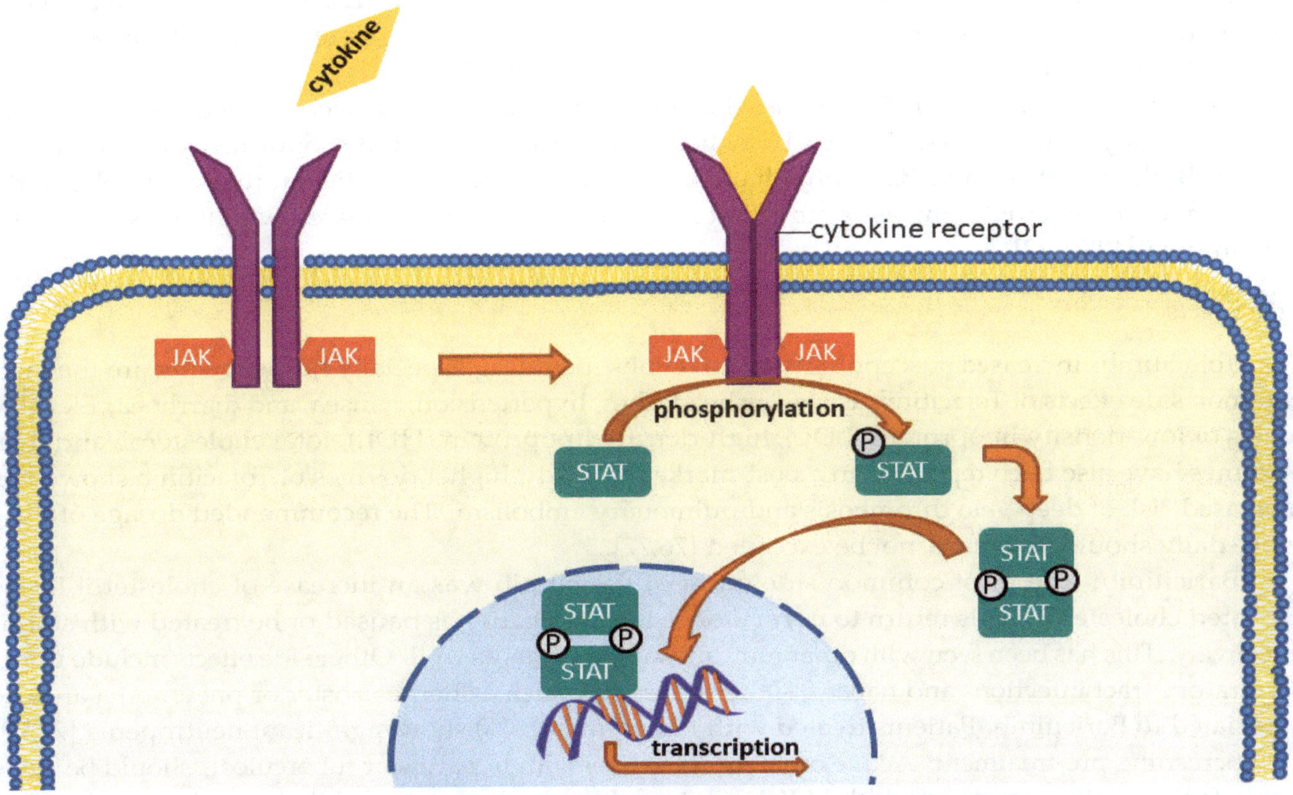

Figure 2. Cytokines bind to the receptors, which then undergo a change in their configuration into a dimeric structure, thereby activating their ability to work as a kinase. Consequently, they phosphorylate the STAT molecules (Signal Transducer and Activator of Transcription). Phosphorylated STATs also form dimeres that travel to the cell core, where they activate transcription processes, which further fuel inflammatory processes.

Pharmacological aspects: JAK-inhibitors are referred to as small molecules, meaning that these compounds carry a low molecular weight and bind to a macromolecular target, altering their activity and function [68,69].

To date, two JAK-inhibitors are approved for therapeutic use in rheumatoid arthritis: Tofacitinib and Baricitinib.

Tofacitinib was approved by the FDA (Food and Drug Administration) in the US in 2012. In 2017, the European Medicines Agency (EMA) approved the drug for use in the European Union. Tofacitinib is an inhibitor of JAK 1 and 3, with only little affinity to JAK 2 and Tyrosine-Kinase 2. It has been shown effective in moderate and severe rheumatoid arthritis in monotherapy or in combination with methotrexate. Several phase III clinical trials showed efficacy in DMARD naïve patients as well as in patients with insufficient responses to csDMARDs and even bDMARDS. Tofacitinib is taken orally twice daily with a dosage of 5 mg. The elimination is mostly hepatic; therefore, an adaption to impaired kidney function is not necessary up to a GFR > 30 mL/min. Consequently, the treatment of patients with end-stage renal failure with a GFR < 30 mL/min with Tofacitinib is possible with reduced dosage [70,71].

The second JAK-inhibitor currently approved is Baricitinib which is an inhibitor of JAK 1 and 2. It was approved by the FDA as well as the EMA in 2017. Baricitinib can be administered as monotherapy or in combination with methotrexate. Several phase III clinical trials showed efficacy in the treatment of DMARD naïve patients as well as in patients with insufficient responses to csDMARDS or even bDMARDS [72–75].

Baricitinib is taken orally once daily. There are two dosages available: 4 mg or 2 mg. The elimination for Baricitinib is mostly renal, which makes it necessary to reduce the dosage for patients with impaired kidney function (estimated GFR 30–60 mL/min) from 4 mg to 2 mg daily. For patients with an estimated GFR < 30 mL/min, the use of Baricitinib is not recommended [2].

According to the EULAR-Guidelines, both JAK-Inhibitors can be used in rheumatoid arthritis once a therapy with csDMARDs has been insufficient or had to be discontinued due to adverse events. Both Tofacitinib and Baricitinib have been shown to be more efficient than a placebo in the treatment of rheumatoid arthritisl; both could show non-inferiority compared with the TNF-inhibitor Adalimumab [2,71,73].

Side Effects

Tofacitinib: Increased susceptibility to infections including especially herpes zoster are the most common side effects of Tofacitinib as well as headaches, hypertension, nausea, and diarrhoea. Elevated levels of low-density lipoprotein (LDL), high-density lipoprotein (HDL), total cholesterol, and liver enzymes have also been reported. In a post-marketing study, higher dosages of Tofacitinib showed an increased risk of deep vein thrombosis and pulmonary embolism. The recommended dosage of 5 mg twice daily should, therefore, not be exceeded [76,77].

Baricitinib: The most common side effect of Baricitinib was an increase of cholesterol levels. Elevated cholesterol levels return to normal once the medication is paused or be treated with statins effectively. This has been seen with other immunosuppressants as well. Other side effects include upper respiratory tract infections and nausea. Other infections, such as herpes zoster or pneumonia are also associated to Baricitinib. Patients treated with Baricitinib (0.3%) show significant neutropenia [78,79].

Screening pre-treatment: Active or latent infections with hepatitis or tuberculosis should be ruled out before initiating treatment with JAK-inhibitors. Blood cell counts and liver and kidney function also need to be evaluated prior to treatment.

Screening during treatment: neutrophil levels, lymphocyte levels, hemoglobin, and kidney and liver function should be screened; 8–12 weeks after the initiation of treatment, HDL, LDL, overall cholesterol, and triglycerides should also be screened.

Contraindications: JAK-inhibitors should not be prescribed for patients with neutropenia (<1/nL), active tuberculosis or severe infections, or severe liver impairment and during pregnancy.

A combination with other bDMARDs or strong immunodepressants as azathioprine, cyclosporine, or tacrolimus should be avoided due to the elevated risk of infection and the lack of experience.

Use during Pregnancy: drugs from the JAK-inhibitor family have not been tested in pregnant women yet. As both drugs are small molecules, it seems likely that cross the placenta. Women taking JAK-inhibitors should be instructed to use safe contraceptive methods throughout the treatment and up to one week (Baricitinib) to four weeks (Tofacitinib) after a discontinuation of the drug.

Perioperative management: Although there are not enough long-term data for a conclusive recommendation on perioperative management, JAK-inhibitors in general have a short elimination-time. It therefore seems possible to continue treatment until shortly before surgery. The therapy should then be paused until proper wound-healing is achieved.

Ongoing development: Two selective JAK-1-Inhibitors are currently undergoing Phase 3 trials for clinical approval: Upadacitinib and Filgotinib. Both drugs show promising results in terms of efficacy and safety. Another JAK-inhibitor currently being evaluated in Phase 3 trials is the selective JAK-3-Inhibitor Peficitinib, with limited data available so far [80,81].

7. Conclusions

The therapeutic strategies of RA have improved dramatically over the past 3 decades. At that time, only a few drugs were available and therapy started late in disease course. With the T2T strategy and the possibility to choose from different mode of actions, the aim of stable remission can be reached and joint destruction can be prevented. Equally important to the choice of drugs is to diagnose the disease early and to start therapy within 6–12 weeks after disease onset. Early arthritis clinics headed by experienced rheumatologists are a good tool to achieve this. T2T further improves the prognosis of RA.

Author Contributions: Concept—H.-M.L., B.M.K., J.G. and D.K. Design—B.M.K., J.G. and D.K. Supervision—H.-M.L.; Literature Search—B.M.K., J.G. and D.K.; Writing Manuscript—B.M.K., J.G. and D.K.; Critical Review—H.-M.L. All authors read and approved the final manuscript.

References

1. Hoes, J.N.; Jacobs, J.W.G.; Boers, M.; Boumpas, D.; Buttgereit, F.; Caeyers, N.; Choy, E.H.; Cutolo, M.; Silva, J.A.P.D.; Esselens, G.; et al. EULAR evidence-based recommendations on the management of systemic glucocorticoid therapy in rheumatic diseases. *Ann. Rheum. Dis.* **2007**, *66*, 1560–1567. [CrossRef] [PubMed]
2. Smolen, J.S.; Landewe, R.; Breedveld, F.C.; Buch, M.; Burmester, G.; Dougados, M.; Emery, P.; Gaujoux-Viala, C.; Gossec, L.; Nam, J.; et al. EULAR recommendations for the management of rheumatoid arthritis with synthetic and biological disease-modifying antirheumatic drugs: 2013 update. *Ann. Rheum. Dis.* **2014**, *73*, 492–509. [CrossRef] [PubMed]
3. Smolen, J.S.; Breedveld, F.C.; Burmester, G.R.; Bykerk, V.; Dougados, M.; Emery, P.; Kvien, T.K.; Navarro-Compan, M.V.; Oliver, S.; Schoels, M.; et al. Treating rheumatoid arthritis to target: 2014 update of the recommendations of an international task force. *Ann. Rheum. Dis.* **2016**, *75*, 3–15. [CrossRef] [PubMed]
4. Aletaha, D.; Smolen, J.S. Diagnosis and management of rheumatoid arthritis: A review. *JAMA* **2018**, *320*, 1360–1372. [CrossRef] [PubMed]
5. Fiehn, C.; Holle, J.; Iking-Konert, C.; Leipe, J.; Weseloh, C.; Frerix, M.; Alten, R.; Behrens, F.; Baerwald, C.; Braun, J.; et al. S2e guideline: Treatment of rheumatoid arthritis with disease-modifying drugs. *Z. Rheumatol.* **2018**, *77*, 3553.
6. Verschueren, P.; De Cock, D.; Corluy, L.; Joos, R.; Langenaken, C.; Taelman, V.; Raeman, F.; Ravelingien, I.; Vandevyvere, K.; Lenaerts, J.; et al. Effectiveness of methotrexate with step-down glucocorticoid remission induction (COBRA Slim) versus other intensive treatment strategies for early rheumatoid arthritis in a treat-to-target approach: 1-year results of CareRA, a randomised pragmatic open-label superiority trial. *Ann. Rheum. Dis.* **2017**, *76*, 511–520. [PubMed]

7. Smolen, J.S.; Kalden, J.R.; Scott, D.L.; Rozman, B.; Kvien, T.K.; Larsen, A.; Loew-Friedrich, I.; Oed, C.; Rosenburg, R. Efficacy and safety of leflunomide compared with placebo and sulphasalazine in active rheumatoid arthritis: A double-blind, randomised, multicentre trial. *Lancet* **1999**, *353*, 259–266. [CrossRef]
8. Brown, P.M.; Pratt, A.G.; Isaacs, J.D. Mechanism of action of methotrexate in rheumatoid arthritis, and the search for biomarkers. *Nat. Rev. Rheumatol.* **2016**, *12*, 731–742. [CrossRef]
9. Kremer, J.M. Major Side Effects of Low-Dose Methotrexate. Available online: www.UpToDate.com (accessed on 2 April 2019).
10. Shea, B.; Swinden, M.V.; Ghogomu, E.T.; Ortiz, Z.; Katchamart, W.; Rader, T.; Bombardier, C.; A Wells, G.; Tugwell, P. Folic acid and folinic acid for reducing side effects in patients receiving methotrexate for rheumatoid arthritis. *Cochrane Database Syst. Rev.* **2013**, CD000951. [CrossRef]
11. Kruger, K.; Albrecht, K.; Rehart, S.; Scholz, R. Recommendations of the German society for rheumatology on the perioperative approach under therapy with DMARDs and biologicals in inflammatory rheumatic diseases. *Z. Rheumatol.* **2014**, *73*, 77–84. [CrossRef]
12. Østensen, M.; Khamashta, M.; Lockshin, M.; Parke, A.; Brucato, A.; Carp, H.; Doria, A.; Rai, R.; Meroni, P.L.; Cetin, I.; et al. Anti-inflammatory and immunosuppressive drugs and reproduction. *Arthritis Res. Ther.* **2006**, *8*, 209. [CrossRef] [PubMed]
13. Breedveld, F.C.; Dayer, J. Leflunomide: Mode of action in the treatment of rheumatoid arthritis. *Ann. Rheum. Dis.* **2000**, *59*, 841–849. [CrossRef] [PubMed]
14. Kruger, K.; Bolten, W. Treatment with leflunomide in rheumatoid arthritis. *Z. Rheumatol.* **2005**, *64*, 96–101. [CrossRef] [PubMed]
15. Fox, R.; Helfgott, S.M. Pharmacology, Dosing, and Adverse Effects of Leflunomide in the Treatment of Rheumatoid Arthritis. Available online: www.UpToDate.com (accessed on 2 April 2019).
16. Smedegård, G.; Björk, J. Sulphasalazine: Mechanism of Action in Rheumatoid Arthritis. *Rheumatology* **1995**, *34*, 7–15. [CrossRef]
17. Michael, H.; Weisman, R.Z.R. Sulfasalazine: Pharmacology, Administration, and Adverse Effects in the Treatment of Rheumatoid Arthritis. Available online: www.UpToDate.com (accessed on 2 April 2019).
18. Pullar, T.; A Box, S. Sulphasalazine in the treatment of rheumatoid arthritis. *Rheumatology* **1997**, *36*, 382–386.
19. Fachinformation Sulfasalazin HEXAL. Available online: https://s3.eu-central-1.amazonaws.com/prod-cerebro-ifap/media_all/72466.pdf (accessed on 2 April 2019).
20. Keffer, J.; Probert, L.; Cazlaris, H.; Georgopoulos, S.; Kaslaris, E.; Kioussis, D.; Kollias, G. Transgenic mice expressing human tumour necrosis factor: A predictive genetic model of arthritis. *EMBO J.* **1991**, *10*, 4025–4031. [CrossRef] [PubMed]
21. Emery, P. Infliximab: A new treatment for rheumatoid arthritis. *Hosp. Med.* **2001**, *62*, 150–152. [CrossRef]
22. Moreland, L.W. Recent advances in anti-tumour necrosis factor (TNF) therapy in rheumatoid arthritis: Focus on the soluble TNF receptor p75 fusion protein, etanercept. *BioDrugs* **1999**, *11*, 201–210. [CrossRef]
23. Mikuls, T.R.; Moreland, L.W. TNF blockade in the treatment of rheumatoid arthritis: Infliximab versus etanercept. *Expert Opin. Pharmacother.* **2001**, *2*, 75–84. [CrossRef]
24. Rau, R. Adalimumab (a fully human anti-tumour necrosis factor alpha monoclonal antibody) in the treatment of active rheumatoid arthritis: The initial results of five trials. *Ann. Rheum. Dis.* **2002**, *61*, 70–73. [CrossRef]
25. Kay, J.; Matteson, E.L.; Dasgupta, B.; Nash, P.; Durez, P.; Hall, S.; Hsia, E.C.; Han, J.; Wagner, C.; Xu, Z.; et al. Golimumab in patients with active rheumatoid arthritis despite treatment with methotrexate: A randomized, double-blind, placebo-controlled, dose-ranging study. *Arthritis Rheum.* **2008**, *58*, 964–975. [CrossRef] [PubMed]
26. Smolen, J.; Landewe, R.B.; Mease, P.; Brzezicki, J.; Mason, D.; Luijtens, K.; van Vollenhoven, R.F.; Kavanaugh, A.; Schiff, M.; Burmester, G.R.; et al. Efficacy and safety of certolizumab pegol plus methotrexate in active rheumatoid arthritis: The RAPID 2 study. A randomised controlled trial. *Ann. Rheum. Dis.* **2009**, *68*, 797–804. [CrossRef] [PubMed]
27. Fleischmann, R.; Vencovsky, J.; van Vollenhoven, R.F.; Borenstein, D.; Box, J.; Coteur, G.; Goel, N.; Brezinschek, H.P.; Innes, A.; Strand, V. Efficacy and safety of certolizumab pegol monotherapy every 4 weeks in patients with rheumatoid arthritis failing previous disease-modifying antirheumatic therapy: The FAST4WARD study. *Ann. Rheum. Dis.* **2009**, *68*, 805–811. [CrossRef]

28. Fleischmann, R.; van Vollenhoven, R.F.; Vencovsky, J.; Alten, R.; Davies, O.; Mountian, I.; de Longueville, M.; Carter, D.; Choy, E. Long-Term Maintenance of Certolizumab Pegol Safety and Efficacy, in Combination with Methotrexate and as Monotherapy, in Rheumatoid Arthritis Patients. *Rheumatol. Ther.* **2017**, *4*, 57–69. [CrossRef] [PubMed]
29. Keystone, E.C.; Breedveld, F.C.; Kupper, H.; Li, Y.; Florentinus, S.; Sainsbury, I. Long-term use of adalimumab as monotherapy after attainment of low disease activity with adalimumab plus methotrexate in patients with rheumatoid arthritis. *RMD Open* **2018**, *4*, e000637. [CrossRef] [PubMed]
30. Narayanan, S.; Lu, Y.; Hutchings, R.; Baynton, E.; Hautamaki, E. Comparison of Disease Status And Outcomes of Patients With Rheumatoid Arthritis (Ra) Receiving Adalimumab or Etanercept Monotherapy In Europe. *Value Heal.* **2014**, *17*, A374. [CrossRef] [PubMed]
31. Gaubitz, M.; Göttl, K.-H.; Behmer, O.; Lippe, R.; Meng, T.; Löschmann, P.-A. Etanercept is effective as monotherapy or in combination with methotrexate in rheumatoid arthritis: Subanalysis of an observational study. *Clin. Rheumatol.* **2017**, *36*, 1989–1996. [CrossRef] [PubMed]
32. Cheifetz, A.; Mayer, L. Monoclonal antibodies, immunogenicity, and associated infusion reactions. *Mount Sinai J. Med.* **2005**, *72*, 250–256.
33. Weinblatt, M.E.; Schiff, M.; Valente, R.; van der Heijde, D.; Citera, G.; Zhao, C.; Maldonado, M.; Fleischmann, R. Head-to-head comparison of subcutaneous abatacept versus adalimumab for rheumatoid arthritis: Findings of a phase IIIb, multinational, prospective, randomized study. *Arthritis Rheum.* **2013**, *65*, 28–38. [CrossRef]
34. Cheifetz, A.; Smedley, M.; Martín, S.; Reiter, M.; Leone, G.; Mayer, L.; Plevy, S. The incidence and management of infusion reactions to infliximab: A large center experience. *Am. J. Gastroenterol.* **2003**, *98*, 1315–1324. [CrossRef]
35. A Wells, G.; Christensen, R.; Ghogomu, E.T.; Maxwell, L.; Macdonald, J.K.; Filippini, G.; Skoetz, N.; Francis, D.K.; Lopes, L.C.; Guyatt, G.H.; et al. Adverse effects of biologics: A network meta-analysis and Cochrane overview. *Cochrane Database Syst. Rev.* **2011**.
36. Calabrese, L.H.; Calabrese, C.; Kirchner, E. The 2015 American College of Rheumatology Guideline for the Treatment of Rheumatoid Arthritis Should Include New Standards for Hepatitis B Screening: Comment on the Article by Singh et al. *Arthritis Rheum.* **2016**, *68*, 723–724. [CrossRef] [PubMed]
37. Hastings, R.; Ding, T.; Butt, S.; Gadsby, K.; Zhang, W.; Moots, R.J.; Deighton, C. Neutropenia in patients receiving anti-tumor necrosis factor therapy. *Arthritis Rheum.* **2010**, *62*, 764–769. [CrossRef] [PubMed]
38. van Oosten, B.W.; Barkhof, F.; Truyen, L.; Boringa, J.B.; Bertelsmann, F.W.; von Blomberg, B.M.; Woody, J.N.; Hartung, H.P.; Polman, C.H. Increased MRI activity and immune activation in two multiple sclerosis patients treated with the monoclonal anti-tumor necrosis factor antibody cA2. *Neurology* **1996**, *47*, 1531–1534. [CrossRef] [PubMed]
39. Kwon, H.J.; Cote, T.R.; Cuffe, M.S.; Kramer, J.M.; Braun, M.M. Case reports of heart failure after therapy with a tumor necrosis factor antagonist. *Ann. Intern. Med.* **2003**, *138*, 807–811. [CrossRef] [PubMed]
40. Gabriel, S.E. Tumor necrosis factor inhibition: A part of the solution or a part of the problem of heart failure in rheumatoid arthritis? *Arthritis Rheum.* **2008**, *58*, 637–640. [CrossRef] [PubMed]
41. Marchioni, R.M.; Lichtenstein, G.R. Tumor necrosis factor-alpha inhibitor therapy and fetal risk: A systematic literature review. *World J. Gastroenterol.* **2013**, *19*, 2591–2602. [CrossRef]
42. Malek, A.; Sager, R.; Schneider, H. Maternal-fetal transport of immunoglobulin-G and its subclasses during the 3rd trimester of human-pregnancy. *Am. J. Reprod. Immunol.* **1994**, *32*, 8–14. [CrossRef]
43. Mahadevan, U.; Wolf, D.C.; Dubinsky, M.; Cortot, A.; Lee, S.D.; Siegel, C.A.; Ullman, T.; Glover, S.; Valentine, J.F.; Rubin, D.T.; et al. Placental transfer of anti-tumor necrosis factor agents in pregnant patients with inflammatory bowel disease. *Clin. Gastroenterol. Hepatol.* **2013**, *11*, 286–292. [CrossRef]
44. Clowse, M.E.B.; Scheuerle, A.E.; Chambers, C.; Afzali, A.; Kimball, A.B.; Cush, J.J.; Cooney, M.; Shaughnessy, L.; Vanderkelen, M.; Forger, F. Pregnancy Outcomes After Exposure to Certolizumab Pegol: Updated Results From a Pharmacovigilance Safety Database. *Arthritis Rheumatol.* **2018**, *70*, 1399–1407. [CrossRef]
45. Konttinen, L.; Kankaanpää, E.; Luosujärvi, R.; Blåfield, H.; Vuori, K.; Hakala, M.; Rantalaiho, V.; Savolainen, E.; Uutela, T.; Nordström, D.; et al. Effectiveness of anakinra in rheumatic disease in patients naive to biological drugs or previously on TNF blocking drugs: An observational study. *Clin. Rheumatol.* **2006**, *25*, 882–884. [CrossRef] [PubMed]
46. Mertens, M.; Singh, J.A. Anakinra for Rheumatoid Arthritis: A Systematic Review. *J. Rheumatol.* **2009**, *36*, 1118–1125. [CrossRef] [PubMed]

47. Eungdamrong, J.; Boyd, K.P.; A Meehan, S.; Latkowski, J.-A. Muckle-Wells treatment with anakinra. *Dermatol. Online J.* **2013**, *19*.
48. Kohler, B.M.; Lorenz, H.-M.; Blank, N. IL1-blocking therapy in colchicine-resistant familial Mediterranean fever. *Eur. J. Rheumatol.* **2018**, *5*, 230–234. [CrossRef] [PubMed]
49. Vounotrypidis, P.; Sakellariou, G.T.; Zisopoulos, D.; Berberidis, C. Refractory relapsing polychondritis: Rapid and sustained response in the treatment with an IL-1 receptor antagonist (anakinra). *Rheumatology* **2006**, *45*, 491–492. [CrossRef] [PubMed]
50. Gratton, S.B.; Scalapino, K.J.; Fye, K.H. Case of anakinra as a steroid-sparing agent for gout inflammation. *Arthritis Rheum.* **2009**, *61*, 1268–1270. [CrossRef] [PubMed]
51. Fleischmann, R.M.; Tesser, J.; Schiff, M.H.; Schechtman, J.; Burmester, G.-R.; Bennett, R.; Modafferi, D.; Zhou, L.; Bell, D.; Appleton, B. Safety of extended treatment with anakinra in patients with rheumatoid arthritis. *Ann. Rheum. Dis.* **2006**, *65*, 1006–1012. [CrossRef] [PubMed]
52. Chang, Z.; Spong, C.Y.; Jesus, A.A.; Davis, M.A.; Plass, N.; Stone, D.L.; Chapelle, D.; Hoffmann, P.; Kastner, D.L.; Barron, K.; et al. Anakinra Use During Pregnancy in Patients with Cryopyrin-Associated Periodic Syndromes (CAPS). *Arthritis Rheumatol.* **2014**, *66*, 3227–3232. [CrossRef] [PubMed]
53. Gabay, C.; Emery, P.; van Vollenhoven, R.; Dikranian, A.; Alten, R.; Pavelka, K.; Klearman, M.; Musselman, D.; Agarwal, S.; Green, J.; et al. Tocilizumab monotherapy versus adalimumab monotherapy for treatment of rheumatoid arthritis (ADACTA): A randomised, double-blind, controlled phase 4 trial. *Lancet* **2013**, *381*, 1541–1550. [CrossRef]
54. Zhang, X.; Chen, Y.-C.; Fettner, S.; Rowell, L.; Gott, T.; Grimsey, P.; Unsworth, A. Pharmacokinetics and pharmacodynamics of tocilizumab after subcutaneous administration in patients with rheumatoid arthritis. *Int. J. Clin. Pharmacol. Ther.* **2013**, *51*, 620–630. [CrossRef]
55. Burmester, G.R.; Lin, Y.; Patel, R.; van Adelsberg, J.; Mangan, E.K.; Graham, N.M.; van Hoogstraten, H.; Bauer, D.; Ignacio Vargas, J.; Lee, E.B. Efficacy and safety of sarilumab monotherapy versus adalimumab monotherapy for the treatment of patients with active rheumatoid arthritis (MONARCH): A randomised, double-blind, parallel-group phase III trial. *Ann. Rheum. Dis.* **2017**, *76*, 840–847. [CrossRef] [PubMed]
56. Genovese, M.C.; Rubbert-Roth, A.; Smolen, J.S.; Kremer, J.; Khraishi, M.; Gómez-Reino, J.; Sebba, A.; Pilson, R.; Williams, S.; Van Vollenhoven, R. Longterm Safety and Efficacy of Tocilizumab in Patients with Rheumatoid Arthritis: A Cumulative Analysis of Up to 4.6 Years of Exposure. *J. Rheumatol.* **2013**, *40*, 768–780. [CrossRef] [PubMed]
57. Saito, J.; Yakuwa, N.; Kaneko, K.; Takai, C.; Goto, M.; Nakajima, K.; Yamatani, A.; Murashima, A. Tocilizumab during pregnancy and lactation: Drug levels in maternal serum, cord blood, breast milk and infant serum. *Rheumatology* **2019**. [CrossRef] [PubMed]
58. Nakajima, K.; Watanabe, O.; Mochizuki, M.; Nakasone, A.; Ishizuka, N.; Murashima, A. Pregnancy outcomes after exposure to tocilizumab: A retrospective analysis of 61 patients in Japan. *Mod. Rheumatol.* **2016**, *26*, 667–671. [CrossRef] [PubMed]
59. Maxwell, L.; Singh, J.A. Abatacept for rheumatoid arthritis. *Cochrane Database Syst. Rev.* **2009**, CD007277. [CrossRef] [PubMed]
60. Herrero-Beaumont, G.; Calatrava, M.J.M.; Castañeda, S. Abatacept Mechanism of Action: Concordance With Its Clinical Profile. *Reumatol. Clínica (Engl. Ed.)* **2012**, *8*, 78–83. [CrossRef]
61. Atzeni, F.; Sarzi-Puttini, P.; Mutti, A.; Bugatti, S.; Cavagna, L.; Caporali, R. Long-term safety of abatacept in patients with rheumatoid arthritis. *Autoimmun. Rev.* **2013**, *12*, 1115–1117. [CrossRef]
62. Smolen, J.S.; Keystone, E.C.; Emery, P.; Breedveld, F.C.; Betteridge, N.; Burmester, G.R.; Dougados, M.; Ferraccioli, G.; Jaeger, U.; Klareskog, L.; et al. Consensus statement on the use of rituximab in patients with rheumatoid arthritis. *Ann. Rheum. Dis.* **2007**, *66*, 143–150. [CrossRef]
63. Harrold, L.R.; John, A.; Best, J.; Zlotnick, S.; Karki, C.; Li, Y.; Greenberg, J.D.; Kremer, J.M. Impact of rituximab on patient-reported outcomes in patients with rheumatoid arthritis from the US Corrona Registry. *Clin. Rheumatol.* **2017**, *36*, 2135–2140. [CrossRef]
64. Chatzidionysiou, K.; Lie, E.; Nasonov, E.; Lukina, G.; Hetland, M.L.; Tarp, U.; Gabay, C.; van Riel, P.L.; Nordstrom, D.C.; Gomez-Reino, J.; et al. Highest clinical effectiveness of rituximab in autoantibody-positive patients with rheumatoid arthritis and in those for whom no more than one previous TNF antagonist has failed: Pooled data from 10 European registries. *Ann. Rheum. Dis.* **2011**, *70*, 1575–1580. [CrossRef]

65. Lee, Y.H.; Bae, S.C.; Song, G.G. The efficacy and safety of rituximab for the treatment of active rheumatoid arthritis: A systematic review and meta-analysis of randomized controlled trials. *Rheumatol. Int.* **2011**, *31*, 1493–1499. [CrossRef] [PubMed]
66. Chakravarty, E.F.; Murray, E.R.; Kelman, A.; Farmer, P. Pregnancy outcomes after maternal exposure to rituximab. *Blood* **2011**, *117*, 1499–1506. [CrossRef] [PubMed]
67. Iwata, S.; Tanaka, Y. Progress in understanding the safety and efficacy of Janus kinase inhibitors for treatment of rheumatoid arthritis. *Expert Rev. Clin. Immunol.* **2016**, *12*, 1047–1057. [CrossRef] [PubMed]
68. Migita, K.; Izumi, Y.; Torigoshi, T.; Satomura, K.; Izumi, M.; Nishino, Y.; Jiuchi, Y.; Nakamura, M.; Kozuru, H.; Nonaka, F.; et al. Inhibition of Janus kinase/signal transducer and activator of transcription (JAK/STAT) signalling pathway in rheumatoid synovial fibroblasts using small molecule compounds. *Clin. Exp. Immunol.* **2013**, *174*, 356–363. [CrossRef] [PubMed]
69. Migita, K.; Koga, T.; Komori, A.; Torigoshi, T.; Maeda, Y.; Izumi, Y.; Sato, J.; Jiuchi, Y.; Miyashita, T.; Yamasaki, S.; et al. Influence of Janus Kinase Inhibition on Interleukin 6-mediated Induction of Acute-phase Serum Amyloid A in Rheumatoid Synovium. *J. Rheumatol.* **2011**, *38*, 2309–2317. [CrossRef] [PubMed]
70. Arkin, M.R.; Wells, J.A. Small-molecule inhibitors of protein–protein interactions: Progressing towards the dream. *Nat. Rev. Drug Discov.* **2004**, *3*, 301–317. [CrossRef] [PubMed]
71. Dhillon, S. Tofacitinib: A Review in Rheumatoid Arthritis. *Drugs* **2017**, *77*, 1987–2001. [CrossRef]
72. Kremer, J.; Li, Z.G.; Hall, S.; Fleischmann, R.; Genovese, M.; Martin-Mola, E.; Isaacs, J.D.; Gruben, D.; Wallenstein, G.; Krishnaswami, S.; et al. Tofacitinib in combination with nonbiologic disease-modifying antirheumatic drugs in patients with active rheumatoid arthritis: A randomized trial. *Ann. Intern. Med.* **2013**, *159*, 253–261. [CrossRef]
73. Taylor, P.C.; Keystone, E.C.; van der Heijde, D.; Weinblatt, M.E.; Del Carmen Morales, L.; Reyes Gonzaga, J.; Yakushin, S.; Ishii, T.; Emoto, K.; Beattie, S.; et al. Baricitinib versus Placebo or Adalimumab in Rheumatoid Arthritis. *N. Engl. J. Med.* **2017**, *376*, 652–662. [CrossRef]
74. Fleischmann, R.; Schiff, M.; van der Heijde, D.; Ramos-Remus, C.; Spindler, A.; Stanislav, M.; Zerbini, C.A.; Gurbuz, S.; Dickson, C.; de Bono, S.; et al. Baricitinib, Methotrexate, or Combination in Patients With Rheumatoid Arthritis and No or Limited Prior Disease-Modifying Antirheumatic Drug Treatment. *Arthritis Rheumatol.* **2017**, *69*, 506–517. [CrossRef]
75. Dougados, M.; van der Heijde, D.; Chen, Y.C.; Greenwald, M.; Drescher, E.; Liu, J.; Beattie, S.; Witt, S.; de la Torre, I.; Gaich, C.; et al. Baricitinib in patients with inadequate response or intolerance to conventional synthetic DMARDs: Results from the RA-BUILD study. *Ann. Rheum. Dis.* **2017**, *76*, 88–95. [CrossRef] [PubMed]
76. Yamaoka, K. Benefit and Risk of Tofacitinib in the Treatment of Rheumatoid Arthritis: A Focus on Herpes Zoster. *Drug Saf.* **2016**, *39*, 823–840. [CrossRef] [PubMed]
77. Cohen, S.B.; Koenig, A.; Wang, L.; Kwok, K.; Mebus, C.A.; Riese, R.; Fleischmann, R. Efficacy and safety of tofacitinib in US and non-US rheumatoid arthritis patients: Pooled analyses of phase II and III. *Clin. Exp. Rheumatol.* **2016**, *34*, 32–36. [PubMed]
78. Keystone, E.C.; Taylor, P.C.; Drescher, E.; Schlichting, D.E.; Beattie, S.D.; Berclaz, P.Y.; Lee, C.H.; Fidelus-Gort, R.K.; Luchi, M.E.; Rooney, T.P.; et al. Safety and efficacy of baricitinib at 24 weeks in patients with rheumatoid arthritis who have had an inadequate response to methotrexate. *Ann. Rheum. Dis.* **2015**, *74*, 333–340. [CrossRef] [PubMed]
79. Smolen, J.S.; Genovese, M.C.; Takeuchi, T.; Hyslop, D.L.; Macias, W.L.; Rooney, T.; Chen, L.; Dickson, C.L.; Riddle Camp, J.; Cardillo, T.E.; et al. Safety Profile of Baricitinib in Patients with Active Rheumatoid Arthritis with over 2 Years Median Time in Treatment. *J. Rheumatol.* **2019**, *46*, 7–18. [CrossRef] [PubMed]
80. Westhovens, R. Clinical efficacy of new JAK inhibitors under development. Just more of the same? *Rheumatology* **2019**, *58* (Suppl. 1), i27–i33. [CrossRef]
81. Serhal, L.; Edwards, C.J. Upadacitinib for the treatment of rheumatoid arthritis. *Expert Rev. Clin. Immunol.* **2018**, *15*, 1–13. [CrossRef]

13

How to Get the Most from Methotrexate (MTX) Treatment for Your Rheumatoid Arthritis Patient?—MTX in the Treat-to-Target Strategy

Peter. C. Taylor [1,*], Alejandro Balsa Criado [2], Anne-Barbara Mongey [3], Jerome Avouac [4], Hubert Marotte [5] and Rudiger B. Mueller [6]

1 Botnar Research Centre, NDORMS, University of Oxford, Windmill Road, Oxford OX3 7LD, UK
2 Rheumatology unit, University Hospital La Paz, Institute for Health Research–IdiPAZ, Universidad Autonoma de Madrid, 28046 Madrid, Spain; alejandro.balsa@salud.madrid.org
3 St. Vincent's University Hospital, Elm Park, Dublin 4, Ireland; anne.b.mongey@ucd.ie
4 Paris Descartes University, Sorbonne Paris Cité, Rheumatology Department, Cochin Hopital, Assistance Publique-Hôpitaux de Paris, 75014 Paris, France; javouac@me.com
5 SAINBIOSE, INSERM U1059, Université de Lyon, Saint-Etienne, France Service de Rhumatologie, CHU Saint-Etienne, 42055 Saint-Etienne, France; Hubert.marotte@chu-st-etienne.fr
6 Division of Rheumatology, Medical University Department, Kantonsspital Aarau, 5001 Aarau, Switzerland; ruediger.mueler@ksa.ch
* Correspondence: peter.taylor@kennedy.ox.ac.uk

Abstract: Methotrexate (MTX) is a remarkable drug with a key role in the management of rheumatoid arthritis (RA) at every stage of its evolution. Its attributes include good overall efficacy for signs and symptoms, inhibition of structural damage and preservation of function with acceptable and manageable safety, a large dose-titratable range, options for either an oral or parenteral route of administration, and currently unrivalled cost-effectiveness. It has a place as a monotherapy and also as an anchor drug that can be safely used in combination with other conventional synthetic disease-modifying antirheumatic drugs (csDMARDs) or used concomitantly with biological DMARDs or targeted synthetic DMARDs. MTX is not without potential issues regarding toxicity, notably hepatotoxicity and bone marrow toxicity, as well as tolerability problems for some, but not all, patients. But many of these issues can be mitigated or managed. In the face of a welcome expansion in available targeted therapies for the treatment of RA, MTX looks set to remain at the foundation of pharmacotherapy for the majority of people living with RA and other inflammatory rheumatic diseases. In this article, we provide an evidence-based discussion as to how to achieve the best outcomes with this versatile drug in the context of a treat-to-target strategy for the management of RA.

Keywords: methotrexate; rheumatoid arthritis; tolerability; efficacy; posology; titration; oral route; subcutaneous route; bioavailability; effectiveness

---

1. Introduction

Rheumatoid arthritis (RA) is a chronic autoimmune disease characterized by inflammation, pain, stiffness, and progressive joint destruction with a detrimental impact on joint function, work ability, and health-related quality of life (HrQoL) [1]. The primary goal of treating patients with RA is to maximize long-term HrQoL through control of symptoms, prevention of structural damage, normalization of function, and participation in social and work-related activities. Abrogation of inflammation is considered the most important way to achieve optimal outcomes [2], and its achievement is facilitated by Treat-to-Target (T2T) recommendations [2].

The T2T paradigm has emerged during the last decade and was incorporated in recommendations issued primarily in 2010 and recently updated [2]. The T2T paradigm relies on five principles: the definition of a treatment target; the close and regular assessment of disease activity using composite measures that include joint counts; the regular adaptation of therapy, if the target is not achieved within a particular timeframe; the consideration of individual patients' aspects; and shared decision-making with the patient. A T2T strategy is more effective in terms of reducing disease activity compared to routine care [3], and has a beneficial effect on working ability. T2T principles underpin the current recommendations of European League Against Rheumatism (EULAR) Task Force [4], American College of Rheumatology (ACR) guidelines [5], and the Canadian Rheumatology Association (CRA) recommendations [6] and the Asian APLAR guidelines [7]. T2T overarching principles affirm the necessity of a shared decision between patient and the whole team involved in the care of RA [2].

The ideal treatment target is remission [8], or, if remission cannot be achieved, low disease activity (LDA). Remission is associated with the best achievable outcomes including limitation or prevention of joint damage [9], preservation of physical function, and work capacity as well as optimizing overall quality of life [10,11]. Furthermore, remission reduces comorbidity risks [12]. Treatment targets should however be adapted according to the presence of comorbidities, individual patient factors and drug-associated risks [2] to ensure the most favorable benefit: risk ratio for any given patient. Treatment should be titrated to the therapeutic response assessed by composite measures of disease activity, ideally with therapy adjustment at least every three months [2] if the patient is not in remission, a recommendation based on evidence provided by clinical trials [13–15], until the desired treatment target is reached.

Early treatment [16] and rapid attainment of the targeted endpoint are critical. Disease-modifying anti-rheumatic drugs (DMARDs) are the main therapy of RA. The most commonly prescribed conventional synthetic (cs) DMARDs are methotrexate (MTX), leflunomide, sulfasalazine, and hydroxychloroquine [6]. Based on its efficacy, safety, large dose-titratable range, options for either an oral or parenteral route of administration, and cost-effectiveness, MTX holds a unique place in the management of RA, with a role at every stage of the evolution of this chronic condition. MTX monotherapy is recommended as an initial pharmacological strategy [4–6], but it can also be used as an "anchor drug" in combination with another conventional synthetic disease-modifying antirheumatic drugs (csDMARD), any biological DMARD (bDMARD), or targeted synthetic DMARD (tsDMARD) [4]. MTX is currently the most commonly used first-line therapy for RA in the world [17].

While recommendations advocate the use of methotrexate at various positions in the contemporary treatment paradigm, the heterogeneity of presentation of RA and versatility of approaches to effective MTX use are such that there is need for evidence- and experience-based supplementary information to enable clinicians to get the most out of MTX for their patients in the T2T era. Notably, this process includes allaying any misconceptions that patients may have concerning this therapy, adapting dose and administration routes for optimal efficacy, mitigating toxicity and tolerability issues, and taking into account the relatively slow kinetic of response, which can be managed by the use of bridging steroids as appropriate.

In this position paper, we address these and other issues regarding the optimal use of MTX in a target population comprising adult (age ≥ 18 years) patients meeting current classification criteria for RA and patients with early inflammatory arthritis suspected of having RA but not yet fulfilling classification criteria.

2. Pharmacology

2.1. Pharmacokinetics

MTX (4-amino-10-methylfolic acid), an antifolate agent that was licensed for a RA indication in the 1980s [18], is a prodrug that becomes active when glutamated within cells, exhibiting a high binding activity for dihydrofolate reductase (DHFR) [19].

Oral MTX is absorbed from the small gut by an active transport mechanism involving the proton-coupled folate transporter. Bioavailability ranges from 30% to 70% [20] and plateaus for single oral dose >15 mg [21], suggesting an absorption limitation [22]. Intracellular MTX is gradually polyglutamated (MTXGlu$_n$). There is a competitive process between glutamation and deglutamation and steady-state levels of intracellular MTX are reached in a median time of 28 weeks with variability between patients due to different polyglutamation rates [23,24]. The major determinants of MTXGlu$_n$ concentrations are age, renal function, and MTX dose [25]. Serum concentration of MTX falls rapidly following an intravenous administration [26]. The plasma half-life is 4.5 h to 10 h [27] but MTX is retained within cells long after its serum clearance. Excretion of MTX is mainly renal, occurring through glomerular filtration and active tubular excretion. Seventy-five percent of MTX is excreted unchanged in the urine with large interpatient variability [28].

The active transport mechanism limits oral MTX absorption resulting in lower bioavailability of higher MTX doses. Interestingly, bioavailability may increase by splitting the oral dose [22] or switching to a parenteral route [22]. Polyglutamation is progressive, explaining the slow onset of the action of MTX [19] and the delay before maximal benefit. In some patients with low glutamation rates, a relatively low dosing strategy will lengthen the time required for adequate drug concentration to be achieved [23]. This may be detrimental, as higher intracellular MTXGlu$_n$ levels have been associated with better clinical response [29]. The subcutaneous (SC) administration route is associated with a significant increase in long-chain MTXGlu$_n$ when compared to the oral route [30]. Renal function impacts the generation of MTXGlu$_n$. The anti-inflammatory effects of MTX in patients with RA are much more prolonged than its plasma half-life might suggests due to the accumulation of polyglutamated metabolites in tissues. Since the MTX excretion mainly involves the kidney, renal failure, or competitive excretion with other drugs in patients receiving multiple treatments will prolong MTX serum half-life [31].

2.2. Mode of Action

The mechanisms by which low-dose MTX exerts its therapeutic effect in RA remain incompletely understood [19]. MTX has several important anti-inflammatory actions mediated through a variety of pathways that do not involve folate antagonism. The main putative mechanisms are the promotion of adenosine release, inhibition of purine and pyrimidine synthesis, inhibition of methyl donors, generation of reactive oxygen species, downregulation of adhesion-molecule expression, modification of cytokine profiles, and downregulation of eicosanoids and matrix metalloproteinases [19]. Adenosine exerts an anti-inflammatory activity by down-regulating the activation and proliferation of T-Lymphocytes. Adenosine receptors are overexpressed on immune cells and synoviocytes of patients with RA, probably because of the high tumor necrosis factor (TNF) levels. Inhibition of DHFR prevents the regeneration from dihydrofolate to tetrahydrofolate, an essential factor for the production of folate cofactors required for purine and pyrimidine synthesis [32]. Inhibition of DHFR also inhibits the production of methyl donors and attenuates the formation of polyamines.

Since the anti-inflammatory properties of MTX are not mediated by folate antagonism, some toxic effects may be prevented or minimized by folic acid supplementation (not taken on the same day as MTX) without loss of therapeutic benefit.

In the future, pharmacogenetic advances may help to predict non-responses to MTX, thus directing patients to combination therapy as initial treatment. Promising results have recently been published [33,34].

3. MTX: A Forefront Position among csDMARDs

3.1. Flexible

More intensive treatment interventions provide the best chance of achieving remission in RA patients [35]. However, potential benefits need to be balanced against potential risks and every effort must be made to ensure acceptable tolerability of any given therapeutic regime. The most frequent strategy for management of early RA is a "step-up" approach, where MTX is initiated at a dose estimated to be well tolerated and then titrated up according to therapeutic response. Current recommendations for management of RA [5,36] advocate the initial use of MTX as a monotherapy with a bridging steroid to give more rapid symptomatic relief before the clinic benefits of MTX become apparent. Some authors have advocated a step-down approach to treatment, initiating MTX at a high dose and arguing that this takes advantage of a "window of opportunity" for best outcomes early in the disease [37]. However, this process has the potential disadvantage of making tolerability issues more challenging to manage. Whatever the strategy, MTX has a central role to play, both as a monotherapy and as an "anchor drug", for many successful DMARD combinations whether conventional, targeted synthetic, or biologic [38]. Some unique attributes of MTX contributing to this versatility include the wide dose titratable range, choice of administration routes, the favorable efficacy:toxicity ratio, utility in DMARD combinations, potential ancillary benefits, and outstanding cost-effectiveness. Unfortunately, despite treatment guidelines, up to 50% of patients [39] do not continue MTX when treatment with a biologic is initiated. Over the last few years there has been a discussion about tsDMARD or bDMARD monotherapy. Some authors suggest that MTX administered in a tolerated dose should be continued as a combination partner until remission is achieved [40]. This process is recommended because the highest benefits for all targeted therapies are generally observed when they are used with concomitant MTX.

MTX is marketed in the form of tablets with increments of 2.5, 5, or 10 mg/tablet, and as prefilled syringes or auto-injectors with various doses per injection, allowing one to finely tune the weekly dose. Oral and (SC) are the most widely routes used in RA patients. SC injections should be considered for weekly doses of 15 mg or higher due to the better bioavailability of MTX when administered parenterally.

3.2. *Clinically Efficient*

The TEAR study has demonstrated that low disease activity illustrated with the Disease Activity Score-28 with the erythrocyte sedimentation rate (DAS28-ESR) can be achieved by 28% of patients with early RA treated with MTX monotherapy [41]. It was a 2 × 2 factorial design comparing four treatment arms (immediate combination of MTX + etanercept (ETN); immediate combination of MTX + hydroxychloquine (HCQ) + sulfasalazine (SSZ)); initial MTX with step-up treatment adding ETN; initial MTX with step-up treatment adding HCQ and SSZ. The study aimed to assess if it was better to intensively treat all early RA cases with drug combinations or to reserve this procedure for those who do not achieve low disease activity (DAS28-ESR < 3.2) after 24 weeks. At week 24, 28% of the patients from step-up groups achieved the treatment target. Similar results were achieved in the BeST study [42]. An even higher rate was demonstrated by Mueller et al in real-life [43]. Moreover, no difference was found between groups with respect to disease activity after 48 weeks and 102 weeks of treatment. Favorable results obtained with initial MTX monotherapy in the step-up groups were maintained until week 102. Moreover, there was no difference in radiologic progression when comparing step-up with combination therapy in a post-hoc analysis [38]. Since differences in outcomes were negligible between patient groups that were started at a baseline on an aggressive combination therapy regimen, or were delayed before stepping up (by 6 months), the authors concluded that there is no penalty for delaying step-up therapy until it is clinically indicated [38]. In comparison with those patients exhibiting a sustained, good response to MTX monotherapy, aggressive combined treatment would only result in a higher risk of side effects and higher costs. Importantly, these results were obtained employing a strict MTX dosage escalation regime (10 mg/w, escalated to 15 mg/w at week 6 and 20 mg/w at week 12, unless the patients had zero tender joints and zero swollen joints at that visit). LDA, but not remission, was the key factor that determined whether to step-up to combination therapy at week 24. The SWEFOT study reported similar results with 29.8% of patients meeting EULAR criteria for response after 3 months of MTX monotherapy [44].

3.3. Ancillary Benefits

Besides its efficacy in ameliorating arthritis, MTX may have ancillary benefits. Patients with RA have a higher risk of cardiovascular disease, infection, and cancer [45–47], resulting in reduced survival. Low-dose MTX is reported to reduce all-cause mortality in RA by 60% and cardiovascular mortality by 70%, while other DMARDs have no effect on mortality. Protective effects appear to be independent of MTX dose [48]. Another study reported that all-cause mortality was reduced by 70% in a vast cohort of RA patients treated with MTX when compared to those receiving other treatments [49]. Protective effects were evident only after one year of MTX use and were independent of the effect on RA activity [49]. The biological mechanisms underpinning this protection are not fully understood. Effects of MTX on the survival of RA patients are likely to be mediated by its anti-inflammatory properties, since MTX failed to demonstrate any protective effects on cardiovascular events in patients with previous myocardial infarction or multivessel coronary disease who additionally had type 2 diabetes or metabolic syndrome but no major inflammation [50].

Interstitial lung disease (ILD) is a common extra-articular manifestation of RA [51], affecting around 10% of patients [52]. Chronic lung disease (CLD) and ILD increase the risk of death in RA patients [53,54]. Methotrexate has been associated with severe lung toxicity, including ILD [55]. However, there is recent data that questions the results of case studies or observational studies linking methotrexate to pulmonary damage. Two meta-analyses also failed to associate methotrexate with ILD; in the first one [56], a meta-analysis of clinical trials (22 studies with 8584 patients with RA), the use of MTX in patients with RA was associated with an increased risk of total respiratory complications (RR 1.10), mainly due to an increased risk of respiratory infections (RR 1.11) and acute pneumonitis (RR: 7.81) but it was not observed that treatment with MTX increased the risk of death due to lung disease (RR 1.53, 0.46–5.01). In the second one [57], a meta-analysis of the clinical trials of psoriasis, psoriatic arthritis, and inflammatory bowel disease, all clinical conditions without pulmonary manifestations, did not find an increase in lung disease in patients treated with MTX. A recent analysis of a large prospective cohort of predominantly male US Veterans showed no increase in mortality risk in RA-CLD patients treated with MTX or biologics [54]. Moreover, in a recent study, MTX was a strong predictor of survival in RA patients with ILD [53].

The role for MTX in the prevention of dementia remains controversial. Inflammation is a common feature of both RA and dementia [58]. Despite the blood brain barrier, systemic inflammation is associated with cerebral inflammation [58]. A retrospective population-based study involving more than 11,000 RA patients, including 70.6% of csDMARD users, revealed that csDMARDs users had a 40% risk reduction of dementia. The strongest effect was with the use of MTX [59].

Felty's syndrome comprises a triad of RA, neutropenia, and splenomegaly, occurring in less than 1% of RA patients. Pseudo Felty's syndrome is characterized by RA, monoclonal expansion of lymphocytes, and neutropenia. The main complication is infection, whose risk increases with the depth and duration of neutropenia [60]. MTX is the first-line treatment of Felty's syndrome and is indicated, despite neutropenia [61,62].

3.4. Cost-Effectiveness

Therapeutic decisions should also be guided by cost-effectiveness considerations. Based on a decision analysis model extended to lifetime duration, early MTX monotherapy was more cost-effective than the early combination of MTX and TNF Inhibitor (TNFi)-based biologics [63]. The cost-effectiveness ratio of the early MTX strategy was less than $5,000/quality-adjusted life year (QALY) and more than $150,000/QALY for TNFis. In patients who failed to respond or to tolerate oral MTX; switching to SC MTX was described as more cost-effective than adding bDMARDs [64], since a large proportion of these patients achieved adequate response with SC MTX and, therefore, did not require more expensive therapy [65]. A cost-minimization analysis based on UK costs indicated that a routine use of SC MTX following oral MTX failure had the potential to save an estimated £7,197 (5536 US$) per patient in the first year of therapy [64]. Prefilled syringes and auto-injectors facilitate self-administration of SC

MTX by the patients, thus increasing costs savings. In addition, in some countries, the prescription of bDMARDs can be reimbursed only if the patient did not adequately respond to at least 2 csDMARDs, if not contra-indicated [66,67].

3.5. Combinable with Other Treatments

MTX is a great combination partner with other csDMARDs and bDMARDs. The most popular csDMARDs combinations are MTX and HCQ and the triple combination of MTX, HCQ, and SSZ. The combination of MTX and HCQ is synergistic and gave better results than MTX alone in a head-to-head comparison after 6 months of treatment, but the difference was no longer significant after 12 months [68]. Combining MTX and HCQ may be useful in patients who have a good response to MTX, attaining LDA but not remission [69]. The efficacy of this combination may be explained by pharmacokinetic interactions. Concomitant administration of HCQ increases the mean area under the curve (AUC) of MTX blood concentration, decreases the maximum MTX concentration (Cmax), and extends the time to reach Cmax [67]. A reduced Cmax may also explain the diminution of acute liver adverse effects. However, extra vigilance for MTX adverse events is recommended, especially in patients with impaired renal function [67]. Triple therapy combining MTX, HCQ, and SSZ may be a valuable alternative to the addition of bDMARDs to MTX, in cases of inadequate response to MTX and in the absence of poor prognosis factors. In a randomized trial comparing a triple combination of csDMARDs versus a regimen of MTX and etanercept (ETN), patients receiving triple therapy adhered for a longer time to their regimen than patients receiving MTX + ETN, despite similar outcomes [70], thus reflecting better acceptability. Infections were more frequent with the MTX+ETN regimen, whereas gastrointestinal side effects were more frequent with the triple combination [71]. Conversely, in a network meta-analysis of 33 studies, the odds of remission were lower with triple therapy than with the combination of MTX and TNFi [72]. However, the analysis considered both patients with inadequate response to MTX and MTX-naïve patients. These results were contested by a recent meta-analysis showing that triple association of csDMARDs and the combination of MTX and bDMARD as a second-line treatment in patients with insufficient response to MTX gave similar results [69]. Nonetheless, this result provides additional evidence supporting conventional combinations over bDMARDs after an inadequate response to MTX.

MTX is also a valuable partner in combined therapy with tsDMARD and bDMARDs. Such combinations have been shown to significantly improve clinical manifestations of RA [73–76]. Around two thirds of patients will have to step-up from MTX monotherapy to combined strategies [41]. In addition, RA patients with severe presentation and poor prognostic factors may require combined therapy upfront to prevent irreversible joint damage and functional impairment. The efficacy of targeted therapies is enhanced when the bDMARD is administered in combination with MTX. This may be due to complementary mechanisms of action, pharmacokinetic interactions, and reduction of the immunogenicity of the biologic agent.

The CONCERTO study was the first blinded, controlled trial to address the relationship between MTX dose and serum drug concentrations in RA patients treated with adalimumab. Steady-state trough serum concentrations of adalimumab were almost two-fold higher in patients concomitantly receiving MTX [77]. Patients were randomized into four groups with an increasing MTX dose (from 2.5/week to 20 mg/week, orally). There was no difference between the two highest MTX doses on clinical, radiographic, and functional response, whereas both doses were associated with better outcomes when comparing to the two lowest doses [77]. In parallel, adalimumab serum concentrations were higher with 10 or 20 mg MTX than with 2.5 or 5 mg MTX, mimicking the clinical findings. These results suggested that MTX at a dose of 10 mg/w reduced the clearance of adalimumab and increased the adalimumab serum level, thereby enhancing its efficacy. The MUSICA study [78] evaluated the effects of low and high MTX doses in combination with the initiation of adalimumab in patients who did not adequately respond to MTX. Patients with a stable MTX dose of at least 15 mg/week prior to screening were randomized to receive blinded MTX, at either 7.5 or 20 mg/week in combination with open-label

40 mg of adalimumab every other week. Since low-doses of MTX associated to adalimumab failed to show non-inferiority as compared to high doses for most clinical, functional, and ultrasound outcomes, the MUSICA study results do not support routine MTX reduction at the moment of adalimumab initiation. However, in a proportion of patients who may need to reduce MTX for toxicity reasons, much of the clinical efficacy in association with adalimumab may be retained, particularly when MTX dose reductions are modest.

Secondary failure to bDMARDs after an initial response can occur in as many as 30% of patients [79]. Development of anti-drug antibodies (ADAb) is one of the main drivers of loss of treatment efficacy [80–84]. ADAb have been described with infliximab, adalimumab, but not with etanercept. In a recent cross-sectional study on Spanish RA patients experiencing secondary failure while receiving TNFi, the prevalence of adalimumab ADAb was 29.3%, the one of infliximab ADA was 27.3%, and none of the patients treated with ETN developed ADAb [84]. Randomized-controlled trials reported ADAb in a small proportion on patients on golimumab and certolizumab [80]. ADAb either neutralize the active drug or decrease the serum drug concentration, resulting in a loss of clinical response [85]. Around 80% of patients who tested positive to ADAb had no detectable drug in the serum [84]. In a retrospective cohort of RA patients who were biologic-naïve at the time of enrolment, and were then treated with infliximab for a median time of 5.75 years, ADAb against infliximab were found in 33% of patients, in 24% of responders, and in all non-responder patients [83].

MTX may prevent [84,86] or reverse [87] the formation of ADAb and so maintain efficacy to TNFi, prolong drug survival, and prevent immune complex-mediated adverse events [80,83]. The pooled risk ratio for the formation of ADAb in patients receiving combined therapy with immunomodulators versus that of patients receiving anti-TNF monotherapy was 0.49 in a meta-analysis of 35 studies involving 6790 patients with inflammatory bowel disease [88]. The development of ADAb is reduced by the concomitant use of MTX in a dose-dependent manner [89]. It is, therefore, desirable to prescribe bDMARDs in combination with concomitant MTX when it is satisfactorily tolerated with toxicity. However, in the event of tolerability issues with MTX, the dose can be lowered while still providing efficacy benefits in combination, as illustrated in the CONCERTO [77] and MUSICA [90] studies.

3.6. Challenges Associated with MTX Use

When prescribing MTX as first-line therapy in RA patients, the physician has to face several challenges, such as explaining the time-course of the clinical benefits to the patient, improving patient compliance and adherence to therapy and monitoring, and avoiding unnecessary premature discontinuation of MTX are at the forefront of physician concerns.

The collective findings of combination therapy studies with MTX monotherapy arms, such as SWEFOT [44], CAMERA [14], TEAR [41], OPTIMA [91], and PREMIER [74], illustrate that, in general, it takes 6 months to see a full response to MTX. In patients with early RA and no poor prognostic factors, the relatively slow onset of action of MTX does not jeopardize clinical or functional outcomes. During this period, and especially during the first months, patients do not experience the full clinical benefit of MTX but are maybe exposed to adverse events. This is a crucial period in which too many patients discontinue MTX. The risk of premature stopping can be mitigated by the provision of clear and complete information to the patient. The slow kinetic of onset of symptomatic improvement with MTX can be mitigated by co-prescription of corticosteroids as a bridging therapy.

The best outcomes with the use of MTX are achieved when a shared decision-making approach to treatment is used in which the patient is an active participant. Patients need to understand and take responsibility for attendance for blood tests to ensure close monitoring of laboratory parameters, as well as following recommendations for folic acid supplementation in order to reduce the likelihood of certain adverse events. Reassuring tolerability and safety of low-dose MTX have recently been studied confirmed in the large placebo-controlled CIRT study aimed at determining if low-dose MTX could reduce the incidence of atherosclerotic events in patients with metabolic disorders and a history of myocardial infarction or multivessel coronary disease [50]. The study included 2391 patients who were allocated to the MTX arm. The median follow-up was 2.3 years before the study was stopped because of its futility. Most frequent AEs were infections, mouth sores and oral pain, unintended weight loss, leukopenia, and elevation of liver enzymes more than three times the normal range. Severe AEs are far less frequent. No case of marrow depletion was reported, even if leukopenia was frequent [50]. However, the report of more non-basal skin cancers in the MTX group was unexpected and deserves further exploration.

Elevations of liver enzymes must alert the physician to potential hepatotoxicity, in which case it may be prudent to temporarily reduce the MTX dose or even to discontinue the drug. Acute elevations of liver enzymes occur relatively frequently but are usually transient and generally resolve spontaneously. Rarely, persistent abnormal liver function tests reveal hepatotoxic effects of MTX, justifying treatment cessation. Among 41 patients receiving low-dose MTX for rheumatic diseases, experiencing elevation of liver enzymes, and underwent liver biopsy, only 2 patients had histological signs of direct hepatic MTX toxicity. Most frequently, liver biopsies revealed autoimmune hepatitis-like lesions, especially in patients with RA [92]. However, it is important to avoid the unnecessarily premature discontinuation of MTX for reasons of small elevations in transaminases. It is important to bear in mind other causes of transaminitis, such as alcohol consumption or over-the-counter use of nonsteroidal anti-inflammatory drugs (NSAIDs). The limited data available on the effects of alcohol consumption on the risk of liver toxicity in patients with RA who are receiving MTX are insufficient to draw firm conclusions on the amount of alcohol that patients receiving MTX can safely consume. International guidelines vary. The American College of Rheumatology recommends that alcohol should be avoided whilst on MTX [93], while EULAR advises avoiding MTX in patients with a history of alcohol abuse, without specifying a restriction of alcohol consumption otherwise [94]. A systematic literature review found little evidence to provide specific guidelines regarding alcohol consumption [95]. Following their analysis, they estimated a 3% risk for the development of severe liver disease in patients who drink over 100 g of alcohol (12.5 units) per week in the absence of additional risk factors such as obesity, diabetes, or hepatitis. The authors advised caution in using MTX in patients with risk factors. A more recent study suggested that a weekly consumption of <14 units of alcohol per week does not appear to be associated with an increased risk of hepatotoxicity as defined by transaminitis based on aspartate transaminase (AST) or alanine transaminase (ALT), >3 times the upper limit of normal. Consuming between 15 and 21 units is associated with a "possible risk", and over 21 units with a significantly increased risk of transaminitis [96]. However, this definition of hepatotoxicity is somewhat arbitrary as it is not supported by the use of hepatic scans or histology. Furthermore, allowing alcohol consumption of up to 14 units/week may place patients at risk of hepatotoxicity, such as hepatic fibrosis and cirrhosis [97]. In practice, many rheumatologists allow patients without additional risk factors for hepatotoxicity to consume small to moderate amounts of alcohol while taking MTX, preferably avoiding alcohol consumption on the days that they take MTX. Decisions regarding alcohol consumption should be made on an individual patient basis after taking into consideration the presence of other risk factors.

The next section of this position-paper will detail how to deal with these challenges in real-life conditions in order to get the most out of MTX as a first-line treatment.

4. How to Get the Most out of MTX as a First-Line Treatment?

Despite the many advantages of MTX, it may still be used suboptimally. Studies indicate that half of patients discontinue oral MTX within 2 years and that MTX is still frequently stopped rather than combined with bDMARDs or tsDMARDs when these target therapies are initiated. The risk of discontinuation is higher in older patients [98–100]. Patients should be treated early since a longer duration of RA decreases the probability of response [101]. Baseline high disease activity increases the probability of non-response in most studies [102,103].

When initiating MTX, the choice of dose, route of administration, and approach to subsequent dose escalation is not an exact science. Choices may depend on several factors, including the age, gender, ethnicity, weight, and renal function of the patient. These choices will be made with the intent to minimize any tolerability issues and drug-related toxicity, as well as to optimize efficacy and maximize adherence to MTX.

4.1. Dealing with Modifiable Predictors of Response to MTX

Some factors have been shown to impact the response to MTX. Of these, many such as age [104], gender [104], and pharmacogenetic profile [34] cannot be modified. However, others such as smoking may be modifiable, and physicians should endeavor to address this.

Smoking may affect the pharmacokinetic and pharmacodynamics properties of MTX [25]. Smoking habits are predictors of poor response [102,104,105] in a dose-dependent manner [103], with heavy smokers being at higher risk of non-response. In addition, given the higher cardiovascular risk attached to RA patients, smoking cessation is highly desirable [106,107]. Even if it is a demanding objective [107], smoking cessation should be a priority for physicians.

Alcohol consumption, particularly when excessive, has been implicated in the risk of inadequate response to MTX [103]. For most patients, a modest alcohol intake is acceptable, provided that hepatic monitoring remains within safe limits.

Setting realistic but positive expectations about the likely magnitude of benefit, speed of onset, and mitigation strategies to limit toxicity and tolerability issues for MTX may favorably influence the drug's efficacy via improved compliance. High quality education plays a crucial role in achieving this goal. The impact of patient anxiety has also been underscored in limiting the potential benefits of MTX and can be accentuated by the ready availability of misinformation through the internet and other sources. In a multivariate model predicting non-response to MTX in a real-life setting, the risk of non-response was higher in patients who were negative for rheumatoid factor, had a higher Health Assessment Questionnaire (HAQ) score, a higher tender joint count, a lower DAS28 score, and a higher anxiety score [108]. Nonetheless, anxiety is a modifiable risk factor. This issue should be addressed during the shared decision-making process. This process should include exploring the patient's expectations regarding the disease and its treatment, providing honest and positive messages about achievable outcomes, and allaying unfounded fears about adverse effects of therapy. Educating the patient may lower the level of anxiety and improve clinical outcomes.

4.2. Choosing the Route of Administration

When starting MTX, the physician has the choice between oral or parenteral administration. Although MTX can be given by intramuscular (IM) injection, the subcutaneous route is the preferred parenteral administration mode.

Depending on the MTX dose, the bioavailability differs between oral and subcutaneous routes. Oral MTX at a dose of 7.5 mg/week has a 100 percent bioavailability. However, bioavailability is reduced by 30% starting at just 15 mg/week due to gut absorption limitations [22,109]. This threshold is also the point where the bioavailability of oral MTX reaches a plateau in RA patients [21,110]. Consequently, for a patient receiving a weekly dose of 20 mg, intestinal absorption may be reduced by 30% and the effective dose actually received by the patients may be only 14 mg/week. Despite this fact, orally administered doses greater than 15 mg/week are frequently used to control disease activity.

By contrast, the bioavailability of SC MTX is greater than that of oral MTX and does not depend on the MTX dose with a linear increase in systemic exposure for increasing doses [21]. The ratio of dose-normalised $AUC_{0\text{–}24\,h}$ of the SC MTX compared to oral MTX was 127.61 (90% CI 122.30 to 133.15) in a cross-over study comparing the two administration routes of the same MTX dose [21]. The AUC ratio between SC and oral MTX increases with higher doses [110]. Therefore, upon switching from an oral to SC MTX formulation, a patient may experience a bioequivalent increase of more than 6 mg MTX per week. The practical implication of this is that for many patients, there may be no advantage to increasing oral MTX dose above 15 mg/week [21]. Rather, RA patients with an inadequate clinical response to orally administered MTX may benefit from the higher drug exposure offered when switched to the SC formulation [21]. Initiating the MTX regimen with SC administration has been associated with better clinical outcomes at the same dosages [111]. Initial treatment with SC MTX has been associated with lower rates of treatment change, no difference in toxicity, and some improvements in disease control compared to oral MTX over the first year, in a large cohort of early RA [112].

4.3. Starting at the Right Dose

As monotherapy, the dose of MTX can range from 7.5 to 25 mg/week, depending on national guidelines and physician's preference. Such a range allows a wide variety of practices. Indeed, considerable heterogeneity exists in rheumatologist prescribing behaviours [113].

The recommended MTX dose at initiation is generally 10–15 mg/week [94] but should be personalized, depending on age, ethnicity, body weight and prior history of intolerance to other medications. In the interventional C-OPERA study involving Japanese patients, the initial MTX dose was 8 mg/week [114]. Considering the average patient body weight in the Japanese population, a MTX dose of 8 mg/week gave a similar MTX dose, per pound of body weight, to a 10 mg MTX dose in the USA or Europe [114]. In the French ESPOIR cohort involving 813 patients recruited in 14 regional centres the median MTX dose at initiation was 12.5 mg/week [113] with two peaks in the distribution at 10 mg and 15 mg/week. An optimal treatment defined by a starting dose of at least 10 mg/week during the first 3 months, with escalation to at least 20 mg/week at 6 months, has been associated with better clinical outcomes at two years in this cohort [113]. Of note, only 26.3% of patients were considered to have had an optimal dose.

Clinical response is associated with longer-chain polyglutamates, which take 3–8 weeks to become detectable in erythrocytes [23]. These data raise the question as to whether a more rapid attainment of a steady state could be achieved with alternative dosing strategies, such as more rapid dose escalation or starting therapy with higher doses. Starting with a high oral dose does not make pharmacologic sense due to the reduced bioavailability of oral MTX above 15 mg/week. Recent trials have used higher initial MTX dosage (20–30 mg/week) [115]. However, combining the results of 31 studies involving 5589 patients, a meta-regression analysis did not support higher effectiveness of increasing MTX dose in monotherapy [116]. In the CONCERTO study which investigated the effects of starting with various dosages of oral MTX in combination with adalimumab 40 mg every other week, there was no difference in clinical or radiographic outcomes of patients starting with a 10 mg/week MTX dose, compared to those starting with a 20 mg/week dose [77]. Starting with higher oral doses may also result in discontinuation due to adverse events, such as nausea.

In patients who reintroduce MTX after previous discontinuation for tolerability problems, the MTX dose selection should be determined by the last tolerated dose.

4.4. Escalating and Adapting the MTX Dose

In the context of a treat-to-target strategy, the large dose-titratable range of MTX offers numerous possibilities of dose adjustment before combining with bDMARDS and tsDMARDs. Around one third of DMARD-naïve patients will respond to MTX monotherapy and maintain favourable outcomes for several years as reported in the SWEFOT study [117]. The MTX dose should be increased until remission or at least LDA. In clinical trials comparing bDMARDs to MTX monotherapy, 25% of the patients allocated to the MTX arm reached ACR70 criterion within 6 months, bringing them in the range of LDA [118]. With the subcutaneous route [111], the proportion of patients reaching LDA was even higher.

Titration is highly influenced by the starting dose and initial response to treatment. An optimal treatment defined by a starting dose of at least 10 mg/week during the first 3 months with escalation to at least 20 mg/week at 6 months has been associated with better clinical outcomes at two years in the ESPOIR cohort [113]. In the C-EARLY study comparing certolizumab + MTX and placebo + MTX in DMARD-RA patients with poor prognostic factors, MTX was started at 10 mg/week and escalated by 5 mg every 2 weeks, if tolerated, to a maximum of 25 mg/week by week 8. In the MTX monotherapy group, 39.4% of patients reached LDA at week 52. Withdrawals due to AEs occurred for 9.2% of patients [119]. These results suggest that the MTX dose should not be less than 10 mg/week and that dose escalation should be as rapid as tolerated. Maximum dose varies according to the region. The usual maximum MTX dose is 25 mg/week in USA and Europe although some patients may benefit from higher doses. The maximum recommended dose in China is 20 mg/week [120] and in Japan, 16 mg/week [114]. In a randomized controlled trial in patients with active RA despite oral MTX, intramuscular (IM) MTX, starting at a dose of 15 mg/week then increasing to 45 mg/week, did not improve disease control; however, higher doses were generally well tolerated [121]. The CRA 2012 Working Group recommends individualized dosing (oral or parenteral) titrated, to a usual maximum dose of 25 mg/week, by rapid escalation [6]. The French Society for Rheumatology recommends rapid dose escalation (e.g., 5 mg increments every 1–4 weeks) reaching an optimal dose of MTX (15 to 25 mg/week) within 4–8 weeks [122], depending on effectiveness and safety, as well as individual characteristics. The use of split oral dosing (2 half-doses at 8 h interval on one day of the week) has been reported to improve bioavailability, tolerance, adherence, and efficacy [123]. Given the higher bioavailability of SC MTX beyond 15 mg/week, as compared to oral MTX, switching to SC MTX before increasing the MTX dose beyond 15 mg/week could be good practice. In addition, switching to SC MTX may also prevent dose-dependent gastrointestinal side effects [124].

When remission without structural progression is achieved in a patient who is not taking glucocorticoid therapy, and sustained for many months or even years, therapy de-escalation according to tight control principles could be considered [122]. However, withdrawing MTX bears the risk of losing the state of remission and difficulties in regaining a good outcome after a post-withdrawal flare [118].

4.5. Switching to SC Route

In patients with an inadequate response or intolerance to oral MTX, parenteral administration should be considered [6]. In Germany, the 2012 adapted EULAR Task Force recommendations and treatment algorithm in RA support optimization of MTX monotherapy with parenteral administration [125]. Similarly, the British Society for Rheumatology 2008 guidelines for DMARD use recommends switching to IM or SC MTX if oral MTX is ineffective or not tolerated [126].

Parenteral administration has been reported to reduce disease activity in patients who have an inadequate response to oral MTX [127]. Conversely, a change from parenteral to oral MTX has been associated with disease flare [128], increased disease activity, and greater frequency of gastrointestinal side effects. Switching back to intramuscular MTX improved disease manifestations and reduced side effects [129].

Switching patients treated with oral MTX to an SC formulation should be considered when the maximum tolerated dose has been reached without achieving LDA. The SC route may also be proposed upfront to the patient at the time of MTX initiation, although this has relatively greater economic implications. However, data from a randomized controlled trial of 375 MTX-naïve RA patients favoured initiation of 15 mg once weekly MTX therapy by the SC route, which resulted in higher ACR20 and 70 response rates than oral MTX with a similar safety profile at 24 weeks [111]. Furthermore, in a large retrospective cohort study, Harris et al. reported that patients taking SC MTX received higher starting and maximum doses than those on oral MTX (>15 mg starting dose and >20 mg maximum dose) [130], perhaps reflecting the better tolerability of the parenterally delivered drug.

There have been advocates in Canada, Germany, and the United Kingdom for the use of SC MTX in order to optimize achievable efficacy of MTX prior to commencing biologic treatment or even to prevent or delay the need for biologic therapy with attendant health economic benefits [6,125,126]. Indeed, multiple lines of evidence suggest that SC MTX, which bypasses first-pass metabolism in the gastrointestinal tract, appears to be an effective option in patients who have had an inadequate response or are intolerant to oral MTX. Switching such patients to SC MTX has been shown to result in higher and more constant bioavailability [22], to be more effective at the same dosage [111], and to have less intense gastrointestinal side effects compared to oral MTX [124]. Higher bioavailability and increased long-chain $MTXGlu_n$ may translate into efficacy [30,65,131,132]. A retrospective population-based study in 156 patients who were intolerant or unresponsive to oral MTX found that switching to SC MTX ($n = 78$) resulted in a decrease in RA disease severity, with good tolerability reported in these patients [65]. In the retrospective analysis of the US Veterans Affairs database of patients treated with injectable MTX after failing prior oral MTX, higher doses of MTX (>20 mg/wk) were achieved more readily with SC administration, and were associated with a significantly longer duration of MTX monotherapy before therapeutic change or the addition of other DMARDs/biologic agents, as compared to the oral formulation [133]. In the previously mentioned clinical trial comparing SC and oral MTX in 375 RA patients, after 16 weeks, patients from the oral group not fulfilling ACR20 criteria were switched from 15 mg of oral MTX to 15 mg of SC MTX following which 30% went on to achieve ACR20 responses [111]. In keeping with this observations, but in a real-world setting, retrospective analysis of 103 RA patients who switched from oral to SC MTX showed significant improvements in DAS-28 scores in patients who switched due to inefficacy or intolerability to prior oral MTX [132].

A prospective survey (i.e., office questionnaires) study evaluating patients ($n = 70$; each serving as their own control) with long-lasting RA who were switched from oral MTX to SC MTX due to side effects reported that when receiving the SC formulation, patients experienced less intense GI side effects, with no patients reporting vomiting or diarrhoea AEs [124].

SC MTX should also be considered in patients with poor compliance to oral MTX. There is currently no clear biomarker available to measure adherence to MTX in daily practice, despite some data suggesting a strong correlation between $MTXGlu_n$ and compliance assessed by the electronic monitoring of treatment intakes with the Medication Event Monitoring System [134].

4.6. Giving Time for MTX to Achieve its Maximum Clinical Benefit and Using Bridge Therapies

Whether MTX is initiated at a higher dose, or a lower dose with upward titration, it will still take up to six months to achieve a maximum clinical benefit. Nevertheless, therapeutic response to MTX should be assessed after 3 months of treatment with the objective of a clinical improvement at least 50% [4]. If this short-term target is not reached, treatment adjustment should be considered.

Intra-articular glucocorticoids or short term systemic glucocorticoids may be used as part of the initial treatment strategy while waiting for MTX to take effect [6]. When MTX and intra-articular glucocorticoids were used with a treat-to-target approach in patients with early RA in the context of a clinical trial, this strategy effectively decreased synovitis, osteitis, and tenosynovitis and halted structural damage progression, as judged by MRI [135]. The EULAR Task Force recommends using glucocorticoids in combination with csDMARDs primarily as bridging therapy until the csDMARD reaches its maximum effect but corticosteroids should be tapered as rapidly as clinically feasible [4,6]. Intra-articular glucocorticoid application may be considered in residually inflamed or reactivated joint [4].

4.7. Preventing or Dealing with Adverse Events by Folic Acid Supplementation

In clinical practice, MTX-related toxicity may limit optimum treatment. Mild toxicity occurs in about 60% of patients and roughly seven to 38% of patients discontinue MTX within the first year of treatment due to toxicity [18,136,137]. Predisposing factors include existing folate deficiency, advanced age, cumulative MTX dose, renal insufficiency, and concomitant use of other folate inhibitors. A folate deficiency may cause side effects, such as mouth sores, abdominal pain, elevation of liver enzymes, or bone marrow depletion. Folate deficiency is frequent in RA patients and even more in those treated with MTX [138]. In a meta-analysis of six clinical studies, RA patients treated with low-dose MTX and "dummy" folic or folinic acid frequently experienced side effects: nausea and vomiting were reported by 35% of patients, abnormal liver blood tests were reported by 21% of patients, 22% of patients experienced mouth sores [139]. By contrast, genuine folic acid and folinic acid supplementation greatly reduced discontinuation of MTX compared to placebo supplementation in a placebo-controlled double-blind clinical trial. This was mainly due to the MTX stopping rules based on elevations of liver enzymes [137]. By delaying or preventing a premature switch from MTX to a far more expensive bDMARD or tsDMARD, folate supplementation may contribute to health costs savings [140].

There is a large variability of folate supplementation practices amongst rheumatologists. In a study of 2467 incident users of MTX in the Veterans Health Administration database, 27% of patients were not prescribed folic acid within 30 days of MTX initiation. After 20 months, only 50% of patients continued to receive folic acid [141].

In a Cochrane review of patients on MTX therapy for RA, folic acid or folinic acid supplementation reduced the risk of gastrointestinal side effects (nausea, vomiting, and abdominal pain) by 26% (not statistically significant); abnormal serum transaminase elevations were decreased by 77%; the risk of premature discontinuations from MTX for any reason was reduced by 61%. A trend towards a reduction in stomatitis was demonstrated but did not reach statistical significance [139]. Folate supplementation did not negatively impact the efficacy of MTX. These results were confirmed by a recent meta-analysis of seven studies involving 709 patients [142]. A third meta-analysis of 68 studies (not limited to RA) of patients taking MTX revealed that MTX increased the risk of nausea and vomiting, elevated transaminase levels, mucosal ulcerations, leucopenia, thrombocytopenia and infectious events. The concomitant prescription of folic acid or folinic acid was associated with a significantly lower risk of any adverse events [143].

No evidence of a significant difference between folic or folinic acid has been reported, but given its low-cost, folic acid may be the most cost-effective therapy [139]. Prescription of at least 5 mg folic acid per week with MTX therapy is strongly recommended [94] to avoid or prevent side effects. Taking folic acid two days before MTX intake may improve its tolerability. Folic acid supplementation can be increased to 5 mg/day, other than the methotrexate dosing day, if needed. However, a pilot study recently compared two folate supplementation regimens with folic acid (5 mg/week and 0.8 mg/week) with similar results [144]. Folinic acid should be administered on a weekly basis the day after MTX. Although daily use of folic acid other than the MTX day does not appear to affect MTX efficacy, dosing of folinic acid close to MTX administration or dose of folinic acid over 7.5 mg/week may hinder MTX efficacy.

4.8. Potential Toxicities

Most frequent adverse events of MTX are gastrointestinal and there is a correlation between the MTX dose and the intensity of side effects [124]. Other possible side effects include anaemia, neutropenia, increased risk of bruising and dermatitis. Gastric side effects can be reduced both by switching patients to the SC route [124] and by folate supplementation [139]. Elevation of transaminases is frequent, but MTX treated patients are not at increased risk of symptomatic or severe liver related adverse events [55]. The incidence of clinically important cytopenia in patients treated with low dose MTX is estimated to be less than 1%. A complete blood count, liver and renal biochemistry, and a chest radiograph should be ordered prior to initiating MTX therapy [6]. Screening for hepatitis B and C should be considered and HIV testing is recommended in high-risk patients [6].

MTX is excreted via the kidneys and is contraindicated in patients with an estimated glomerular filtration rate of less than 30 mL/min. Patients with impaired renal function should be closely monitored particularly for hematologic toxicity.

Concomitant intake of NSAIDs may reduce renal function, thereby increasing MTX bioavailability. In a registry-based analysis, concomitant use of NSAIDs and MTX increased the risk of serious adverse events with a higher risk of renal failure and cytopenia [145]. However, it should be remembered that NSAIDs, per se, may increase liver enzymes. Therefore, if raised transaminases are observed in patients taking concomitant MTX and NSAIDs, it is worth considering a decrease (or cessation) in the dose of NSAIDs rather than diminishing the MTX dose. The physician should pay attention to self-medication with NSAIDs. MTX should not be used with trimethoprim-sulfamethoxazole when used in a twice-daily regimen for treatment of an infection since the combination may result in significant bone marrow toxicity. However, it can be used for patients taking prophylactic doses of trimethoprim-sulfamethoxazole (dosed three times per week) for prevention of *Pneumocysis Carinii*. The main drug interactions are summarized in Table 1.

Table 1. Drug interactions. MTX, methotrexate.

Interactions	Source of Interactions
Increase MTX levels	• Allopurinol, triamterene • Decrease renal MTX clearance: ciprofloxacin, cephalothin, penicillin, probenecid, sulfonamides • Decrease MTX excretion: diuretics, proton pump inhibitors • Increase MTX reabsorption by the kidney tubule: probenecid
Decrease MTX levels	• Decrease intestinal absorption of MTX: chloramphenicol, tetracyclines
Increase the risk of bone marrow suppression	• Chloramphenicol, co-trimoxazole, pyrimethamine, sulfonamides, trimethoprine-sulfamethoxazole
Increase liver toxicity	• Alcohol, leflunomide

MTX-induced pneumonitis is a potentially life-threatening adverse effect [146]. It is an idiosyncratic hypersensitivity reaction due to activated T-cell-mediated (CD4 and CD8) stimulation of type 2 alveolar cells to release cytokines which lead to the recruitment of inflammatory cells, resulting in alveolitis. Acute or subacute pneumonitis related to methotrexate usually occurs during the first year of treatment [55,147]. It appears rapidly with low grade fever or high fever, nonproductive cough, and dyspnea that usually progresses to respiratory failure. The presence of eosinophilia in peripheral blood but not in bronchoalveolar lavage is common (50%). A diffuse interstitial pattern or a mixed interstitial-alveolar pattern (nodular or patchy infiltrates) is observed in the chest radiograph and high-resolution CT usually reveals the pattern of a usual interstitial pneumonia or a nonspecific interstitial pneumonia. Risk factors for this complication are age (>60 years), previous use of other DMARDs, hypoalbuminemia, the presence of diabetes mellitus, and a history of pleural disease and/or prior ILD related to AR (OR: 7.1), the latter being a great confounding factor when establishing a causal relationship with the drug [148]. It could be difficult to distinguish MTX-induced pneumonitis and pneumonitis related to *Pneumocystis* [149]. In a systematic review, 15 of 3463 RA patients (0.43%) who were receiving MTX developed MTX-induced pneumonitis [150]. Even if rare, this complication needs to be known and should not be neglected. Its treatment includes withdrawal of MTX, supportive therapy, and adjunctive steroids. The outcome is good if the condition is recognized early, and if appropriate treatment is given [146].

Although the overall benefit:risk ratio for MTX is remarkably favourable, as with any drug, adverse events can occur. Based on known adverse events of MTX treatment, we propose that it is good practice to assess the patient for several potential risk factors (Table 2). Among these precautions are the assessment of pre-existing infections, immunosuppression, haematological, kidney or liver diseases, neoplasms, the cardiovascular risks, potential interactions with concomitant therapies. In parallel the psychological status of the patient should be judged or assessed including the coping strategies and the internal resilience.

Table 2. Preparation of MTX therapy.

Diagnosis of rheumatoid/inflammatory arthritis and/or need for treatment
Diagnosis of chronic kidney or liver diseases
Assessment of cardiovascular risks
Assessment of a neoplastic disease
Discussion on smoking habits and the advantage of smoking cessation
Evaluation/judging of depression and resilience/coping strategies
Assessment of anemia, leukopenia, or thrombocytopenia
Documentation of concomitant drug therapy
Defining therapeutic aim
Shared decision making with the patient
Evaluation of alcohol-consumption
Diagnosis of active/chronic infection with herpes zoster, tuberculosis, hepatitis, HIV, relevant fungal infection
Diagnosis of immunodeficiency
Documentation of vaccination status
Consider testing for tuberculosis
Anticonception/assessing wish of conception/family planning

4.9. Placing MTX as an Anchor Drug

MTX is considered the initial drug of choice in RA pharmacotherapy with subsequent use as an anchor drug when used in combination due to its efficacy (when used optimally), safety, large dose-titratable range, and cost-effectiveness [4,5,94].

If the patient is unable to achieve treatment targets on maximally tolerated doses of oral MTX, and after a switch to the SC route, other treatment strategies must be considered. These include adding other csDMARDs, and adding or switching to biologic therapies or tsDMARDs, depending on the absence or presence of poor prognostic factors [4]. In routine practice, several combinations can be considered with some variations in preference according to country. As an example, physicians may take advantage of the combination with probenecid [151], the synergistic action of MTX and HCQ [69], or the triple combination MTX, HCQ, and SSZ [69,70]. In UK or Canada, rheumatologists are required to use at least two csDMARDs before the application of bDMARDs is approved by the payers [4]. The EULAR Task Force strongly recommends that bDMARDs and tsDMARDs should primarily be added to csDMARDs, such as MTX, since all bDMARDs have better efficacy when combined with MTX than as monotherapy [4]. This may be due to complementary mechanisms of action, pharmacokinetic interactions, and reduction of immunogenicity of the administered biologic agent.

If MTX is well tolerated in combination with concomitant csDMARDs or targeted therapies, the dose does not need to be tapered while waiting to achieve the desired treatment target. In case of poor tolerability, MTX can be used at 7.5–10 mg/week to provide additional efficacy to TNF-inhibitors [77] and intolerance at these low doses leading to discontinuation is very rare. Stopping MTX should be limited to patients with contraindications or very poor tolerance to MTX.

Current application of these guidelines is far from optimal. Analysing a database of 35,640 US patients with RA starting oral MTX, Rohr et al. [152] reported that over the 20,041 patients who had to change the treatment over a 5 year follow-up, only 13% switched to SC MTX. In those who added or switched to a biologic, only 37% were on >15 mg/week of oral MTX when a biologic was started. The addition or switch to a biologic occurred in the first 3 months of MTX therapy in 41% of patients, and in the first 6 months in 51% of patients. As stated by the authors, this study revealed that the MTX was dramatically underutilized as an efficacious anchor drug in clinical practice

4.10. Conception and Pregnancy

This section applies to RA patients who are planning to become pregnant and/or breastfeeding, men planning to conceive and patients who have accidentally conceived while taking MTX.

MTX is pro-abortive and teratogenic but does not decrease fertility [153]. Therefore, MTX at any dose should be avoided during pregnancy [154]. The optimal delay between the last MTX dose and conception is still a matter of debate and may vary between countries. Guidelines from the British Society for Rheumatology (BSR) and the British Health Professionals Society in Rheumatology recommend to stop MTX three months in advance of conception [154]. On the other hand, MTX is recommended to be stopped between 48 h and 6 months before conception, in France and in Spain, respectively. Thus, to avoid medicolegal issues, we recommend following the legal label of your country. In the case of accidental pregnancy on low-dose MTX, the drug should be stopped immediately [154].

MTX cannot be recommended in breastfeeding because [154] MTX is excreted into breast milk and may be toxic for the neonate.

If a woman has received MTX within 3 months prior to conception, or in the case of accidental pregnancy on MTX, folate supplementation should be continued prior to and throughout pregnancy at a dose of 5 mg/day [154].

Data regarding preconception exposure to MTX in men are reassuring, and, indeed, recent BSR guidelines state there is no need for men wishing to father children to stop MTX [154]. A study involving a very large cohort concluded that paternal exposure to MTX within 90 days before pregnancy was not associated with congenital malformations, stillbirths, and preterm birth [155]. Older recommendations suggest to stop MTX three months prior to conception, but this is not evidenced by an understanding of the impact of MTX on spermatogenesis or paternal-mediated teratogenicity, but rather relies on the timeframe of spermatogenesis [156].

4.11. Vaccinations

RA patients are more prone to infections than healthy subjects due to the immune dysfunction associated with the condition. DMARDs inhibit cellular and humoral immunity, thus aggravating the susceptibility to infections. For these reasons, vaccines against preventable diseases should be counselled in patients with RA. Influenza, pneumococcal, and shingles are important for all patients with RA whereas human papilloma virus, hepatitis B virus, and yellow fever (YF) vaccines are relevant only in selected patients, such as those living in or traveling to a YF-endemic country [157]. Protection is far from optimal. In 2012, in the United States, only 28.5% of patients older than 60 with rheumatic diseases were vaccinated against pneumococcal pneumonia; 45.8% were optimally vaccinated against influenza, and only 4.0% of patients were vaccinated against shingles [158].

MTX significantly decreases vaccine response to pneumococcal [159,160] and seasonal influenza vaccines [159] in a dose-dependent manner [161]. A recent randomized controlled trial showed that, in order to impair the response to vaccines, MTX had to be present just before or at the same time of vaccination [162]. It is, therefore, recommended that vaccination be done before a DMARD is started, where practically feasible [5]. However, it may be necessary to prioritize control of the disease. In such circumstances, and for seasonal vaccinations, MTX dosing can be temporarily interrupted. In a prospective randomized parallel-group trial, patients with RA taking a stable dose of MTX were randomly assigned at a ratio of 1:1:1:1 to continue MTX (group 1), suspend MTX for 4 weeks before vaccination (group 2), suspend MTX for 2 weeks before and 2 weeks after vaccination (group 3), or suspend MTX for 4 weeks after vaccination (group 4). All participants were vaccinated with trivalent influenza vaccine. Temporary MTX discontinuation improved the immunogenicity of vaccination. No difference was found between groups three and four [162]. These results were confirmed in another study [161] that demonstrated improvement in immunogenicity of seasonal influenza vaccination in patients receiving methotrexate in whom the drug was withheld for 2 weeks immediately after immunisation, compared with those who continued to receive methotrexate with a satisfactory vaccine response seen in 76% of the former compared with 55% of the latter group. However, there was a slightly higher incidence of flares in those patients who withheld methotrexate compared with those who had remained on methotrexate (11% vs. 5%). Therefore, suspending MTX administration for 2 weeks after the vaccination seems to be good practice.

Shingles vaccine can be used safely with low-dose MTX (i.e., up to 25 mg/week) [157].

Live vaccines, such as yellow fever, measles/mumps/rubella, varicella, and oral typhoid vaccinations, are contra-indicated in patients receiving MTX. Information remains too scarce to question the current guidelines.

4.12. No Need for MTX Discontinuation in Case of Surgery

Despite the efficacy of DMARDs, 58% of RA patients will ultimately undergo orthopaedic surgery, with nearly 24% undergoing large-joint arthroplasty [163]. Patients receiving DMARD are potentially at higher risk of infections and delay in wound healing due to the anti-inflammatory properties of these compounds. A study involving 388 patients with RA who underwent surgery found that patients who continued MTX through surgery had fewer complications, infections, and RA flares than patients who discontinued MTX for 2 weeks before and after surgery [164]. A special consideration should be given to patients who develop renal dysfunction postoperatively, since the risk of MTX toxicity is increased in cases of renal failure.

4.13. Sharing the Decision Making with the Patient

Adherence to treatment has been shown to depend on the level of appropriate information provided to patients and the amount of good interaction with the rheumatologist [165]. Non-adherent patients flare four times more frequently than adherent patients [100]. Most arthritis patients prefer to be involved in decisions about their medication [166], and this has been linked to higher patient satisfaction.

Patients exhibit a complex range of beliefs related to DMARD therapy [167]. Furthermore, the degree to which patients desire to be directed by their physician regarding treatment choice varies tremendously and may evolve over time to become more collaborative [168]. Sympathetic understanding will facilitate the provision of appropriate information to allow the patient to make informed decisions [169]. Furthermore, it is crucial to educate patients about the importance of a T2T strategy, since it has been shown that patient preference is among the leading barriers to treatment adjustment to T2T in RA [170].

The EULAR Task Force recently reiterated the relative safety of MTX and recommended that the frequent fears of patients after reading the package insert should be addressed by providing appropriate information [4]. The overemphasis on the risk of side effects that are widely spread on social media can generally be overcome by an open, balanced, and reassuring discussion regarding the benefits/risks and risk mitigation at the time of the first prescription. The other crucial points to address are the importance of maintained therapy, especially in those patients in remission who want to stop MTX, and patient adherence (in particular, for patients who tell their practitioner that they are taking MTX when, actually, this is not the case). Available data suggest that adherence to RA therapy does not exceed 66% [171], but this proportion is enhanced by the belief in the necessity of the medication. For this reason, when explaining the achievable goals of treatment to the patient, the rheumatologist should emphasise the availability of long-term observational data demonstrating the numerous benefits and good overall tolerability of MTX.

When initiating MTX, we recommend that rheumatologists adopt a shared decision-making approach to the recommended regime. Key points to be emphasised in dialogue with the patient are summarized on Table 3.

Table 3. Key points patients will need to be counselled about when rheumatologists adopt a shared decision-making approach to the recommended regime. NSAIDs, non-steroidal anti-inflammatory drugs.

Topics to Discuss with Patients
• The choice of routes of administration and the advantages of each
• Expected time to experiencing benefits (this is very important as a patient may experience transient tolerability problems such as nausea prior to experiencing and improvement in symptoms and there will therefore be a danger of non-adherence if there has not been appropriate counselling)
• Potential toxicities with reassurance about the capability to mitigate these risks through regular and appropriate blood monitoring
• The potential tolerability issues, especially nausea with appropriate reassurance that this can be lessened or mitigated with use of folic acid supplementation or parenteral administration
• Women of childbearing potential need to be counselled about pregnancy and family planning.
• Vaccinations and how to ensure optimum outcomes of vaccination
• Alcohol consumption
• Interactions between MTX and other medication with particular advice about NSAIDs

5. Conclusions

In conclusion, MTX is a remarkable drug with a unique place in the pharmacotherapeutic management of RA. Key recommendations for clinical use are listed in Table 4. In the last 2 decades, the cumulative experience of rheumatologists has helped to refine the possibility of achieving the best outcomes with MTX. It has a large dose titratable range and can be administered as a once weekly dose regimen by either oral or subcutaneous routes. Parenteral administration of MTX has the advantages of maximising bioavailability, reducing gastrointestinal intolerance, and potentially enhancing compliance and adherence. MTX is recommended as the first-line csDMARD treatment for RA and can also be used in combination with other csDMARDs, bDMARDs, or tsDMARDs. In the case of concomitant use with targeted therapies, MTX facilitates optimum achievable efficacy, and also has the advantage, when used with bDMARDs, of reducing ADAb responses to administered biologic. MTX is also highly cost-effective and has a favourable benefit/risk profile overall. Nonetheless, adverse events associated with MTX are well-described and tolerability issues can be a troublesome complication of this treatment. However, with appropriate risk-mitigation strategies, including folic acid supplementation, blood monitoring, and patient education, one can optimise achievable outcomes.

Table 4. Key recommendations for clinical use of MTX. csDMARD, conventional synthetic disease-modifying antirheumatic drugs; bDMARDs, biological DMARDs; tsDMARDs, targeted synthetic DMARDs; SC, subcutaneous.

Key Points for Clinical Use of MTX
Modify predictors of response to MTX
Encourage smoking cessation
Limit alcohol consumption
Ensure appropriate education on how to optimise outcomes
Manage anxiety and depression
Start at the right dose
Generally 10–15 mg/week, but should be personalized There is no need to start with higher dose
Choose between oral and parenteral route.

Table 4. *Cont.*

Key Points for Clinical Use of MTX
Escalate as quickly as tolerated
Titrate dose according to individual clinical response Generally aim to reach a dose of at least 20 mg/week after 6 months Consider local recommendations and clinical context
Switch to SC route for doses higher than 15 mg/week to enhance MTX bioavailability
Prevent side effects
Start folic acid supplementation at a dose of at least 5 mg/week and up to 5 mg/day other than the day of methotrexate (or folinic acid at a dose lower than 7.5 mg/week)
Instruct the patient to not take folic acid on the day of MTX administration
Folinic acid should be administered on a weekly basis the day after MTX administration
Counsel patients about risk mitigation through blood monitoring according to local protocols
Be aware of potential drug to drug interactions
Instruct the patients to seek advice from their rheumatologist about compatibility with methotrexate of self-medicated drugs or drugs prescribed by another physician
In case of poor tolerability
Diminish gastrointestinal side effects by switching to SC route
In case of inadequate response
Enhance MTX bioavailability by splitting oral dose or switching to SC route
Consider combination with csDMARD, bDMARDs or tsDMARDs Do not stop MTX nor reduce MTX dose unless there are toxicity or tolerability concerns
Give time for MTX achieving maximum clinical benefit
Use intra-articular or systemic glucocorticoids as bridging therapies
Educate the patient and adopt a shared decision-making approach

Author Contributions: Conceptualization P.C.T., A.B.C., A.B.M., J.A., H.M., R.B.M., Funding acquisition P.C.T., A.B.C., A.B.M., J.A., H.M., R.B.M., Investigation P.C.T., A.B.C., A.B.M., J.A., H.M., R.B.M., Validation P.C.T., A.B.C., A.B.M., J.A., H.M., R.B.M., Writing, original draft P.C.T., R.B.M., Writing, review and editing P.C.T., A.B.C., A.B.M., J.A., H.M., R.B.M.

Acknowledgments: The authors thanks Pierre Clerson and Yann Fardini (Soladis Clinical Studies) for assistance in the preparation of the manuscript. This assistance was funded by Nordic Pharma SAS. PCT would like to thank Oxford BRC and AR UK for support.

Conflicts of Interest: P.C.T. has received research grants from Celgene, Galapagos Lilly and Janssen and served as a consultant to AbbVie, Biogen, Gilead, GlaxoSmithKline, Janssen, Lilly, Pfizer, Roche, Fresenius, Sandoz, Sanofi, Nordic Pharma and UCB; A.B.C. has/ahd consultancy relationship and/or has received research funding from AbbVie, Pfizer, Novartis, Nordic Pharma, Sanofi, Bristol Myers Squibb, Sandoz, Lilly, UCB; A.B.M. declares no conflict of interest; J.A. has/had consultancy relationship and/or has received research funding from Boehringer, Bristol Myers Squibb, Nordic Pharma, Pfizer and Sanofi; H.M. has/had consultancy relationship and/or has received research funding from Pfizer, AbbVie, Nordic Pharma, MSD, UCB, Bristol Myers Squibb, Novartis, Roche-Chugai, Janssen, Biogen, Biogaran, Sanofi; R.M. has/had consultancy relationship with Nordic Pharma and has received research funding from Gebro; The funders had no role in the writing of the manuscript, or in the decision to publish the results.

References

1. Heinimann, K.; von Kempis, J.; Sauter, R.; Schiff, M.; Sokka-Isler, T.; Schulze-Koops, H.; Muller, R. Long-Term Increase of Radiographic Damage and Disability in Patients with RA in Relation to Disease Duration in the Era of Biologics. Results from the SCQM Cohort. *J. Clin. Med.* **2018**, *7*, 57. [CrossRef] [PubMed]
2. Smolen, J.S.; Breedveld, F.C.; Burmester, G.R.; Bykerk, V.; Dougados, M.; Emery, P.; Kvien, T.K.; Navarro-Compan, M.V.; Oliver, S.; Schoels, M.; et al. Treating rheumatoid arthritis to target: 2014 update of the recommendations of an international task force. *Ann. Rheum. Dis.* **2016**, *75*, 3–15. [CrossRef]
3. Brinkmann, G.H.; Norvang, V.; Norli, E.S.; Grovle, L.; Haugen, A.J.; Lexberg, A.S.; Rodevand, E.; Bakland, G.; Nygaard, H.; Kroll, F.; et al. Treat to target strategy in early rheumatoid arthritis versus routine care—A comparative clinical practice study. *Semin. Arthritis Rheum.* **2018**. [CrossRef]
4. Smolen, J.S.; Landewe, R.; Bijlsma, J.; Burmester, G.; Chatzidionysiou, K.; Dougados, M.; Nam, J.; Ramiro, S.; Voshaar, M.; van Vollenhoven, R.; et al. EULAR recommendations for the management of rheumatoid arthritis with synthetic and biological disease-modifying antirheumatic drugs: 2016 update. *Ann. Rheum. Dis.* **2017**, *76*, 960–977. [CrossRef]
5. Singh, J.A.; Saag, K.G.; Bridges, S.L., Jr.; Akl, E.A.; Bannuru, R.R.; Sullivan, M.C.; Vaysbrot, E.; McNaughton, C.; Osani, M.; Shmerling, R.H.; et al. 2015 American College of Rheumatology Guideline for the Treatment of Rheumatoid Arthritis. *Arthritis Care Res. (Hoboken)* **2016**, *68*, 1–25. [CrossRef] [PubMed]
6. Bykerk, V.P.; Akhavan, P.; Hazlewood, G.S.; Schieir, O.; Dooley, A.; Haraoui, B.; Khraishi, M.; Leclercq, S.A.; Legare, J.; Mosher, D.P.; et al. Canadian Rheumatology Association recommendations for pharmacological management of rheumatoid arthritis with traditional and biologic disease-modifying antirheumatic drugs. *J. Rheumatol.* **2012**, *39*, 1559–1582. [CrossRef]
7. Lau, C.S.; Chia, F.; Harrison, A.; Hsieh, T.Y.; Jain, R.; Jung, S.M.; Kishimoto, M.; Kumar, A.; Leong, K.P.; Li, Z.; et al. APLAR rheumatoid arthritis treatment recommendations. *Int. J. Rheum. Dis.* **2015**, *18*, 685–713. [CrossRef] [PubMed]
8. Felson, D.T.; Smolen, J.S.; Wells, G.; Zhang, B.; van Tuyl, L.H.; Funovits, J.; Aletaha, D.; Allaart, C.F.; Bathon, J.; Bombardieri, S.; et al. American College of Rheumatology/European League against Rheumatism provisional definition of remission in rheumatoid arthritis for clinical trials. *Ann. Rheum. Dis.* **2011**, *70*, 404–413. [CrossRef]
9. Kavanaugh, A.; Fleischmann, R.M.; Emery, P.; Kupper, H.; Redden, L.; Guerette, B.; Santra, S.; Smolen, J.S. Clinical, functional and radiographic consequences of achieving stable low disease activity and remission with adalimumab plus methotrexate or methotrexate alone in early rheumatoid arthritis: 26-week results from the randomised, controlled OPTIMA study. *Ann. Rheum. Dis.* **2013**, *72*, 64–71. [CrossRef]
10. Radner, H.; Smolen, J.S.; Aletaha, D. Remission in rheumatoid arthritis: Benefit over low disease activity in patient-reported outcomes and costs. *Arthritis Res. Ther.* **2014**, *16*, R56. [CrossRef]
11. Linde, L.; Hetland, M.L.; Ostergaard, M. Drug survival and reasons for discontinuation of intramuscular methotrexate: A study of 212 consecutive patients switching from oral methotrexate. *Scand. J. Rheumatol.* **2006**, *35*, 102–106. [CrossRef]
12. Thiele, K.; Huscher, D.; Bischoff, S.; Spathling-Mestekemper, S.; Backhaus, M.; Aringer, M.; Kohlmann, T.; Zink, A.; German Collaborative Arthritis Centres. Performance of the 2011 ACR/EULAR preliminary remission criteria compared with DAS28 remission in unselected patients with rheumatoid arthritis. *Ann. Rheum. Dis.* **2013**, *72*, 1194–1199. [CrossRef]
13. Grigor, C.; Capell, H.; Stirling, A.; McMahon, A.D.; Lock, P.; Vallance, R.; Kincaid, W.; Porter, D. Effect of a treatment strategy of tight control for rheumatoid arthritis (the TICORA study): A single-blind randomised controlled trial. *Lancet* **2004**, *364*, 263–269. [CrossRef]
14. Verstappen, S.M.; Jacobs, J.W.; van der Veen, M.J.; Heurkens, A.H.; Schenk, Y.; ter Borg, E.J.; Blaauw, A.A.; Bijlsma, J.W.; The Utrecht Rheumatoid Arthritis Cohort Study Group. Intensive treatment with methotrexate in early rheumatoid arthritis: Aiming for remission. Computer Assisted Management in Early Rheumatoid Arthritis (CAMERA, an open-label strategy trial). *Ann. Rheum. Dis.* **2007**, *66*, 1443–1449. [CrossRef]
15. Mueller, R.B.; Spaeth, M.; von Restorff, C.; Ackerman, C.; Schulze-Koops, H.; Von Kempis, J. Superiority of a Treat-to Target Strategy over conventional treatment with csDMARD and corticosteroids: A multi-center randomized controlled trial in RA patients with an inadequate response to conventional synthetic DMARDs, and new therapy with certolizumab pegol. *J. Clin. Med.* **2019**, *8*, 302.

16. Kyburz, D.; Gabay, C.; Michel, B.A.; Finckh, A. The long-term impact of early treatment of rheumatoid arthritis on radiographic progression: A population-based cohort study. *Rheumatology (Oxford)* **2011**, *50*, 1106–1110. [CrossRef]
17. Weinblatt, M.E. Methotrexate in rheumatoid arthritis: A quarter century of development. *Trans. Am. Clin. Climatol. Assoc.* **2013**, *124*, 16–25.
18. Weinblatt, M.E.; Coblyn, J.S.; Fox, D.A.; Fraser, P.A.; Holdsworth, D.E.; Glass, D.N.; Trentham, D.E. Efficacy of low-dose methotrexate in rheumatoid arthritis. *N. Engl. J. Med.* **1985**, *312*, 818–822. [CrossRef]
19. Brown, P.M.; Pratt, A.G.; Isaacs, J.D. Mechanism of action of methotrexate in rheumatoid arthritis, and the search for biomarkers. *Nat. Rev. Rheumatol.* **2016**, *12*, 731–742. [CrossRef]
20. Lebbe, C.; Beyeler, C.; Gerber, N.J.; Reichen, J. Intraindividual variability of the bioavailability of low dose methotrexate after oral administration in rheumatoid arthritis. *Ann. Rheum. Dis.* **1994**, *53*, 475–477. [CrossRef]
21. Schiff, M.H.; Jaffe, J.S.; Freundlich, B. Head-to-head, randomised, crossover study of oral versus subcutaneous methotrexate in patients with rheumatoid arthritis: Drug-exposure limitations of oral methotrexate at doses >/=15 mg may be overcome with subcutaneous administration. *Ann. Rheum. Dis.* **2014**, *73*, 1549–1551. [CrossRef]
22. Hoekstra, M.; Haagsma, C.; Neef, C.; Proost, J.; Knuif, A.; van de Laar, M. Bioavailability of higher dose methotrexate comparing oral and subcutaneous administration in patients with rheumatoid arthritis. *J. Rheumatol.* **2004**, *31*, 645–648.
23. Dalrymple, J.M.; Stamp, L.K.; O'Donnell, J.L.; Chapman, P.T.; Zhang, M.; Barclay, M.L. Pharmacokinetics of oral methotrexate in patients with rheumatoid arthritis. *Arthritis Rheum.* **2008**, *58*, 3299–3308. [CrossRef]
24. Dervieux, T.; Greenstein, N.; Kremer, J. Pharmacogenomic and metabolic biomarkers in the folate pathway and their association with methotrexate effects during dosage escalation in rheumatoid arthritis. *Arthritis Rheum.* **2006**, *54*, 3095–3103. [CrossRef]
25. Stamp, L.K.; O'Donnell, J.L.; Chapman, P.T.; Zhang, M.; Frampton, C.; James, J.; Barclay, M.L. Determinants of red blood cell methotrexate polyglutamate concentrations in rheumatoid arthritis patients receiving long-term methotrexate treatment. *Arthritis Rheum.* **2009**, *60*, 2248–2256. [CrossRef]
26. Tishler, M.; Caspi, D.; Graff, E.; Segal, R.; Peretz, H.; Yaron, M. Synovial and serum levels of methotrexate during methotrexate therapy of rheumatoid arthritis. *Br. J. Rheumatol.* **1989**, *28*, 422–423. [CrossRef]
27. Herman, R.A.; Veng-Pedersen, P.; Hoffman, J.; Koehnke, R.; Furst, D.E. Pharmacokinetics of low-dose methotrexate in rheumatoid arthritis patients. *J. Pharm. Sci.* **1989**, *78*, 165–171. [CrossRef]
28. Chladek, J.; Martinkova, J.; Simkova, M.; Vaneckova, J.; Koudelkova, V.; Nozickova, M. Pharmacokinetics of low doses of methotrexate in patients with psoriasis over the early period of treatment. *Eur. J. Clin. Pharmacol.* **1998**, *53*, 437–444. [CrossRef]
29. Dervieux, T.; Furst, D.; Lein, D.O.; Capps, R.; Smith, K.; Caldwell, J.; Kremer, J. Pharmacogenetic and metabolite measurements are associated with clinical status in patients with rheumatoid arthritis treated with methotrexate: Results of a multicentred cross sectional observational study. *Ann. Rheum. Dis.* **2005**, *64*, 1180–1185. [CrossRef]
30. Stamp, L.K.; Barclay, M.L.; O'Donnell, J.L.; Zhang, M.; Drake, J.; Frampton, C.; Chapman, P.T. Effects of changing from oral to subcutaneous methotrexate on red blood cell methotrexate polyglutamate concentrations and disease activity in patients with rheumatoid arthritis. *J. Rheumatol.* **2011**, *38*, 2540–2547. [CrossRef]
31. Bressolle, F.; Bologna, C.; Kinowski, J.M.; Sany, J.; Combe, B. Effects of moderate renal insufficiency on pharmacokinetics of methotrexate in rheumatoid arthritis patients. *Ann. Rheum. Dis.* **1998**, *57*, 110–113. [CrossRef] [PubMed]
32. Chan, E.S.; Cronstein, B.N. Methotrexate—How does it really work? *Nat. Rev. Rheumatol.* **2010**, *6*, 175–178. [CrossRef] [PubMed]
33. Wessels, J.A.; van der Kooij, S.M.; le Cessie, S.; Kievit, W.; Barerra, P.; Allaart, C.F.; Huizinga, T.W.; Guchelaar, H.J.; Pharmacogenetics Collaborative Research, G. A clinical pharmacogenetic model to predict the efficacy of methotrexate monotherapy in recent-onset rheumatoid arthritis. *Arthritis Rheum.* **2007**, *56*, 1765–1775. [CrossRef] [PubMed]
34. Lopez-Rodriguez, R.; Ferreiro-Iglesias, A.; Lima, A.; Bernardes, M.; Pawlik, A.; Paradowska-Gorycka, A.; Swierkot, J.; Slezak, R.; Gonzalez-Alvaro, I.; Narvaez, J.; et al. Evaluation of a clinical pharmacogenetics model to predict methotrexate response in patients with rheumatoid arthritis. *Pharmacogenom. J.* **2018**, *18*, 539–545. [CrossRef] [PubMed]

35. Hughes, C.D.; Scott, D.L.; Ibrahim, F.; Investigators, T.P. Intensive therapy and remissions in rheumatoid arthritis: A systematic review. *BMC Musculoskelet. Disord.* **2018**, *19*, 389. [CrossRef] [PubMed]
36. Smolen, J.S.; Aletaha, D.; Bijlsma, J.W.; Breedveld, F.C.; Boumpas, D.; Burmester, G.; Combe, B.; Cutolo, M.; de Wit, M.; Dougados, M.; et al. Treating rheumatoid arthritis to target: Recommendations of an international task force. *Ann. Rheum. Dis.* **2010**, *69*, 631–637. [CrossRef]
37. Van Nies, J.A.; Tsonaka, R.; Gaujoux-Viala, C.; Fautrel, B.; van der Helm-van Mil, A.H. Evaluating relationships between symptom duration and persistence of rheumatoid arthritis: Does a window of opportunity exist? Results on the Leiden early arthritis clinic and ESPOIR cohorts. *Ann. Rheum. Dis.* **2015**, *74*, 806–812. [CrossRef] [PubMed]
38. O'Dell, J.R.; Curtis, J.R.; Mikuls, T.R.; Cofield, S.S.; Bridges, S.L., Jr.; Ranganath, V.K.; Moreland, L.W.; Investigators, T.T. Validation of the methotrexate-first strategy in patients with early, poor-prognosis rheumatoid arthritis: Results from a two-year randomized, double-blind trial. *Arthritis Rheum.* **2013**, *65*, 1985–1994. [CrossRef]
39. O'Dell, J.R.; Cohen, S.B.; Thorne, J.C.; Kremer, J. Treatment of rheumatoid arthritis in the USA: Premature use of tumor necrosis factor inhibition and underutilization of concomitant methotrexate. *Open Access Rheumatol.* **2018**, *10*, 97–101. [CrossRef]
40. Mueller, R.B.; Graninger, W.; Sidiropoulos, P.; Goger, C.; von Kempis, J. Median time to low disease activity is shorter in tocilizumab combination therapy with csDMARDs as compared to tocilizumab monotherapy in patients with active rheumatoid arthritis and inadequate responses to csDMARDs and/or TNF inhibitors: Sub-analysis of the Swiss and Austrian patients from the ACT-SURE study. *Clin. Rheumatol.* **2017**, *36*, 2187–2192. [CrossRef]
41. Moreland, L.W.; O'Dell, J.R.; Paulus, H.E.; Curtis, J.R.; Bathon, J.M.; St Clair, E.W.; Bridges, S.L., Jr.; Zhang, J.; McVie, T.; Howard, G.; et al. A randomized comparative effectiveness study of oral triple therapy versus etanercept plus methotrexate in early aggressive rheumatoid arthritis: The treatment of Early Aggressive Rheumatoid Arthritis Trial. *Arthritis Rheum.* **2012**, *64*, 2824–2835. [CrossRef]
42. Goekoop-Ruiterman, Y.P.; de Vries-Bouwstra, J.K.; Allaart, C.F.; van Zeben, D.; Kerstens, P.J.; Hazes, J.M.; Zwinderman, A.H.; Ronday, H.K.; Han, K.H.; Westedt, M.L.; et al. Clinical and radiographic outcomes of four different treatment strategies in patients with early rheumatoid arthritis (the BeSt study): A randomized, controlled trial. *Arthritis Rheum.* **2005**, *52*, 3381–3390. [CrossRef]
43. Muller, R.B.; von Kempis, J.; Haile, S.R.; Schiff, M.H. Effectiveness, tolerability, and safety of subcutaneous methotrexate in early rheumatoid arthritis: A retrospective analysis of real-world data from the St. Gallen cohort. *Semin. Arthritis Rheum.* **2015**, *45*, 28–34. [CrossRef]
44. Van Vollenhoven, R.F.; Ernestam, S.; Geborek, P.; Petersson, I.F.; Coster, L.; Waltbrand, E.; Zickert, A.; Theander, J.; Thorner, A.; Hellstrom, H.; et al. Addition of infliximab compared with addition of sulfasalazine and hydroxychloroquine to methotrexate in patients with early rheumatoid arthritis (Swefot trial): 1-year results of a randomised trial. *Lancet* **2009**, *374*, 459–466. [CrossRef]
45. Gabriel, S.E.; Michaud, K. Epidemiological studies in incidence, prevalence, mortality, and comorbidity of the rheumatic diseases. *Arthritis Res. Ther.* **2009**, *11*, 229. [CrossRef]
46. Young, A.; Koduri, G.; Batley, M.; Kulinskaya, E.; Gough, A.; Norton, S.; Dixey, J.; Early Rheumatoid Arthritis Study (ERAS) Group. Mortality in rheumatoid arthritis. Increased in the early course of disease, in ischaemic heart disease and in pulmonary fibrosis. *Rheumatology (Oxford)* **2007**, *46*, 350–357. [CrossRef]
47. Gonzalez, A.; Maradit Kremers, H.; Crowson, C.S.; Nicola, P.J.; Davis, J.M., 3rd; Therneau, T.M.; Roger, V.L.; Gabriel, S.E. The widening mortality gap between rheumatoid arthritis patients and the general population. *Arthritis Rheum.* **2007**, *56*, 3583–3587. [CrossRef]
48. Choi, H.K.; Hernan, M.A.; Seeger, J.D.; Robins, J.M.; Wolfe, F. Methotrexate and mortality in patients with rheumatoid arthritis: A prospective study. *Lancet* **2002**, *359*, 1173–1177. [CrossRef]
49. Wasko, M.C.; Dasgupta, A.; Hubert, H.; Fries, J.F.; Ward, M.M. Propensity-adjusted association of methotrexate with overall survival in rheumatoid arthritis. *Arthritis Rheum.* **2013**, *65*, 334–342. [CrossRef]
50. Ridker, P.M.; Everett, B.M.; Pradhan, A.; MacFadyen, J.G.; Solomon, D.H.; Zaharris, E.; Mam, V.; Hasan, A.; Rosenberg, Y.; Iturriaga, E.; et al. Low-Dose Methotrexate for the Prevention of Atherosclerotic Events. *N. Engl. J. Med.* **2019**, *380*, 752–762. [CrossRef]
51. Atzeni, F.; Boiardi, L.; Salli, S.; Benucci, M.; Sarzi-Puttini, P. Lung involvement and drug-induced lung disease in patients with rheumatoid arthritis. *Expert Rev. Clin. Immunol.* **2013**, *9*, 649–657. [CrossRef]
52. Suda, T. Up-to-Date Information on Rheumatoid Arthritis-Associated Interstitial Lung Disease. *Clin. Med. Insights Circ. Respir. Pulm. Med.* **2015**, *9*, 155–162. [CrossRef]

53. Rojas-Serrano, J.; Herrera-Bringas, D.; Perez-Roman, D.I.; Perez-Dorame, R.; Mateos-Toledo, H.; Mejia, M. Rheumatoid arthritis-related interstitial lung disease (RA-ILD): Methotrexate and the severity of lung disease are associated to prognosis. *Clin. Rheumatol.* **2017**, *36*, 1493–1500. [CrossRef]
54. England, B.R.; Sayles, H.; Michaud, K.; Thiele, G.M.; Poole, J.A.; Caplan, L.; Sauer, B.C.; Cannon, G.W.; Reimold, A.; Kerr, G.S.; et al. Chronic lung disease in U.S. Veterans with rheumatoid arthritis and the impact on survival. *Clin. Rheumatol.* **2018**, *37*, 2907–2915. [CrossRef]
55. Conway, R.; Carey, J.J. Methotrexate and lung disease in rheumatoid arthritis. *Panminerva Med.* **2017**, *59*, 33–46. [CrossRef]
56. Conway, R.; Low, C.; Coughlan, R.J.; O'Donnell, M.J.; Carey, J.J. Methotrexate and lung disease in rheumatoid arthritis: A meta-analysis of randomized controlled trials. *Arthritis Rheumatol.* **2014**, *66*, 803–812. [CrossRef]
57. Conway, R.; Low, C.; Coughlan, R.J.; O'Donnell, M.J.; Carey, J.J. Methotrexate use and risk of lung disease in psoriasis, psoriatic arthritis, and inflammatory bowel disease: Systematic literature review and meta-analysis of randomised controlled trials. *BMJ* **2015**, *350*, h1269. [CrossRef]
58. Mason, A.; Holmes, C.; Edwards, C.J. Inflammation and dementia: Using rheumatoid arthritis as a model to develop treatments? *Autoimmun. Rev.* **2018**, *17*, 919–925. [CrossRef]
59. Judge, A.; Garriga, C.; Arden, N.K.; Lovestone, S.; Prieto-Alhambra, D.; Cooper, C.; Edwards, C.J. Protective effect of antirheumatic drugs on dementia in rheumatoid arthritis patients. *Alzheimers Dement. (N. Y.)* **2017**, *3*, 612–621. [CrossRef]
60. Lazaro, E.; Morel, J. Management of neutropenia in patients with rheumatoid arthritis. *Jt. Bone Spine* **2015**, *82*, 235–239. [CrossRef]
61. Allen, L.S.; Groff, G. Treatment of Felty's syndrome with low-dose oral methotrexate. *Arthritis Rheum.* **1986**, *29*, 902–905. [CrossRef]
62. Isasi, C.; Lopez-Martin, J.A.; Angeles Trujillo, M.; Andreu, J.L.; Palacio, S.; Mulero, J. Felty's syndrome: Response to low dose oral methotrexate. *J. Rheumatol.* **1989**, *16*, 983–985. [PubMed]
63. Finckh, A.; Bansback, N.; Marra, C.A.; Anis, A.H.; Michaud, K.; Lubin, S.; White, M.; Sizto, S.; Liang, M.H. Treatment of very early rheumatoid arthritis with symptomatic therapy, disease-modifying antirheumatic drugs, or biologic agents: A cost-effectiveness analysis. *Ann. Intern. Med.* **2009**, *151*, 612–621. [CrossRef]
64. Fitzpatrick, R.; Scott, D.G.; Keary, I. Cost-minimisation analysis of subcutaneous methotrexate versus biologic therapy for the treatment of patients with rheumatoid arthritis who have had an insufficient response or intolerance to oral methotrexate. *Clin. Rheumatol.* **2013**, *32*, 1605–1612. [CrossRef]
65. Mainman, H.; McClaren, E.; Heycock, C.; Saravanan, V.; Hamilton, J.; Kelly, C. When should we use parenteral methotrexate? *Clin. Rheumatol.* **2010**, *29*, 1093–1098. [CrossRef]
66. Deighton, C.; Hyrich, K.; Ding, T.; Ledingham, J.; Lunt, M.; Luqmani, R.; Kiely, P.; Bukhari, M.; Abernethy, R.; Ostor, A.; et al. BSR and BHPR rheumatoid arthritis guidelines on eligibility criteria for the first biological therapy. *Rheumatology (Oxford)* **2010**, *49*, 1197–1199. [CrossRef]
67. Carmichael, S.J.; Beal, J.; Day, R.O.; Tett, S.E. Combination therapy with methotrexate and hydroxychloroquine for rheumatoid arthritis increases exposure to methotrexate. *J. Rheumatol.* **2002**, *29*, 2077–2083. [PubMed]
68. Schapink, L.; van den Ende, C.H.M.; Gevers, L.; van Ede, A.E.; den Broeder, A.A. The effects of methotrexate and hydroxychloroquine combination therapy vs methotrexate monotherapy in early rheumatoid arthritis patients. *Rheumatology (Oxford)* **2018**, *58*, 131–134. [CrossRef]
69. Hazlewood, G.S.; Barnabe, C.; Tomlinson, G.; Marshall, D.; Devoe, D.J.; Bombardier, C. Methotrexate monotherapy and methotrexate combination therapy with traditional and biologic disease modifying anti-rheumatic drugs for rheumatoid arthritis: A network meta-analysis. *Cochrane Database Syst. Rev.* **2016**, CD010227. [CrossRef]
70. Peper, S.M.; Lew, R.; Mikuls, T.; Brophy, M.; Rybin, D.; Wu, H.; O'Dell, J. Rheumatoid Arthritis Treatment After Methotrexate: The Durability of Triple Therapy Versus Etanercept. *Arthritis Care Res. (Hoboken)* **2017**, *69*, 1467–1472. [CrossRef] [PubMed]
71. Quach, L.T.; Chang, B.H.; Brophy, M.T.; Soe Thwin, S.; Hannagan, K.; O'Dell, J.R. Rheumatoid arthritis triple therapy compared with etanercept: Difference in infectious and gastrointestinal adverse events. *Rheumatology (Oxford)* **2017**, *56*, 378–383. [CrossRef]
72. Fleischmann, R.; Tongbram, V.; van Vollenhoven, R.; Tang, D.H.; Chung, J.; Collier, D.; Urs, S.; Ndirangu, K.; Wells, G.; Pope, J. Systematic review and network meta-analysis of the efficacy and safety of tumour necrosis

factor inhibitor-methotrexate combination therapy versus triple therapy in rheumatoid arthritis. *RMD Open* **2017**, *3*, e000371. [CrossRef]

73. Bathon, J.M.; Martin, R.W.; Fleischmann, R.M.; Tesser, J.R.; Schiff, M.H.; Keystone, E.C.; Genovese, M.C.; Wasko, M.C.; Moreland, L.W.; Weaver, A.L.; et al. A comparison of etanercept and methotrexate in patients with early rheumatoid arthritis. *N. Engl. J. Med.* **2000**, *343*, 1586–1593. [CrossRef]
74. Breedveld, F.C.; Weisman, M.H.; Kavanaugh, A.F.; Cohen, S.B.; Pavelka, K.; van Vollenhoven, R.; Sharp, J.; Perez, J.L.; Spencer-Green, G.T. The PREMIER study: A multicenter, randomized, double-blind clinical trial of combination therapy with adalimumab plus methotrexate versus methotrexate alone or adalimumab alone in patients with early, aggressive rheumatoid arthritis who had not had previous methotrexate treatment. *Arthritis Rheum.* **2006**, *54*, 26–37. [CrossRef]
75. Emery, P.; Breedveld, F.C.; Hall, S.; Durez, P.; Chang, D.J.; Robertson, D.; Singh, A.; Pedersen, R.D.; Koenig, A.S.; Freundlich, B. Comparison of methotrexate monotherapy with a combination of methotrexate and etanercept in active, early, moderate to severe rheumatoid arthritis (COMET): A randomised, double-blind, parallel treatment trial. *Lancet* **2008**, *372*, 375–382. [CrossRef]
76. Emery, P.; Fleischmann, R.; van der Heijde, D.; Keystone, E.C.; Genovese, M.C.; Conaghan, P.G.; Hsia, E.C.; Xu, W.; Baratelle, A.; Beutler, A.; et al. The effects of golimumab on radiographic progression in rheumatoid arthritis: Results of randomized controlled studies of golimumab before methotrexate therapy and golimumab after methotrexate therapy. *Arthritis Rheum.* **2011**, *63*, 1200–1210. [CrossRef] [PubMed]
77. Burmester, G.R.; Kivitz, A.J.; Kupper, H.; Arulmani, U.; Florentinus, S.; Goss, S.L.; Rathmann, S.S.; Fleischmann, R.M. Efficacy and safety of ascending methotrexate dose in combination with adalimumab: The randomised CONCERTO trial. *Ann. Rheum. Dis.* **2015**, *74*, 1037–1044. [CrossRef]
78. Kaeley, G.S.; MacCarter, D.K.; Goyal, J.R.; Liu, S.; Chen, K.; Griffith, J.; Kupper, H.; Garg, V.; Kalabic, J. Similar Improvements in Patient Reported Outcomes Among Rheumatoid Arthritis Patients Treated with Two Different Doses of Methotrexate in Combination with Adalimumab: Results From the MUSICA Trial. *Rheumatol. Ther.* **2018**, *5*, 123–134. [CrossRef]
79. Bandres Ciga, S.; Salvatierra, J.; Lopez-Sidro, M.; Garcia-Sanchez, A.; Duran, R.; Vives, F.; Raya-Alvarez, E. An examination of the mechanisms involved in secondary clinical failure to adalimumab or etanercept in inflammatory arthropathies. *J. Clin. Rheumatol.* **2015**, *21*, 115–119. [CrossRef]
80. Jani, M.; Barton, A.; Warren, R.B.; Griffiths, C.E.; Chinoy, H. The role of DMARDs in reducing the immunogenicity of TNF inhibitors in chronic inflammatory diseases. *Rheumatology (Oxford)* **2014**, *53*, 213–222. [CrossRef]
81. Jani, M.; Chinoy, H.; Warren, R.B.; Griffiths, C.E.; Plant, D.; Fu, B.; Morgan, A.W.; Wilson, A.G.; Isaacs, J.D.; Hyrich, K.; et al. Clinical utility of random anti-tumor necrosis factor drug-level testing and measurement of antidrug antibodies on the long-term treatment response in rheumatoid arthritis. *Arthritis Rheumatol.* **2015**, *67*, 2011–2019. [CrossRef]
82. Bartelds, G.M.; Krieckaert, C.L.; Nurmohamed, M.T.; van Schouwenburg, P.A.; Lems, W.F.; Twisk, J.W.; Dijkmans, B.A.; Aarden, L.; Wolbink, G.J. Development of antidrug antibodies against adalimumab and association with disease activity and treatment failure during long-term follow-up. *JAMA* **2011**, *305*, 1460–1468. [CrossRef]
83. Pascual-Salcedo, D.; Plasencia, C.; Ramiro, S.; Nuno, L.; Bonilla, G.; Nagore, D.; Ruiz Del Agua, A.; Martinez, A.; Aarden, L.; Martin-Mola, E.; et al. Influence of immunogenicity on the efficacy of long-term treatment with infliximab in rheumatoid arthritis. *Rheumatology (Oxford)* **2011**, *50*, 1445–1452. [CrossRef]
84. Balsa, A.; Sanmarti, R.; Rosas, J.; Martin, V.; Cabez, A.; Gomez, S.; Montoro, M. Drug immunogenicity in patients with inflammatory arthritis and secondary failure to tumour necrosis factor inhibitor therapies: The REASON study. *Rheumatology (Oxford)* **2018**, *57*, 688–693. [CrossRef] [PubMed]
85. Vogelzang, E.H.; Kneepkens, E.L.; Nurmohamed, M.T.; van Kuijk, A.W.; Rispens, T.; Wolbink, G.; Krieckaert, C.L. Anti-adalimumab antibodies and adalimumab concentrations in psoriatic arthritis; an association with disease activity at 28 and 52 weeks of follow-up. *Ann. Rheum. Dis.* **2014**, *73*, 2178–2182. [CrossRef]
86. Bartelds, G.M.; Wijbrandts, C.A.; Nurmohamed, M.T.; Stapel, S.; Lems, W.F.; Aarden, L.; Dijkmans, B.A.; Tak, P.P.; Wolbink, G.J. Clinical response to adalimumab: Relationship to anti-adalimumab antibodies and serum adalimumab concentrations in rheumatoid arthritis. *Ann. Rheum. Dis.* **2007**, *66*, 921–926. [CrossRef]

87. Ungar, B.; Kopylov, U.; Engel, T.; Yavzori, M.; Fudim, E.; Picard, O.; Lang, A.; Williet, N.; Paul, S.; Chowers, Y.; et al. Addition of an immunomodulator can reverse antibody formation and loss of response in patients treated with adalimumab. *Aliment. Pharmacol. Ther.* **2017**, *45*, 276–282. [CrossRef]
88. Qiu, Y.; Mao, R.; Chen, B.L.; Zhang, S.H.; Guo, J.; He, Y.; Zeng, Z.R.; Ben-Horin, S.; Chen, M.H. Effects of Combination Therapy With Immunomodulators on Trough Levels and Antibodies Against Tumor Necrosis Factor Antagonists in Patients With Inflammatory Bowel Disease: A Meta-analysis. *Clin. Gastroenterol. Hepatol.* **2017**, *15*, 1359.e6–1372.e6. [CrossRef]
89. Krieckaert, C.L.; Nurmohamed, M.T.; Wolbink, G.J. Methotrexate reduces immunogenicity in adalimumab treated rheumatoid arthritis patients in a dose dependent manner. *Ann. Rheum. Dis.* **2012**, *71*, 1914–1915. [CrossRef] [PubMed]
90. Kaeley, G.S.; Evangelisto, A.M.; Nishio, M.J.; Goss, S.L.; Liu, S.; Kalabic, J.; Kupper, H. Methotrexate dosage reduction upon adalimumab initiation: Clinical and ultrasonographic outcomes from the randomized noninferiority MUSICA trial. *J. Rheumatol.* **2016**, *43*, 1480–1489. [CrossRef] [PubMed]
91. Klareskog, L.; van der Heijde, D.; de Jager, J.P.; Gough, A.; Kalden, J.; Malaise, M.; Martin Mola, E.; Pavelka, K.; Sany, J.; Settas, L.; et al. Therapeutic effect of the combination of etanercept and methotrexate compared with each treatment alone in patients with rheumatoid arthritis: Double-blind randomised controlled trial. *Lancet* **2004**, *363*, 675–681. [CrossRef]
92. Quintin, E.; Scoazec, J.Y.; Marotte, H.; Miossec, P. Rare incidence of methotrexate-specific lesions in liver biopsy of patients with arthritis and elevated liver enzymes. *Arthritis Res. Ther.* **2010**, *12*, R143. [CrossRef]
93. Simms, R.W.; Kwoh, C.K.; Anderson, L.G.; Erlandson, D.M.; Greene, J.M.; Kelleher, M.; O'Dell, J.R.; Partridge, A.J.; Roberts, W.N.; Robbins, M.L. Guidelines for monitoring drug therapy in rheumatoid arthritis: American College of Rheumatology Ad Hoc Committee on Clinical Guidelines. *Arthritis Rheum.* **1996**, *39*, 723–731.
94. Visser, K.; Katchamart, W.; Loza, E.; Martinez-Lopez, J.; Salliot, C.; Trudeau, J.; Bombardier, C.; Carmona, L.; Van der Heijde, D.; Bijlsma, J.; et al. Multinational evidence-based recommendations for the use of methotrexate in rheumatic disorders with a focus on rheumatoid arthritis: Integrating systematic literature research and expert opinion of a broad international panel of rheumatologists in the 3E Initiative. *Ann. Rheum. Dis.* **2009**, *68*, 1086–1093.
95. Price, S.; James, C.; Deighton, C. Methotrexate use and alcohol. *Clin. Exp. Rheumatol.* **2010**, *28*, S114–S116.
96. Humphreys, J.H.; Warner, A.; Costello, R.; Lunt, M.; Verstappen, S.M.M.; Dixon, W.G. Quantifying the hepatotoxic risk of alcohol consumption in patients with rheumatoid arthritis taking methotrexate. *Ann. Rheum. Dis.* **2017**, *76*, 1509–1514. [CrossRef]
97. Kremer, J.M.; Weinblatt, M.E. Quantifying the hepatotoxic risk of alcohol consumption in patients with rheumatoid arthritis taking methotrexate. *Ann. Rheum. Dis.* **2018**, *77*, e4. [CrossRef]
98. Bernatsky, S.; Ehrmann Feldman, D. Discontinuation of methotrexate therapy in older patients with newly diagnosed rheumatoid arthritis: Analysis of administrative health databases in Quebec, Canada. *Drugs Aging* **2008**, *25*, 879–884. [CrossRef]
99. Van den Bemt, B.J.F.; van den Hoogen, F.H.J.; Benraad, B.; Hekster, Y.A.; van Riel, P.L.C.M.; van Lankveld, W. Adherence Rates and Associations with Nonadherence in Patients with Rheumatoid Arthritis Using Disease Modifying Antirheumatic Drugs. *J. Rheumatol.* **2009**, *36*, 2164–2170. [CrossRef]
100. Contreras-Yanez, I.; Ponce De Leon, S.; Cabiedes, J.; Rull-Gabayet, M.; Pascual-Ramos, V. Inadequate therapy behavior is associated to disease flares in patients with rheumatoid arthritis who have achieved remission with disease-modifying antirheumatic drugs. *Am. J. Med. Sci.* **2010**, *340*, 282–290. [CrossRef]
101. Anderson, J.J.; Wells, G.; Verhoeven, A.C.; Felson, D.T. Factors predicting response to treatment in rheumatoid arthritis: The importance of disease duration. *Arthritis Rheum.* **2000**, *43*, 22–29. [CrossRef]
102. Saevarsdottir, S.; Wallin, H.; Seddighzadeh, M.; Ernestam, S.; Geborek, P.; Petersson, I.F.; Bratt, J.; van Vollenhoven, R.F.; SWEFOT Trial Investigators Group. Predictors of response to methotrexate in early DMARD naive rheumatoid arthritis: Results from the initial open-label phase of the SWEFOT trial. *Ann. Rheum. Dis.* **2011**, *70*, 469–475. [CrossRef]
103. Teitsma, X.M.; Jacobs, J.W.G.; Welsing, P.M.J.; de Jong, P.H.P.; Hazes, J.M.W.; Weel, A.; Petho-Schramm, A.; Borm, M.E.A.; van Laar, J.M.; Lafeber, F.; et al. Inadequate response to treat-to-target methotrexate therapy in patients with new-onset rheumatoid arthritis: Development and validation of clinical predictors. *Ann. Rheum. Dis.* **2018**, *77*, 1261–1267. [CrossRef]

104. Romao, V.C.; Canhao, H.; Fonseca, J.E. Old drugs, old problems: Where do we stand in prediction of rheumatoid arthritis responsiveness to methotrexate and other synthetic DMARDs? *BMC Med.* **2013**, *11*, 17. [CrossRef]

105. Saevarsdottir, S.; Wedren, S.; Seddighzadeh, M.; Bengtsson, C.; Wesley, A.; Lindblad, S.; Askling, J.; Alfredsson, L.; Klareskog, L. Patients with early rheumatoid arthritis who smoke are less likely to respond to treatment with methotrexate and tumor necrosis factor inhibitors: Observations from the Epidemiological Investigation of Rheumatoid Arthritis and the Swedish Rheumatology Register cohorts. *Arthritis Rheum.* **2011**, *63*, 26–36. [CrossRef]

106. Crowson, C.S.; Rollefstad, S.; Ikdahl, E.; Kitas, G.D.; van Riel, P.; Gabriel, S.E.; Matteson, E.L.; Kvien, T.K.; Douglas, K.; Sandoo, A.; et al. Impact of risk factors associated with cardiovascular outcomes in patients with rheumatoid arthritis. *Ann. Rheum. Dis.* **2018**, *77*, 48–54. [CrossRef]

107. Joseph, R.M.; Movahedi, M.; Dixon, W.G.; Symmons, D.P. Smoking-Related Mortality in Patients With Early Rheumatoid Arthritis: A Retrospective Cohort Study Using the Clinical Practice Research Datalink. *Arthritis Care Res. (Hoboken)* **2016**, *68*, 1598–1606. [CrossRef]

108. Sergeant, J.C.; Hyrich, K.L.; Anderson, J.; Kopec-Harding, K.; Hope, H.F.; Symmons, D.P.M.; Co-Investigators, R.; Barton, A.; Verstappen, S.M.M. Prediction of primary non-response to methotrexate therapy using demographic, clinical and psychosocial variables: Results from the UK Rheumatoid Arthritis Medication Study (RAMS). *Arthritis Res. Ther.* **2018**, *20*, 147. [CrossRef]

109. Hamilton, R.A.; Kremer, J.M. Why intramuscular methotrexate may be more efficacious than oral dosing in patients with rheumatoid arthritis. *Br. J. Rheumatol.* **1997**, *36*, 86–90. [CrossRef]

110. Pichlmeier, U.; Heuer, K.U. Subcutaneous administration of methotrexate with a prefilled autoinjector pen results in a higher relative bioavailability compared with oral administration of methotrexate. *Clin. Exp. Rheumatol.* **2014**, *32*, 563–571.

111. Braun, J.; Kastner, P.; Flaxenberg, P.; Wahrisch, J.; Hanke, P.; Demary, W.; von Hinuber, U.; Rockwitz, K.; Heitz, W.; Pichlmeier, U.; et al. Comparison of the clinical efficacy and safety of subcutaneous versus oral administration of methotrexate in patients with active rheumatoid arthritis: Results of a six-month, multicenter, randomized, double-blind, controlled, phase IV trial. *Arthritis Rheum.* **2008**, *58*, 73–81. [CrossRef]

112. Hazlewood, G.S.; Thorne, J.C.; Pope, J.E.; Lin, D.; Tin, D.; Boire, G.; Haraoui, B.; Hitchon, C.A.; Keystone, E.C.; Jamal, S.; et al. The comparative effectiveness of oral versus subcutaneous methotrexate for the treatment of early rheumatoid arthritis. *Ann. Rheum. Dis.* **2016**, *75*, 1003–1008. [CrossRef]

113. Gaujoux-Viala, C.; Rincheval, N.; Dougados, M.; Combe, B.; Fautrel, B. Optimal methotrexate dose is associated with better clinical outcomes than non-optimal dose in daily practice: Results from the ESPOIR early arthritis cohort. *Ann. Rheum. Dis.* **2017**, *76*, 2054–2060. [CrossRef]

114. Atsumi, T.; Yamamoto, K.; Takeuchi, T.; Yamanaka, H.; Ishiguro, N.; Tanaka, Y.; Eguchi, K.; Watanabe, A.; Origasa, H.; Yasuda, S.; et al. The first double-blind, randomised, parallel-group certolizumab pegol study in methotrexate-naive early rheumatoid arthritis patients with poor prognostic factors, C-OPERA, shows inhibition of radiographic progression. *Ann. Rheum. Dis.* **2016**, *75*, 75–83. [CrossRef]

115. Wevers-de Boer, K.; Visser, K.; Heimans, L.; Ronday, H.K.; Molenaar, E.; Groenendael, J.H.; Peeters, A.J.; Westedt, M.L.; Collee, G.; de Sonnaville, P.B.; et al. Remission induction therapy with methotrexate and prednisone in patients with early rheumatoid and undifferentiated arthritis (the IMPROVED study). *Ann. Rheum. Dis.* **2012**, *71*, 1472–1477. [CrossRef]

116. Bergstra, S.A.; Allaart, C.F.; Stijnen, T.; Landewe, R.B.M. Meta-Regression of a Dose-Response Relationship of Methotrexate in Mono- and Combination Therapy in Disease-Modifying Antirheumatic Drug-Naive Early Rheumatoid Arthritis Patients. *Arthritis Care Res. (Hoboken)* **2017**, *69*, 1473–1483. [CrossRef]

117. Rezaei, H.; Saevarsdottir, S.; Forslind, K.; Albertsson, K.; Wallin, H.; Bratt, J.; Ernestam, S.; Geborek, P.; Pettersson, I.F.; van Vollenhoven, R.F. In early rheumatoid arthritis, patients with a good initial response to methotrexate have excellent 2-year clinical outcomes, but radiological progression is not fully prevented: Data from the methotrexate responders population in the SWEFOT trial. *Ann. Rheum. Dis.* **2012**, *71*, 186–191. [CrossRef]

118. Smolen, J.S.; Aletaha, D. Rheumatoid arthritis therapy reappraisal: Strategies, opportunities and challenges. *Nat. Rev. Rheumatol.* **2015**, *11*, 276–289. [CrossRef]

119. Emery, P.; Bingham, C.O., 3rd; Burmester, G.R.; Bykerk, V.P.; Furst, D.E.; Mariette, X.; van der Heijde, D.; van Vollenhoven, R.; Arendt, C.; Mountian, I.; et al. Certolizumab pegol in combination with dose-optimised methotrexate

in DMARD-naive patients with early, active rheumatoid arthritis with poor prognostic factors: 1-year results from C-EARLY, a randomised, double-blind, placebo-controlled phase III study. *Ann. Rheum. Dis.* **2017**, *76*, 96–104. [CrossRef]

120. Li, R.; Zhao, J.X.; Su, Y.; He, J.; Chen, L.N.; Gu, F.; Zhao, C.; Deng, X.R.; Zhou, W.; Hao, Y.J.; et al. High remission and low relapse with prolonged intensive DMARD therapy in rheumatoid arthritis (PRINT): A multicenter randomized clinical trial. *Medicine (Baltimore)* **2016**, *95*, e3968. [CrossRef]
121. Lambert, C.M.; Sandhu, S.; Lochhead, A.; Hurst, N.P.; McRorie, E.; Dhillon, V. Dose escalation of parenteral methotrexate in active rheumatoid arthritis that has been unresponsive to conventional doses of methotrexate: A randomized, controlled trial. *Arthritis Rheum.* **2004**, *50*, 364–371. [CrossRef]
122. Daien, C.; Hua, C.; Gaujoux-Viala, C.; Cantagrel, A.; Dubremetz, M.; Dougados, M.; Fautrel, B.; Mariette, X.; Nayral, N.; Richez, C.; et al. Update of French Society for Rheumatology Recommendations for Managing Rheumatoid Arthritis. *Jt. Bone Spine* **2019**, *86*, 135–150. [CrossRef]
123. Dhaon, P.; Das, S.K.; Srivastava, R.; Agarwal, G.; Asthana, A. Oral Methotrexate in split dose weekly versus oral or parenteral Methotrexate once weekly in Rheumatoid Arthritis: A short-term study. *Int. J. Rheum. Dis.* **2018**, *21*, 1010–1017. [CrossRef]
124. Rutkowska-Sak, L.; Rell-Bakalarska, M.; Lisowska, B. Oral vs. subcutaneous low-dose methotrexate treatment in reducing gastrointestinal side effects. *Reumatol./Rheumatol.* **2009**, *47*, 207–211.
125. Kruger, K.; Wollenhaupt, J.; Albrecht, K.; Alten, R.; Backhaus, M.; Baerwald, C.; Bolten, W.; Braun, J.; Burkhardt, H.; Burmester, G.; et al. German 2012 guidelines for the sequential medical treatment of rheumatoid arthritis. Adapted EULAR recommendations and updated treatment algorithm. *Z. Rheumatol.* **2012**, *71*, 592–603. [CrossRef]
126. Chakravarty, K.; McDonald, H.; Pullar, T.; Taggart, A.; Chalmers, R.; Oliver, S.; Mooney, J.; Somerville, M.; Bosworth, A.; Kennedy, T.; et al. BSR/BHPR guideline for disease-modifying anti-rheumatic drug (DMARD) therapy in consultation with the British Association of Dermatologists. *Rheumatology (Oxford)* **2008**, *47*, 924–925. [CrossRef]
127. Bingham, S.J.; Buch, M.H.; Lindsay, S.; Pollard, A.; White, J.; Emery, P. Parenteral methotrexate should be given before biological therapy. *Rheumatology (Oxford)* **2003**, *42*, 1009–1010. [CrossRef]
128. Rozin, A.; Schapira, D.; Balbir-Gurman, A.; Braun-Moscovici, Y.; Markovits, D.; Militianu, D.; Nahir, M.A. Relapse of rheumatoid arthritis after substitution of oral for parenteral administration of methotrexate. *Ann. Rheum. Dis.* **2002**, *61*, 756–757. [CrossRef]
129. Wegrzyn, J.; Adeleine, P.; Miossec, P. Better efficacy of methotrexate given by intramuscular injection than orally in patients with rheumatoid arthritis. *Ann. Rheum. Dis.* **2004**, *63*, 1232–1234. [CrossRef]
130. Harris, E.; Ng, B. Using subcutaneous methotrexate to prolong duration of methotrexate therapy in rheumatoid arthritis. *Eur. J. Rheumatol.* **2018**, *5*, 85–91. [CrossRef]
131. Bakker, M.F.; Jacobs, J.W.; Welsing, P.M.; van der Werf, J.H.; Linn-Rasker, S.P.; van der Veen, M.J.; Lafeber, F.P.; Bijlsma, J.W.; Utrecht Arthritis Cohort Study Group. Are switches from oral to subcutaneous methotrexate or addition of ciclosporin to methotrexate useful steps in a tight control treatment strategy for rheumatoid arthritis? A post hoc analysis of the CAMERA study. *Ann. Rheum. Dis.* **2010**, *69*, 1849–1852. [CrossRef] [PubMed]
132. Hameed, B.; Jones, H. Subcutaneous methotrexate is well tolerated and superior to oral methotrexate in the treatment of rheumatoid arthritis. *Int. J. Rheum. Dis.* **2010**, *13*, e83–e84. [CrossRef] [PubMed]
133. Ng, B.; Chu, A. Factors associated with methotrexate dosing and therapeutic decisions in veterans with rheumatoid arthritis. *Clin. Rheumatol.* **2014**, *33*, 21–30. [CrossRef] [PubMed]
134. Pasma, A.; den Boer, E.; van't Spijker, A.; Timman, R.; van den Bemt, B.; Busschbach, J.J.; Hazes, J.M. Nonadherence to disease modifying antirheumatic drugs in the first year after diagnosis: Comparing three adherence measures in early arthritis patients. *Rheumatology (Oxford)* **2016**, *55*, 1812–1819. [CrossRef] [PubMed]
135. Axelsen, M.B.; Eshed, I.; Horslev-Petersen, K.; Stengaard-Pedersen, K.; Hetland, M.L.; Moller, J.; Junker, P.; Podenphant, J.; Schlemmer, A.; Ellingsen, T.; et al. A treat-to-target strategy with methotrexate and intra-articular triamcinolone with or without adalimumab effectively reduces MRI synovitis, osteitis and tenosynovitis and halts structural damage progression in early rheumatoid arthritis: Results from the OPERA randomised controlled trial. *Ann. Rheum. Dis.* **2015**, *74*, 867–875. [CrossRef] [PubMed]
136. Alarcon, G.S.; Tracy, I.C.; Blackburn, W.D., Jr. Methotrexate in rheumatoid arthritis. Toxic effects as the major factor in limiting long-term treatment. *Arthritis Rheum.* **1989**, *32*, 671–676. [CrossRef]

137. Van Ede, A.E.; Laan, R.F.; Rood, M.J.; Huizinga, T.W.; van de Laar, M.A.; van Denderen, C.J.; Westgeest, T.A.; Romme, T.C.; de Rooij, D.J.; Jacobs, M.J.; et al. Effect of folic or folinic acid supplementation on the toxicity and efficacy of methotrexate in rheumatoid arthritis: A forty-eight week, multicenter, randomized, double-blind, placebo-controlled study. *Arthritis Rheum.* **2001**, *44*, 1515–1524. [CrossRef]
138. Leeb, B.F.; Witzmann, G.; Ogris, E.; Studnicka-Benke, A.; Andel, I.; Schweitzer, H.; Smolen, J.S. Folic acid and cyanocobalamin levels in serum and erythrocytes during low-dose methotrexate therapy of rheumatoid arthritis and psoriatic arthritis patients. *Clin. Exp. Rheumatol.* **1995**, *13*, 459–463. [PubMed]
139. Shea, B.; Swinden, M.V.; Tanjong Ghogomu, E.; Ortiz, Z.; Katchamart, W.; Rader, T.; Bombardier, C.; Wells, G.A.; Tugwell, P. Folic acid and folinic acid for reducing side effects in patients receiving methotrexate for rheumatoid arthritis. *Cochrane Database Syst. Rev.* **2013**, CD000951. [CrossRef] [PubMed]
140. Hartman, M.; van Ede, A.; Severens, J.L.; Laan, R.F.; van de Putte, L.; van der Wilt, G.J. Economic evaluation of folate supplementation during methotrexate treatment in rheumatoid arthritis. *J. Rheumatol.* **2004**, *31*, 902–908.
141. Schmajuk, G.; Tonner, C.; Miao, Y.; Yazdany, J.; Gannon, J.; Boscardin, W.J.; Daikh, D.I.; Steinman, M.A. Folic Acid Supplementation Is Suboptimal in a National Cohort of Older Veterans Receiving Low Dose Oral Methotrexate. *PLoS ONE* **2016**, *11*, e0168369. [CrossRef] [PubMed]
142. Liu, L.; Liu, S.; Wang, C.; Guan, W.; Zhang, Y.; Hu, W.; Zhang, L.; He, Y.; Lu, J.; Li, T.; et al. Folate Supplementation for Methotrexate Therapy in Patients With Rheumatoid Arthritis: A Systematic Review. *J Clin. Rheumatol.* **2018**. [CrossRef] [PubMed]
143. Mazaud, C.; Fardet, L. Relative risk of and determinants for adverse events of methotrexate prescribed at a low dose: A systematic review and meta-analysis of randomized placebo-controlled trials. *Br. J. Dermatol.* **2017**, *177*, 978–986. [CrossRef] [PubMed]
144. Stamp, L.K.; O'Donnell, J.L.; Frampton, C.; Drake, J.; Zhang, M.; Barclay, M.; Chapman, P.T. A Pilot Randomized Controlled Double-Blind Trial of High- Versus Low-Dose Weekly Folic Acid in People With Rheumatoid Arthritis Receiving Methotrexate. *J. Clin. Rheumatol.* **2018**. [CrossRef]
145. Svanstrom, H.; Lund, M.; Melbye, M.; Pasternak, B. Concomitant use of low-dose methotrexate and NSAIDs and the risk of serious adverse events among patients with rheumatoid arthritis. *Pharmacoepidemiol. Drug Saf.* **2018**, *27*, 885–893. [CrossRef]
146. Iyyadurai, R.; Carey, R.A.; Satyendra, S. Low-dose methotrexate-induced acute interstitial pneumonitis: Report of two cases from South India and review of literature. *J. Fam. Med. Prim. Care* **2016**, *5*, 875–878. [CrossRef]
147. Kremer, J.M.; Alarcon, G.S.; Weinblatt, M.E.; Kaymakcian, M.V.; Macaluso, M.; Cannon, G.W.; Palmer, W.R.; Sundy, J.S.; St Clair, E.W.; Alexander, R.W.; et al. Clinical, laboratory, radiographic, and histopathologic features of methotrexate-associated lung injury in patients with rheumatoid arthritis: A multicenter study with literature review. *Arthritis Rheum.* **1997**, *40*, 1829–1837. [CrossRef]
148. Alarcon, G.S.; Kremer, J.M.; Macaluso, M.; Weinblatt, M.E.; Cannon, G.W.; Palmer, W.R.; St Clair, E.W.; Sundy, J.S.; Alexander, R.W.; Smith, G.J.; et al. Risk factors for methotrexate-induced lung injury in patients with rheumatoid arthritis. A multicenter, case-control study. *Ann. Intern. Med.* **1997**, *127*, 356–364. [CrossRef]
149. Tokuda, H.; Sakai, F.; Yamada, H.; Johkoh, T.; Imamura, A.; Dohi, M.; Hirakata, M.; Yamada, T.; Kamatani, N.; Kikuchi, Y.; et al. Clinical and radiological features of Pneumocystis pneumonia in patients with rheumatoid arthritis, in comparison with methotrexate pneumonitis and Pneumocystis pneumonia in acquired immunodeficiency syndrome: A multicenter study. *Intern. Med.* **2008**, *47*, 915–923. [CrossRef]
150. Maetzel, A.; Wong, A.; Strand, V.; Tugwell, P.; Wells, G.; Bombardier, C. Meta-analysis of treatment termination rates among rheumatoid arthritis patients receiving disease-modifying anti-rheumatic drugs. *Rheumatology (Oxford)* **2000**, *39*, 975–981. [CrossRef]
151. Furst, D.E. Practical clinical pharmacology and drug interactions of low-dose methotrexate therapy in rheumatoid arthritis. *Br. J. Rheumatol.* **1995**, *34* (Suppl. 2), 20–25. [CrossRef]
152. Rohr, M.K.; Mikuls, T.R.; Cohen, S.B.; Thorne, J.C.; O'Dell, J.R. Underuse of Methotrexate in the Treatment of Rheumatoid Arthritis: A National Analysis of Prescribing Practices in the US. *Arthritis Care Res. (Hoboken)* **2017**, *69*, 794–800. [CrossRef]
153. Boots, C.E.; Gustofson, R.L.; Feinberg, E.C. Does methotrexate administration for ectopic pregnancy after in vitro fertilization impact ovarian reserve or ovarian responsiveness? *Fertil. Steril.* **2013**, *100*, 1590–1593. [CrossRef]

154. Flint, J.; Panchal, S.; Hurrell, A.; van de Venne, M.; Gayed, M.; Schreiber, K.; Arthanari, S.; Cunningham, J.; Flanders, L.; Moore, L.; et al. BSR and BHPR guideline on prescribing drugs in pregnancy and breastfeeding—Part I: Standard and biologic disease modifying anti-rheumatic drugs and corticosteroids. *Rheumatology (Oxford)* **2016**, *55*, 1693–1697. [CrossRef]
155. Eck, L.K.; Jensen, T.B.; Mastrogiannis, D.; Torp-Pedersen, A.; Askaa, B.; Nielsen, T.K.; Poulsen, H.E.; Jimenez-Solem, E.; Andersen, J.T. Risk of Adverse Pregnancy Outcome After Paternal Exposure to Methotrexate Within 90 Days Before Pregnancy. *Obstet. Gynecol.* **2017**, *129*, 707–714. [CrossRef]
156. Gutierrez, J.C.; Hwang, K. The toxicity of methotrexate in male fertility and paternal teratogenicity. *Expert Opin. Drug Metab. Toxicol.* **2017**, *13*, 51–58. [CrossRef]
157. Friedman, M.A.; Winthrop, K.L. Vaccines and Disease-Modifying Antirheumatic Drugs: Practical Implications for the Rheumatologist. *Rheum. Dis. Clin. N. Am.* **2017**, *43*, 1–13. [CrossRef]
158. Hmamouchi, I.; Winthrop, K.; Launay, O.; Dougados, M. Low rate of influenza and pneumococcal vaccine coverage in rheumatoid arthritis: Data from the international COMORA cohort. *Vaccine* **2015**, *33*, 1446–1452. [CrossRef]
159. Hua, C.; Barnetche, T.; Combe, B.; Morel, J. Effect of methotrexate, anti-tumor necrosis factor alpha, and rituximab on the immune response to influenza and pneumococcal vaccines in patients with rheumatoid arthritis: A systematic review and meta-analysis. *Arthritis Care Res. (Hoboken)* **2014**, *66*, 1016–1026. [CrossRef]
160. Van Aalst, M.; Langedijk, A.C.; Spijker, R.; de Bree, G.J.; Grobusch, M.P.; Goorhuis, A. The effect of immunosuppressive agents on immunogenicity of pneumococcal vaccination: A systematic review and meta-analysis. *Vaccine* **2018**, *36*, 5832–5845. [CrossRef]
161. Park, J.K.; Lee, Y.J.; Shin, K.; Ha, Y.J.; Lee, E.Y.; Song, Y.W.; Choi, Y.; Winthrop, K.L.; Lee, E.B. Impact of temporary methotrexate discontinuation for 2 weeks on immunogenicity of seasonal influenza vaccination in patients with rheumatoid arthritis: A randomised clinical trial. *Ann. Rheum. Dis.* **2018**, *77*, 898–904. [CrossRef]
162. Park, J.K.; Lee, M.A.; Lee, E.Y.; Song, Y.W.; Choi, Y.; Winthrop, K.L.; Lee, E.B. Effect of methotrexate discontinuation on efficacy of seasonal influenza vaccination in patients with rheumatoid arthritis: A randomised clinical trial. *Ann. Rheum. Dis.* **2017**, *76*, 1559–1565. [CrossRef]
163. Goodman, S.M. Rheumatoid arthritis: Perioperative management of biologics and DMARDs. *Semin. Arthritis Rheum.* **2015**, *44*, 627–632. [CrossRef]
164. Grennan, D.M.; Gray, J.; Loudon, J.; Fear, S. Methotrexate and early postoperative complications in patients with rheumatoid arthritis undergoing elective orthopaedic surgery. *Ann. Rheum. Dis.* **2001**, *60*, 214–217. [CrossRef]
165. Viller, F.; Guillemin, F.; Briancon, S.; Moum, T.; Suurmeijer, T.; van den Heuvel, W. Compliance to drug treatment of patients with rheumatoid arthritis: A 3 year longitudinal study. *J. Rheumatol.* **1999**, *26*, 2114–2122.
166. Nota, I.; Drossaert, C.H.; Taal, E.; Vonkeman, H.E.; van de Laar, M.A. Patient participation in decisions about disease modifying anti-rheumatic drugs: A cross-sectional survey. *BMC Musculoskelet. Disord.* **2014**, *15*, 333. [CrossRef]
167. Fraenkel, L.; Nowell, W.B.; Michel, G.; Wiedmeyer, C. Preference phenotypes to facilitate shared decision-making in rheumatoid arthritis. *Ann. Rheum. Dis.* **2018**, *77*, 678–683. [CrossRef]
168. Mathews, A.L.; Coleska, A.; Burns, P.B.; Chung, K.C. Evolution of Patient Decision-Making Regarding Medical Treatment of Rheumatoid Arthritis. *Arthritis Care Res. (Hoboken)* **2016**, *68*, 318–324. [CrossRef]
169. Fraenkel, L.; Peters, E.; Charpentier, P.; Olsen, B.; Errante, L.; Schoen, R.T.; Reyna, V. Decision tool to improve the quality of care in rheumatoid arthritis. *Arthritis Care Res. (Hoboken)* **2012**, *64*, 977–985. [CrossRef]
170. Zak, A.; Corrigan, C.; Yu, Z.; Bitton, A.; Fraenkel, L.; Harrold, L.; Smolen, J.S.; Solomon, D.H. Barriers to treatment adjustment within a treat to target strategy in rheumatoid arthritis: A secondary analysis of the TRACTION trial. *Rheumatology (Oxford)* **2018**, *57*, 1933–1937. [CrossRef]
171. Scheiman-Elazary, A.; Duan, L.; Shourt, C.; Agrawal, H.; Ellashof, D.; Cameron-Hay, M.; Furst, D.E. The Rate of Adherence to Antiarthritis Medications and Associated Factors among Patients with Rheumatoid Arthritis: A Systematic Literature Review and Metaanalysis. *J. Rheumatol.* **2016**, *43*, 512–523. [CrossRef]

14

Effect of Baricitinib and Adalimumab in Reducing Pain and Improving Function in Patients with Rheumatoid Arthritis in Low Disease Activity: Exploratory Analyses from RA-BEAM

Bruno Fautrel [1,2,*], Bruce Kirkham [3], Janet E. Pope [4], Tsutomu Takeuchi [5], Carol Gaich [6], Amanda Quebe [6], Baojin Zhu [6], Inmaculada de la Torre [6], Francesco De Leonardis [6] and Peter C. Taylor [7]

1 Rheumatology Dept, Institut Pierre Louis d'Epidémiologie et de Santé Publique, Sorbonne Université-Assistance Publique Hôpitaux de Paris, 75013 Paris, France
2 Department of Rheumatology, Pitié-Salpêtrière Hospital, Assistance Publique-Hôpitaux de Paris, 83 bd de l'hôpital, 75013 Paris, France
3 Department of Rheumatology, Guys and St Thomas' NHS Trust, Great Maze Pond, London SE1 9RT, UK
4 Department of Medicine, Division of Rheumatology, University of Western Ontario, 1151 Richmond St, London, ON N6A 3K7, Canada
5 Keio University School of Medicine, 35 Shinanomachi, Shinjuku-ku, Tokyo 160-8582, Japan
6 Eli Lilly and Company, Indianapolis, IN 46285, USA
7 Botnar Research Centre, NDORMS, University of Oxford, Old Road, Oxford OX3 7LD, UK
* Correspondence: Bruno.fautrel@aphp.fr

Abstract: Patients with rheumatoid arthritis (RA) may experience residual pain and functional impairment despite good control of disease activity. This study compared improvements in pain and physical function in patients with well-controlled RA after 24 weeks' treatment with baricitinib, adalimumab or placebo in the 52-week RA-BEAM phase III study. Adults with active RA and inadequate response to methotrexate received baricitinib 4 mg once daily, adalimumab 40 mg every two weeks or placebo, with background methotrexate. Patients (N = 1010) were categorised as in remission, in remission or low disease activity, or not in remission or low disease activity at week 24. For patients in remission or low disease activity (n = 310), improvements in mean pain and physical function scores at week 24 were significantly greater with baricitinib than placebo ($p < 0.001$ and $p < 0.01$, respectively) and adalimumab ($p < 0.05$ for both). For both outcomes, differences between adalimumab and placebo were not significant. The proportions of patients in remission or low disease activity with minimal or no pain and with normalised physical function were numerically greater with baricitinib than placebo. Baricitinib 4 mg once daily provided enhanced improvement in pain and physical function in patients with well-controlled RA, suggesting it may produce effects beyond immunomodulation.

Keywords: rheumatoid arthritis; baricitinib; pain; recovery of function; fatigue; productivity

1. Introduction

A major goal in the contemporary treatment of rheumatoid arthritis (RA) is to achieve remission or low disease activity, with the aim of reducing inflammation to prevent joint damage and physical disability [1,2]. However, achieving this objective target is not always associated with a corresponding improvement in disability (Health Assessment Questionnaire (HAQ)) scores and other patient-reported outcomes (PROs): In a study of the Leiden Early Arthritis Clinic cohort, for example, patients with

RA were now diagnosed after a shorter duration of symptoms and with less inflammation than they were 20 years ago, but HAQ results remained stable over this time while PROs worsened [3]. Indeed, residual pain and functional impairment can persist despite ongoing treatment and can negatively affect quality of life [4,5]. Control of pain and maintenance of physical function are priorities for patients with RA [5–9]. Improvement in PROs should, therefore, be considered an important treatment goal, in addition to reducing inflammation, for improving the health outcomes of such patients [10].

Baricitinib is an oral selective inhibitor of Janus kinase (JAK)1 and JAK2 [11], which are essential for the intracellular signalling of various cytokines associated with inflammation in RA [12,13]. It is approved for the treatment of moderately to severely active RA in adults in over 50 countries, including the USA, Europe and Japan [14–16]. The efficacy and safety of baricitinib as a treatment for RA were established in four phase III, randomised, double-blind, multicentre studies in patients with active disease [17–20].

The objective of these post-hoc analyses was to compare improvements in pain, physical function, fatigue and work productivity/loss between baricitinib, adalimumab and placebo, all given with background methotrexate, in patients with well-controlled RA (in remission or low disease activity) at week 24 in RA-BEAM.

2. Materials and Methods

2.1. RA-BEAM Study Design

RA-BEAM (NCT01710358) was a phase III, double-blind, placebo- and active-controlled study in which patients with active RA were randomised to treatment with baricitinib 4 mg, adalimumab or placebo in addition to background methotrexate for 52 weeks (24 weeks for placebo). All patients had an inadequate response to stable doses of methotrexate before study entry. The study design has been described in detail previously [20]. In brief, 1305 adult patients (aged ≥18 years) with moderately to severely active RA were randomised and treated with either baricitinib 4 mg once daily (N = 487), adalimumab 40 mg once every two weeks (N = 330) or once-daily placebo (N = 488) for 52 weeks (24 weeks for placebo) in addition to stable background methotrexate.

RA-BEAM was conducted in accordance with the ethical principles of the 1964 Declaration of Helsinki and its later amendments, and Good Clinical Practice guidelines, and was approved by each centre's institutional review board or ethics committee. Informed consent was obtained from all individual participants included in the study.

2.2. Outcomes Relevant to the Post-Hoc Analyses

Pain was assessed throughout the study, including at week 24, using a pain visual analogue scale (VAS, 0–100 mm), whereas physical function was assessed using the HAQ-Disability Index (HAQ-DI) [21]. Additional PROs assessed at baseline and week 24 included fatigue, measured using the Functional Assessment of Chronic Illness Therapy-Fatigue (FACIT-F) scale [22], and work absenteeism, presenteeism, productivity loss and activity impairment, measured using the Work Productivity and Activity Impairment Questionnaire-RA [23].

2.3. Statistical Analysis

Patients from all treatment groups were categorised as being in remission, being in remission or low disease activity, or not being in remission or low disease activity at week 24 (Table 1). Remission was defined as Disease Activity Score for 28-joint count with erythrocyte sedimentation rate (DAS28-ESR) <2.6 and low disease activity as DAS28-ESR ≥2.6 and ≤3.2. Not being in remission or low disease activity was defined as DAS28-ESR >3.2 based on observed data. Changes from baseline to week 24 in pain VAS, HAQ-DI and FACIT-F scores and work-related outcomes were compared between baricitinib, adalimumab and placebo according to remission or low disease activity status. Comparisons were made using analysis of covariance (ANCOVA) adjusted for randomisation variables (region and baseline joint erosion status (1–2 or ≥3)) and baseline score. The proportions of patients achieving minimal or no pain and those achieving normalisation of physical function at week 24 were also compared descriptively between treatment groups according to remission status. Minimal or no pain was defined as a VAS score of ≤10 mm, and normalisation of physical function was defined as a HAQ-DI score of <0.5 (including patients with a baseline HAQ-DI score of <0.5). For all outcome measures, missing values were imputed using modified last observation carried forward (mLOCF) as per the original predefined study analyses [20]. Analyses were not controlled for multiple testing.

For changes from baseline to week 24 in pain and HAQ-DI scores, sensitivity analyses were conducted for patients in remission or low disease activity according to DAS28 with high-sensitivity C-reactive protein (DAS28-hsCRP), Simplified Disease Activity Index (SDAI) or Clinical Disease Activity Index (CDAI) criteria (Table 1).

Table 1. Remission and remission or low disease activity rates at week 24 in patients with moderately to severely active rheumatoid arthritis from RA-BEAM [14,20].

Treatment ¥	BARI 4 mg	ADA 40 mg Q2W	Placebo
n	487	330	488
Remission rates (%)			
DAS28-ESR <2.6	18 ***	18 ***	5
DAS28-hsCRP <2.6	34 ***	32 ***	8
SDAI ≤3.3	16 ***	14 ***	3
CDAI ≤2.8	16 ***	12 ***	4
Remission or low disease activity rates (%)			
DAS28-ESR ≤3.2	32 ***	34 ***	10
DAS28-hsCRP ≤3.2	52 ***	48 ***	19
DAS28-ESR ≥2.6 and ≤3.2	14	16	5
DAS28-hsCRP ≥2.6 and ≤3.2	18	16	11
SDAI >3.3 and ≤11	35	34	17
CDAI >2.8 and ≤10	34	36	16

¥ Patients remained on background methotrexate throughout the study; all patients were bDMARD naïve. *** $p < 0.001$ vs. placebo. ADA adalimumab, BARI baricitinib, CDAI Clinical Disease Activity Index, bDMARD biologic disease-modifying antirheumatic drug, DAS28-ESR Disease Activity Score for 28-joint count with erythrocyte sedimentation rate, DAS28-hsCRP Disease Activity Score for 28-joint count with high-sensitivity C-reactive protein, Q2W once every two weeks, SDAI Simplified Disease Activity Index.

3. Results

Baseline characteristics of 1305 randomised and treated patients in RA-BEAM are shown in Table 2. Characteristics were similar across the treatment groups, including the proportions taking steroids and/or concomitant conventional synthetic disease-modifying antirheumatic drugs. Of these patients, 1010 were included in the current analyses—168 (baricitinib, $n = 87$; adalimumab, $n = 57$; placebo, $n = 24$) were in remission, 310 (baricitinib, $n = 154$; adalimumab, $n = 110$; placebo, $n = 46$) were in remission or low disease activity and 700 (baricitinib, $n = 267$; adalimumab, $n = 157$; placebo, $n = 276$) were not in remission or low disease activity at week 24, according to DAS28-ESR criteria.

Table 2. Baseline characteristics of 1305 randomised and treated patients in RA-BEAM, and the 168 patients in remission (DAS28-ESR <2.6) at week 24 [20].

Characteristic	All Randomised and Treated Patients (*N* = 1305)			Patients in Remission at Week 24 (*N* = 168)		
	Placebo (*N* = 488)	Baricitinib 4 mg (*N* = 487)	Adalimumab (*N* = 330)	Placebo (*N* = 24)	Baricitinib 4 mg (*N* = 87)	Adalimumab (*N* = 57)
Age (years)	53 ± 12	54 ± 12	53 ± 12	52 ± 12	52 ± 13	53 ± 13
Female	382 (78)	375 (77)	251 (76)	15 (63)	62 (71)	41 (72)
Time from symptom onset (years)	10.4 ± 9	10.3 ± 9	9.6 ± 9	9.1 ± 6	8.9 ± 9	8.1 ± 8
ACPA positive	424 (87)	427 (88)	295 (89)	22 (92)	75 (86)	52 (91)
RF positive	451 (92)	439 (90)	301 (91)	22 (92)	76 (87)	49 (86)
≥3 erosions	371 (76)	371 (76)	245 (75)	17 (71)	66 (77)	41 (75)
mTSS total score	45 ± 50	43 ± 50	44 ± 51	36 ± 41	39 ± 43	37 ± 42
Erosion score	26.8 ± 29	25.1 ± 28	26.4 ± 29	22.5 ± 24	24.4 ± 26	22.7 ± 23
Joint space narrowing score	18.2 ± 23	17.3 ± 23	18.0 ± 24	13.1 ± 18	14.6 ± 19	14.7 ± 20
Concomitant corticosteroid use	290 (59)	275 (56)	201 (61)	13 (54)	50 (58)	39 (68)
Type of csDMARD currently used						
MTX only	398 (82)	413 (85)	277 (84)	20 (83)	71 (82)	49 (86)
MTX + other csDMARD	89 (18)	74 (15)	53 (16)	4 (17)	16 (18)	8 (14)
MTX weekly dose in mg	15 ± 5	15 ± 5	15 ± 4	15 ± 4	14 ± 5	14 ± 5
DAS28-hsCRP	5.7 ± 1.0	5.8 ± 0.9	5.8 ± 0.9	5.0 ± 0.8	5.3 ± 1.0	5.2 ± 0.9
DAS28-ESR	6.4 ± 1.0	6.5 ± 0.9	6.4 ± 1.0	5.4 ± 0.8	5.9 ± 1.0	5.8 ± 0.9
CDAI score	38 ± 13	38 ± 12	38 ± 13	30 ± 10	33 ± 12	32 ± 12
Pain VAS score (0–100 mm) ¥	60 ± 23	62 ± 22	61 ± 23	44 ± 21	57 ± 23	48 ± 23
HAQ-DI ¶	1.6 ± 0.7	1.6 ± 0.7	1.6 ± 0.7	1.1 ± 0.5	1.3 ± 0.6	1.1 ± 0.7
FACIT-F $	28.6 ± 10.7	28.1 ± 10.7	27.6 ± 11.4	32.8 ± 7.9	32.5 ± 10.0	35.7 ± 9.1

Data are presented as mean ± standard deviation or *n* (%). ¥ Higher scores indicate more severe pain. ¶ Score range 0–3, with higher scores indicating greater disability [21]. $ Score range 0–52, with lower scores indicating greater fatigue [22]. ACPA anti-citrullinated protein antibody (positivity >10 units/mL), CDAI Clinical Disease Activity Index, csDMARD conventional synthetic disease-modifying antirheumatic drug, DAS28-hsCRP Disease Activity Score in 28 joints using the high-sensitivity C-reactive protein level, DAS28-ESR Disease Activity Score for 28-joint count with erythrocyte sedimentation rate, FACIT-F Functional Assessment of Chronic Illness Therapy-Fatigue, HAQ-DI Health Assessment Questionnaire-Disability Index, mTSS van der Heijde modified total Sharp score, MTX methotrexate, RF rheumatoid factor (positivity >14 units/mL), VAS visual analogue scale.

3.1. Change in Pain VAS Scores

For patients in remission, change from baseline in mean pain VAS score at week 24 with baricitinib was significantly greater than that with placebo ($p < 0.01$) and greater than that achieved with adalimumab, although the difference between baricitinib and adalimumab was not statistically significant (Figure 1). There was no significant difference between adalimumab and placebo. For patients in remission or low disease activity, change from baseline in mean pain VAS score at week 24 was significantly greater with baricitinib than with placebo ($p < 0.001$) and adalimumab ($p < 0.05$). The difference between adalimumab and placebo was not statistically significant. Results of sensitivity analyses using other disease activity measures were consistent with these findings. For patients not in remission or low disease activity, change from baseline in mean pain VAS score at week 24 was significantly greater with baricitinib and adalimumab than with placebo ($p < 0.0001$ and $p = 0.0130$, respectively). There was no significant difference between baricitinib and adalimumab.

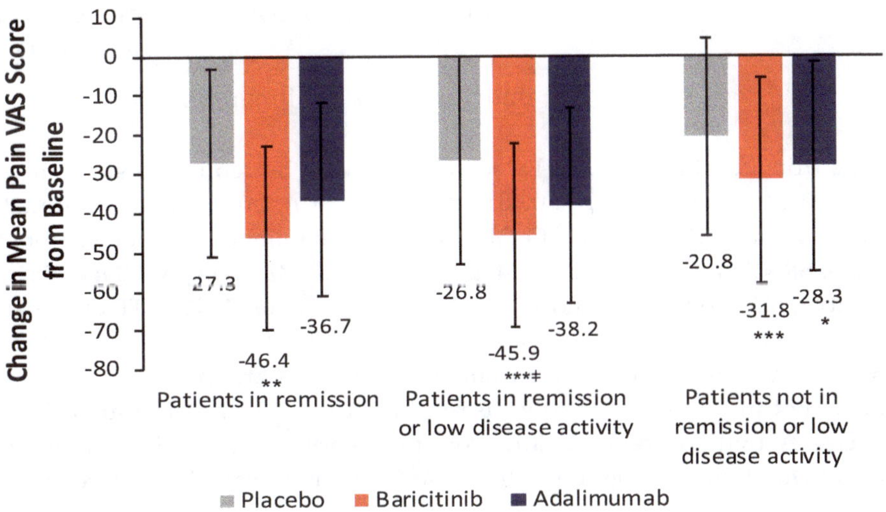

Figure 1. Change from baseline in pain VAS score at week 24 by remission status in patients from RA-BEAM. * $p < 0.05$, ** $p < 0.01$, *** $p < 0.001$ vs. placebo; ‡ $p < 0.05$ vs. adalimumab. Error bars indicate standard deviation. Change in pain VAS score based on numbers of patients from RA-BEAM in remission (DAS28-ESR <2.6): PBO+MTX $n = 24$, BARI+MTX $n = 87$, ADA+MTX $n = 57$; in remission or low disease activity (DAS28-ESR ≥2.6 and ≤3.2): PBO+MTX $n = 46$, BARI+MTX $n = 154$, ADA+MTX $n = 110$; and not in remission or low disease activity: PBO+MTX $n = 276$, BARI+MTX $n = 266$, ADA+MTX $n = 157$. One patient was missing from the BARI+MTX group for patients not in remission or low disease activity. *ADA* adalimumab, *BARI* baricitinib, *DAS28-ESR* Disease Activity Score for 28-joint count with erythrocyte sedimentation rate, *PBO* placebo, *MTX* methotrexate, *VAS* visual analogue scale.

3.2. Change in HAQ-DI Scores

For patients in remission, change from baseline in mean HAQ-DI score at week 24 was significantly greater with baricitinib and adalimumab than with placebo ($p < 0.01$ and $p < 0.05$, respectively) (Figure 2). The difference between baricitinib and adalimumab was not statistically significant. For patients in remission or low disease activity, change from baseline in HAQ-DI score at week 24 was significantly greater with baricitinib than with placebo ($p < 0.01$) and adalimumab ($p < 0.05$). There was no significant difference between adalimumab and placebo. Results of sensitivity analyses using other disease activity measures were consistent with these findings (data not shown). For patients not in remission or low disease activity, change from baseline in mean HAQ-DI score at week 24 was significantly greater with baricitinib and adalimumab than with placebo ($p < 0.0001$ and $p = 0.0014$, respectively). The difference between baricitinib and adalimumab was not statistically significant.

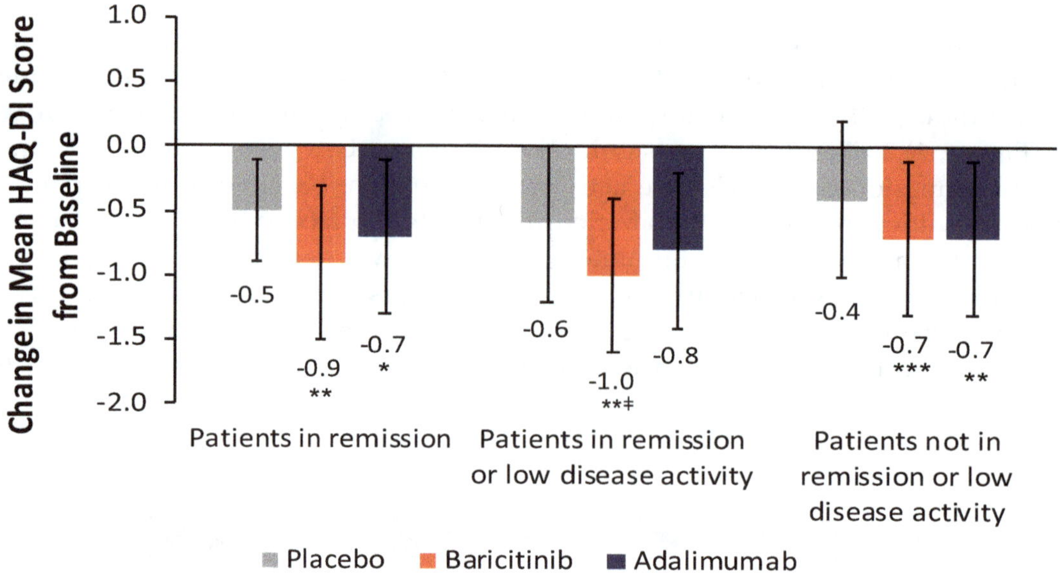

Figure 2. Change from baseline in HAQ-DI score at week 24 by remission status in patients from RA-BEAM. * $p < 0.05$, ** $p < 0.01$, *** $p < 0.001$ vs. placebo; ‡ $p < 0.05$ vs. adalimumab. Error bars indicate standard deviation. Change in HAQ-DI score based on numbers of patients from RA-BEAM in remission (DAS28-ESR <2.6): PBO+MTX $n = 24$, BARI+MTX $n = 87$, ADA+MTX $n = 57$; in remission or low disease activity (DAS28-ESR ≥2.6 and ≤3.2): PBO+MTX $n = 46$, BARI+MTX $n = 154$, ADA+MTX $n = 110$; and not in remission or low disease activity: PBO+MTX $n = 276$, BARI+MTX $n = 266$, ADA+MTX $n = 156$. One patient was missing from the BARI+MTX group and one from the ADA+MTX group for patients not in remission or low disease activity. *ADA* adalimumab, *BARI* baricitinib, *DAS28-ESR* Disease Activity Score for 28-joint count with erythrocyte sedimentation rate, *HAQ-DI* Health Assessment Questionnaire-Disability Index, *MTX* methotrexate, *PBO* placebo.

3.3. Proportion of Patients Achieving Minimal or No Pain and Proportion Achieving Normalisation of Physical Function

The proportion of patients in remission who achieved minimal or no pain at week 24 was 65.5% (57/87) for baricitinib, 61.4% (35/57) for adalimumab and 41.7% (10/24) for placebo (Figure 3a). The proportion of patients in remission who achieved normalised physical function at week 24 was 75.9% (66/87) for baricitinib, 70.2% (40/57) for adalimumab and 50.0% (12/24) for placebo (Figure 3b). Trends were the same, although proportions achieving these endpoints were slightly lower, for patients in remission or low disease activity.

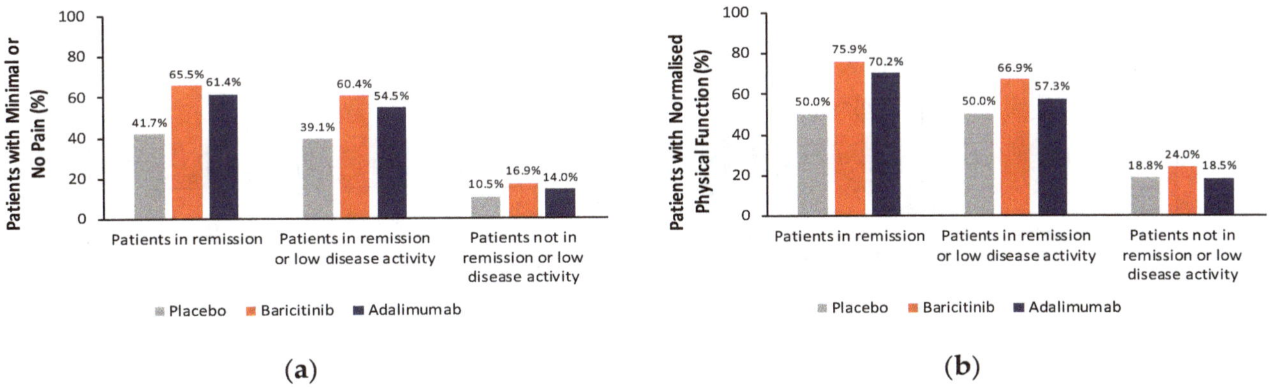

Figure 3. Patients from RA-BEAM with (**a**) minimal/no pain and (**b**) normalised physical function at week 24, by remission status. Proportions of patients from RA-BEAM with (**a**) minimal or no pain (pain VAS ≤10 mm) and (**b**) normalised physical function (HAQ-DI <0.5) based on numbers of patients in remission (DAS28-ESR <2.6): PBO+MTX $n = 24$, BARI+MTX $n = 87$, ADA+MTX $n = 57$; in remission or low disease activity (DAS28-ESR ≥2.6 and ≤3.2): PBO+MTX $n = 46$, BARI+MTX $n = 154$, ADA+MTX $n = 110$; and not in remission or low disease activity (DAS28-ESR >3.2): PBO+MTX $n = 276$, BARI+MTX $n = 266$, ADA+MTX $n = 156$. One patient was missing from the BARI+MTX group and one from the ADA+MTX group for patients not in remission or low disease activity. For the pain analysis, the number of patients not in remission or low disease activity was PBO+MTX $n = 276$, BARI+MTX $n = 210$, ADA+MTX $n = 120$. *ADA* adalimumab, *BARI* baricitinib, *DAS28-ESR* Disease Activity Score for 28-joint count with erythrocyte sedimentation rate, *HAQ-DI* Health Assessment Questionnaire-Disability Index, *MTX* methotrexate, *PBO* placebo, *VAS* visual analogue scale.

3.4. Changes in Other Patient-Reported Outcomes

Despite meeting DAS28-ESR criteria for remission or low disease activity, patients continued to experience fatigue, although FACIT-F scores were <36 in all treatment groups (Figure 4). Work productivity of working patients generally improved in all treatment groups, including those not in remission or low disease activity (Supplementary Table S1). For working patients in remission, improvements in work-related measures were numerically greater with both active treatments than with placebo. For those in remission or low disease activity, improvement in activity impairment was significantly greater with baricitinib than placebo, whereas the difference between adalimumab and placebo was not statistically significant. For working patients not in remission or low disease activity, improvements in the proportion of patients present at work, productivity loss and activity impairment were significantly greater with both active treatments than with placebo.

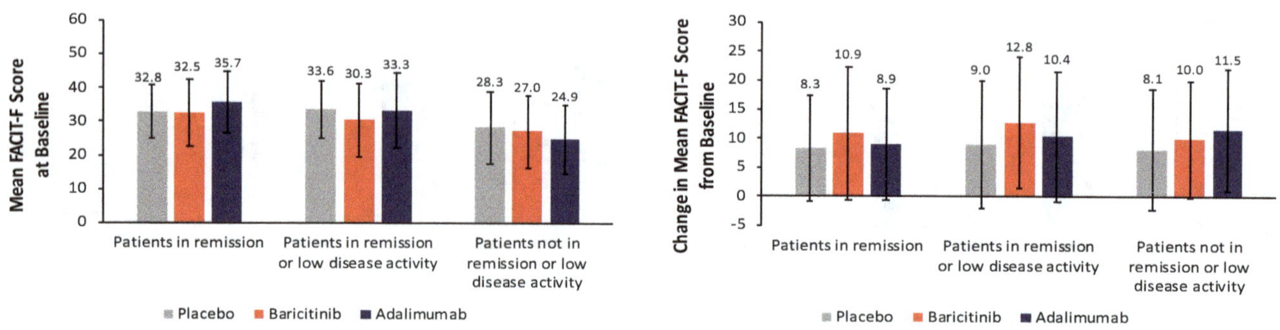

(**a**) (**b**)

Figure 4. FACIT-F scores in patients from RA-BEAM by remission status (**a**) at baseline and (**b**) change at week 24. Error bars indicate standard deviation. FACIT-F scores at baseline and change in FACIT-F scores based on numbers of patients from RA-BEAM in remission (DAS28-ESR <2.6): PBO+MTX $n = 24$, BARI+MTX $n = 87$, ADA+MTX $n = 57$; in remission or low disease activity (DAS28-ESR ≥2.6 and ≤3.2): PBO+MTX $n = 46$, BARI+MTX $n = 154$, ADA+MTX $n = 110$; and not in remission or low disease activity (DAS28-ESR >3.2): PBO+MTX $n = 276$, BARI+MTX $n = 266$, ADA+MTX $n = 156$. One patient was missing from the BARI+MTX group and one from the ADA+MTX group for patients not in remission or low disease activity. *ADA* adalimumab, *BARI* baricitinib, *DAS28-ESR* Disease Activity Score for 28-joint count with erythrocyte sedimentation rate, *FACIT-F* Functional Assessment of Chronic Illness Therapy-Fatigue, *MTX* methotrexate, *PBO* placebo.

4. Discussion

Residual pain and impaired function persist in many patients with RA despite the achievement of disease control [4,5,24]. This residual pain may be non-inflammatory in origin, caused by sensitisation of nociceptors or peripheral joint damage; or it may be due to central sensitisation [25–27]. Results of the post-hoc analyses reported here suggest that, in patients with moderately to severely active RA and an inadequate response to methotrexate, addition of baricitinib may be more effective than adalimumab and placebo in improving pain and physical function in patients with a good level of disease control (i.e., in remission or low disease activity). Among patients in remission, significantly greater improvements in pain and physical function were observed with baricitinib than with continued methotrexate alone (placebo group). Among patients in remission or low disease activity, greater improvements in pain and physical function were observed with the addition of baricitinib than with the addition of adalimumab or with continued methotrexate alone. Notably, both active treatments were significantly more effective than placebo at improving pain and physical function in patients who did not achieve controlled disease during the study (not in remission or low disease activity).

Another analysis of data from RA-BEAM also showed that, among patients with varying levels of inflammation, patients treated with baricitinib achieved consistent pain relief regardless of the CRP level at week 24 [28]. Furthermore, patients treated with baricitinib achieved greater and more rapid pain relief than those receiving adalimumab or placebo. Using CRP levels as a surrogate for inflammation, baricitinib plus methotrexate was associated with greater relief from the non-inflammatory component of RA-associated pain than adalimumab plus methotrexate or placebo plus methotrexate [28].

The mechanisms underlying the effect of baricitinib on non-inflammatory pain are not understood. As reviewed by Taylor et al. [28], it is possible that inhibition of JAK1 and JAK2 also produces anti-nociceptive effects that are not related to inflammation, such as inhibition of the JAK2-dependent cytokine granulocyte-macrophage colony-stimulating factor, which may be involved in the pathophysiology of pain [29], and/or inhibition of the JAK2-dependent signal transducer and activator of transcription (STAT)3 phosphorylation pathway [30]. Further studies to elucidate the underlying mechanisms are warranted.

Both greater disease activity and longer disease duration have been shown to increase the likelihood of a patient retiring early or stopping work because of RA [31]. In RA-BEAM, work productivity generally improved in all working patients, including those who did not achieve remission or low disease activity, but not all work-related problems were resolved (Supplementary Table S1). Control of all aspects of the disease, including reduction of pain and fatigue and maintenance of function, is an important goal of RA treatment, and patients generally consider these specified outcomes more essential than control of inflammation [10]. Pain and physical function have been identified as key unmet needs, both clinically and for patients themselves, that can adversely affect a patient's ability to function normally and their overall well-being [5].

Control of pain in patients with RA is important, since pain has been shown to contribute to worse long-term outcomes. For example, high pain levels at disease onset have been identified as a risk factor for being in the most disabled tertile of RA patients 5–18 years after disease onset [32]. High baseline pain scores were also shown to predict suboptimal mental health ($p = 0.02$) in a cohort of South African patients with early RA [33].

Maintenance of normal physical function is also important in patients with RA. Data from the Dutch DREAM registry showed that having better physical function (measured using the HAQ-DI) was associated with work participation (odds ratio (OR) 0.32, $p = 0.000$) and with starting work after 2 years of treatment with tumour necrosis factor inhibitors (OR 0.58, $p < 0.1$) [34]. Similarly, a survey of patients with RA from France showed a high correlation between deteriorating function and work capacity, such that only 15% of patients with a HAQ score of ≥2 were working, compared with 63% of patients with a HAQ score of <1 [35]. Poor physical function can also affect health-related quality of life [33].

The assessment of PROs, such as pain and function, in RA should help clinicians to focus more on the impact of the disease on patients themselves and how they are feeling rather than solely on the inflammatory component of the disease [10]. This is likely to aid in shared decision-making discussions between patients and clinicians, enabling clinicians to provide more effective and efficient patient care [25]. Indeed, it has been recommended that assessment of the PROs of pain and physical function (HAQ) be added to the current core set of treatment targets to achieve greater patient involvement in the RA treatment process [10]. Our results suggest that patients who do not respond to treatment, as measured using inflammation-associated endpoints, may still experience treatment benefit, and may, therefore, choose to continue with treatment.

Despite major advances in the treatment of RA, predicting remission a priori at the start of disease-modifying treatment remains a clinical conundrum. Nevertheless, in line with recent treatment recommendations for a treat-to-target approach, the aim of any treating rheumatologist should be to help their patients achieve remission or at least low disease activity [1,2]. With respect to this, it could be of clinical relevance to know if differences exist between agents in treating residual symptoms (such as pain) once inflammation is well controlled. Since baricitinib has demonstrated more effective pain control than adalimumab [28], we were interested in investigating whether this benefit persists even when a good level of disease control has been achieved. The post-hoc analyses reported here are not, on their own, intended to inform clinical practice, but to help towards better defining current evidence for the pain-relieving benefits of baricitinib compared to tumour necrosis factor inhibitors.

Limitations of the current analysis include that post-hoc analyses are exploratory by nature, aimed at creating hypotheses rather than clearly demonstrable facts; the sample sizes for patients achieving remission or low disease activity and working patients were small; and generalisability of the results to patients in routine care who receive baricitinib or adalimumab is uncertain. In addition, analyses were not adjusted for multiple testing.

5. Conclusions

Treatment with baricitinib 4 mg once daily or adalimumab 40 mg every other week resulted in improvements in pain, physical function, fatigue and work productivity/impairment in patients with

RA, independent of the impact on inflammation, measured using DAS28-ESR. Among patients in remission or low disease activity, greater improvements in pain and physical function were observed with baricitinib than with adalimumab and placebo. Research to better understand the role of JAK1/JAK2 pathways in the control of pain beyond the regulation of inflammation is underway to help clarify the differential effects of baricitinib relative to adalimumab on pain.

Author Contributions: Conceptualisation, Methodology and Formal Analysis, C.G., A.Q., B.Z., I.d.l.T., F.D.L. and P.C.T.; Data Curation, B.Z.; Investigation, B.F., B.K., J.E.P.; T.T., C.G., A.Q., B.Z., I.d.l.T., F.D.L. and P.C.T.; Writing—Original Draft Preparation, P.C.T.; Writing—Review and Editing, B.F., B.K., J.E.P., T.T., C.G., A.Q., B.Z., I.d.l.T., F.D.L. and P.C.T.; Supervision, I.d.l.T.; Project Administration, F.D.L.

Acknowledgments: The authors would like to acknowledge JS Smolen for critical review of the manuscript, and Sue Chambers and Caroline Spencer (Rx Communications, Mold, UK) for medical writing assistance with the preparation of this manuscript, funded by Eli Lilly and Company. PCT would like to acknowledge support from the National Institute for Health Research (NIHR) Oxford Biomedical Research Centre (BRC) and from Arthritis Research UK.

Conflicts of Interest: B.F. reports grants from AbbVie, Eli Lilly and Company, MSD, and Pfizer, and personal fees from AbbVie, Biogen, BMS, Celgene, Janssen-Cilag, Eli Lilly and Company, Medac, MSD, NORDIC Pharma, Novartis, Pfizer, Roche, Sanofi-Aventis, SOBI and UCB. B.K. reports grants and personal fees from Eli Lilly and Company, Janssen, Novartis and UCB. T.T. reports grants and personal fees from Astellas Pharma Inc., Chugai Pharmaceutical Co. Ltd., Daiichi Sankyo Co., Takeda Pharmaceutical Co. Ltd., AbbVie GK, Asahikasei Pharma Corp., Mitsubishi Tanabe Pharma Co., Pfizer Japan Inc., Eisai Co. Ltd., AYUMI Pharmaceutical Corporation, Nipponkayaku Co. Ltd., Novartis Pharma K.K., Bristol–Myers K.K., Astra Zeneca K.K., Eli Lilly Japan K.K., Taisho Toyama Pharmaceutical Co., Ltd., GlaxoSmithKline K.K., UCB Japan Co. Ltd. and Taiho Pharmaceutical Co. Ltd. C.G. is an employee and stockholder of Eli Lilly and Company. A.Q. is an employee and stockholder of Eli Lilly and Company. I.d.l.T. is an employee and stockholder of Eli Lilly and Company. B.Z. is an employee and stockholder of Eli Lilly and Company. F.D.L. is an employee and stockholder of Eli Lilly and Company. P.C.T. reports grants from Eli Lilly and Company, and Galapagos, and personal fees from Eli Lilly and Company, AbbVie, Gilead, and Pfizer.

References

1. Singh, J.A.; Saag, K.G.; Bridges, S.L., Jr.; Akl, E.A.; Bannuru, R.R.; Sullivan, M.C.; Vaysbrot, E.; McNaughton, C.; Osani, M.; Shmerling, R.H.; et al. 2015 American College of Rheumatology guideline for the treatment of rheumatoid arthritis. *Arthritis Rheumatol.* **2016**, *68*, 1–26. [CrossRef]
2. Smolen, J.S.; Landewé, R.; Bijlsma, J.; Burmester, G.; Chatzidionysiou, K.; Dougados, M.; Nam, J.; Ramiro, S.; Voshaar, M.; Van Vollenhoven, R.; et al. EULAR recommendations for the management of rheumatoid arthritis with synthetic and biological disease-modifying antirheumatic drugs: 2016 update. *Ann. Rheum. Dis.* **2017**, *76*, 960–977. [CrossRef]
3. Nieuwenhuis, W.P.; De Wit, M.P.; Boonen, A.; Van Der Helm-Van Mil, A.H. Changes in the clinical presentation of patients with rheumatoid arthritis from the early 1990s to the years 2010: Earlier identification but more severe patient reported outcomes. *Ann. Rheum. Dis.* **2016**, *75*, 2054–2056. [CrossRef]
4. Ishiguro, N.; Dougados, M.; Cai, Z.; Zhu, B.; Ishida, M.; Sato, M.; Gaich, C.; Quebe, A.; Stoykov, I.; Tanaka, Y. Relationship between disease activity and patient-reported outcomes in rheumatoid arthritis: Post hoc analyses of overall and Japanese results from two phase 3 clinical trials. *Mod. Rheumatol.* **2018**, *28*, 950–959. [CrossRef]
5. Taylor, P.C.; Moore, A.; Vasilescu, R.; Alvir, J.; Tarallo, M. A structured literature review of the burden of illness and unmet needs in patients with rheumatoid arthritis: A current perspective. *Rheumatol. Int.* **2016**, *36*, 685–695. [CrossRef]
6. Gossec, L.; Dougados, M.; Rincheval, N.; Balanescu, A.; Boumpas, D.T.; Canadelo, S.; Carmona, L.; Daurès, J.P.; de Wit, M.; Dijkmans, B.A.; et al. Elaboration of the preliminary Rheumatoid Arthritis Impact of Disease (RAID) score: A EULAR initiative. *Ann. Rheum. Dis.* **2009**, *68*, 1680–1685. [CrossRef]

7. Khan, N.A.; Spencer, H.J.; Abda, E.; Aggarwal, A.; Alten, R.; Ancuta, C.; Andersone, D.; Bergman, M.; Craig-Muller, J.; Detert, J.; et al. Determinants of discordance in patients' and physicians' rating of rheumatoid arthritis disease activity. *Arthritis Care Res.* **2012**, *64*, 206–214. [CrossRef]
8. Wen, H.; Ralph Schumacher, H.; Li, X.; Gu, J.; Ma, L.; Wei, H.; Yokogawa, N.; Shiroto, K.; Baker, J.F.; Dinnella, J.; et al. Comparison of expectations of physicians and patients with rheumatoid arthritis for rheumatology clinic visits: A pilot, multicenter, international study. *Int. J. Rheum. Dis.* **2012**, *15*, 380–389. [CrossRef]
9. Van Tuyl, L.H.; Sadlonova, M.; Hewlett, S.; Davis, B.; Flurey, C.; Goel, N.; Gossec, L.; Brahe, C.H.; Hill, C.L.; Hoogland, W.; et al. The patient perspective on absence of disease activity in rheumatoid arthritis: A survey to identify key domains of patient-perceived remission. *Ann. Rheum. Dis.* **2017**, *76*, 855–861. [CrossRef]
10. Fautrel, B.; Alten, R.; Kirkham, B.; De La Torre, I.; Durand, F.; Barry, J.; Holzkaemper, T.; Fakhouri WTaylor, P.C. Call for action: How to improve use of patient-reported outcomes to guide clinical decision making in rheumatoid arthritis. *Rheumatol. Int.* **2018**, *38*, 935–947. [CrossRef]
11. Fridman, J.S.; Scherle, P.A.; Collins, R.; Burn, T.C.; Li, Y.; Li, J.; Covington, M.B.; Thomas, B.; Collier, P.; Favata, M.F.; et al. Selective inhibition of JAK1 and JAK2 is efficacious in rodent models of arthritis: Preclinical characterization of INCB028050. *J. Immunol.* **2010**, *184*, 5298–5307. [CrossRef]
12. O'Shea, J.J.; Kontzias, A.; Yamaoka, K.; Tanaka, Y.; Laurence, A. Janus kinase inhibitors in autoimmune diseases. *Ann. Rheum. Dis.* **2013**, *72*, ii111–ii115. [CrossRef]
13. Choy, E.H.S.; Miceli-Richard, C.; González-Gay, M.A.; Sinigaglia, L.; Schlichting, D.E.; Meszaros, G.; de la Torre, I.; Schulze-Koops, H. The effect of JAK/JAK2 inhibition in rheumatoid arthritis: Efficacy and safety of baricitinib. *RMD Open* **2019**, *5*, e000798. [CrossRef]
14. European Medicines Agency. Olumiant 2 mg and 4 mg Film-Coated Tablets. Summary of Product Characteristics. 2018. Available online: http://www.ema.europa.eu/docs/en_GB/document_library/EPAR_-_Product_Information/human/004085/WC500223723.pdf (accessed on 11 April 2018).
15. Food and Drug Administration. Olumiant (Baricitinib) Tablets, for Oral Use. Prescribing Information; 2018. Available online: https://www.accessdata.fda.gov/drugsatfda_docs/label/2018/207924s000lbl.pdf (accessed on 21 June 2018).
16. Pharmaceutical and Medical Devices Agency. Report on the Deliberation Results. Olumiant Tablets 2 mg, Olumiant Tablets 4 mg. 2017. Available online: http://www.pmda.go.jp/files/000226301.pdf (accessed on 21 June 2018).
17. Genovese, M.C.; Kremer, J.; Zamani, O.; Ludivico, C.; Krogulec, M.; Xie, L.; Beattie, S.D.; Koch, A.E.; Cardillo, T.E.; Rooney, T.P.; et al. Baricitinib in patients with refractory rheumatoid arthritis. *N. Engl. J. Med.* **2016**, *374*, 1243–1252. [CrossRef]
18. Dougados, M.; van der Heijde, D.; Chen, Y.C.; Greenwald, M.; Drescher, E.; Liu, J.; Beattie, S.; Witt, S.; de la Torre, I.; Gaich CRooney, T. Baricitinib in patients with inadequate response or intolerance to conventional synthetic DMARDs: Results from the RA-BUILD study. *Ann. Rheum. Dis.* **2017**, *76*, 88–95. [CrossRef]
19. Fleischmann, R.; Schiff, M.; van der Heijde, D.; Ramos-Remus, C.; Spindler, A.; Stanislav, M.; Zerbini, C.A.; Gurbuz, S.; Dickson, C.; de Bono, S.; et al. Baricitinib, methotrexate, or combination in patients with rheumatoid arthritis and no or limited prior disease-modifying antirheumatic drug treatment. *Arthritis Rheumatol.* **2017**, *69*, 506–517. [CrossRef]
20. Taylor, P.C.; Keystone, E.C.; van der Heijde, D.; Weinblatt, M.E.; del Carmen Morales, L.; Reyes Gonzaga, J.; Yakushin, S.; Ishii, T.; Emoto, K.; Beattie, S.; et al. Baricitinib versus placebo or adalimumab in rheumatoid arthritis. *N. Engl. J. Med.* **2017**, *376*, 652–662. [CrossRef]
21. Fries, J.F.; Spitz, P.W.; Young, D.Y. The dimensions of health outcomes: The health assessment questionnaire, disability and pain scales. *J. Rheumatol.* **1982**, *9*, 789–793.
22. Cella, D.; Yount, S.; Sorensen, M.; Chartash, E.; Sengupta, N.; Grober, J. Validation of the Functional Assessment of Chronic Illness Therapy Fatigue Scale relative to other instrumentation in patients with rheumatoid arthritis. *J. Rheumatol.* **2005**, *32*, 811–819.
23. Reilly, M.C.; Zbrozek, A.S.; Dukes, E.M. The validity and reproducibility of a work productivity and activity impairment instrument. *Pharmacoeconomics* **1993**, *4*, 353–365. [CrossRef]
24. Ishida, M.; Kuroiwa, Y.; Yoshida, E.; Sato, M.; Krupa, D.; Henry, N.; Ikeda, K.; Kaneko, Y. Residual symptoms and disease burden among patients with rheumatoid arthritis in remission or low disease activity: A systematic literature review. *Mod. Rheumatol.* **2018**, *28*, 789–799. [CrossRef]

25. Taylor, P.; Manger, B.; Alvaro-Gracia, J.; Johnstone, R.; Gomez-Reino, J.; Eberhardt, E.; Wolfe, F.; Schwartzman, S.; Furfaro, N.; Kavanaugh, A. Patient perceptions concerning pain management in the treatment of rheumatoid arthritis. *J. Int. Med. Res.* **2010**, *38*, 1213–1224. [CrossRef]
26. Walsh, D.A.; Mcwilliams, D.F. Mechanisms, impact and management of pain in rheumatoid arthritis. *Nat. Rev. Rheumatol.* **2014**, *10*, 581–592. [CrossRef]
27. Boyden, S.D.; Hossain, I.N.; Wohlfahrt, A.; Lee, Y.C. Non-inflammatory causes of pain in patients with rheumatoid arthritis. *Curr. Rheumatol. Rep.* **2016**, *18*, 30. [CrossRef]
28. Taylor, P.C.; Lee, Y.C.; Fleischmann, R.; Takeuchi, T.; Perkins, E.L.; Fautrel, B.; Zhu, B.; Quebe, A.K.; Gaich, C.L.; Zhang, X.; et al. Achieving pain control in rheumatoid arthritis with baricitinib or adalimumab plus methotrexate: Results from the RA-BEAM trial. *J. Clin. Med.* **2019**, *8*, 831. [CrossRef]
29. Cook, A.D.; Pobjoy, J.; Steidl, S.; Dürr, M.; Braine, E.L.; Turner, A.L.; Lacey, D.C.; Hamilton, J.A. Granulocyte-macrophage colony-stimulating factor is a key mediator in experimental osteoarthritis pain and disease development. *Arthritis Res. Ther.* **2012**, *14*, R199. [CrossRef]
30. Dominguez, E.; Rivat, C.; Pommier, B.; Mauborgne, A.; Pohl, M. JAK/STAT3 pathway is activated in spinal cord microglia after peripheral nerve injury and contributes to neuropathic pain development in rat. *J. Neurochem.* **2008**, *107*, 50–60. [CrossRef]
31. Capron, J.; De Leonardis, F.; Fakhouri, W.; Burke, T.; Rose, A.; Jacob, I. The impact of rheumatoid arthritis (RA) on a patient's ability to stay in work and level of pain experienced. *Value Health* **2017**, *20*, A531–A532. [CrossRef]
32. Malm, K.; Bergman, S.; Andersson, M.; Bremander, A.; BARFOT Study Group. Predictors of severe self-reported disability in RA in a long-term follow-up study. *Disabil. Rehabil.* **2015**, *37*, 686–691. [CrossRef]
33. Hodkinson, B.; Musenge, E.; Ally, M.; Meyer, P.W.; Anderson, R.; Tikly, M. Functional disability and health-related quality of life in South Africans with early rheumatoid arthritis. *Scand. J. Rheumatol.* **2012**, *41*, 366–374. [CrossRef]
34. Manders, S.H.; Kievit, W.; Braakman-Jansen, A.L.; Brus, H.L.; Hendriks, L.; Fransen, J.; van de Laar, M.A.; van Riel, P.L. Determinants associated with work participation in patients with established rheumatoid arthritis taking tumor necrosis factor inhibitors. *J. Rheumatol.* **2014**, *41*, 1263–1269. [CrossRef]
35. Kobelt, G.; Woronoff, A.S.; Richard, B.; Peeters, P.; Sany, J. Disease status, costs and quality of life of patients with rheumatoid arthritis in France: The ECO-PR study. *Jt. Bone Spine* **2008**, *75*, 408–415. [CrossRef]

15

Maintained Clinical Remission in Ankylosing Spondylitis Patients Switched from Reference Infliximab to its Biosimilar: An 18-Month Comparative Open-Label Study

Evripidis Kaltsonoudis, Eleftherios Pelechas, Paraskevi V. Voulgari and Alexandros A. Drosos *

Rheumatology Clinic, Department of Internal Medicine, Medical School, University of Ioannina, 45110 Ioannina, Greece
* Correspondence: adrosos@cc.uoi.gr

Abstract: Background: Switching from reference infliximab (RI) to biosimilar infliximab (BI) had no detrimental effects on efficacy and safety. However, long-term follow-up data is missing. Objective: To evaluate patients with Ankylosing Spondylitis (AS) in clinical remission who were switching from RI to BI, in terms of the safety and efficacy of this, in a long-term fashion. Methods: One hundred and nine consecutive unselected AS patients were investigated. All were naïve to other biologics and were followed-up at predefined times receiving RI. Patients in clinical remission were asked to switch from RI to BI. Those who switched to BI were compared with a matched control-group receiving continuous RI. During follow-up, several parameters were recorded for at least 18 months. Disease activity was measured using the Bath Ankylosing Spondylitis disease activity index (BASDAI), and the Ankylosing Spondylitis disease activity score (ASDAS), using the C-reactive protein. Remission was defined as BASDAI < 4 and ASDAS < 1.3. Results: Eighty-eight patients were evaluated (21 excluded for different reasons). From those, 45 switched to BI, while 43 continued receiving RI. No differences between groups regarding demographic, clinical and laboratory parameters were observed. All patients were in clinical remission. During follow-up, five patients from the BI-group and three from the maintenance-group discontinued the study (4 patients nocebo effect, 1 loss of efficacy). After 18 months of treatment, all patients in both groups remained in clinical remission. No significant adverse events were noted between groups. Conclusion: BI is equivalent to RI in maintaining AS in clinical remission for at least 18 months.

Keywords: ankylosing spondylitis; infliximab; biosimilar; switching

---

1. Introduction

CTP-13 (Inflectra®, Remsima®) the biosimilar infliximab (BI) has been granted all indications, including Ankylosing Spondylitis (AS), of the reference infliximab (RI) in several countries [1]. Clinical evidence for the approval of BI has been obtained from pivotal studies on patients with AS (PLANETAS) [2] and rheumatoid arthritis (RA) (PLANETRA) [3]. Switching from RI to its biosimilar had no detrimental effects on efficacy, safety or immunogenicity compared with continuous RI therapy [4,5]. Therefore, BI is an efficacious alternative to RI in patients with inflammatory arthritis [6]. On the other hand, there are reports emphasizing the role of shared-decision making with patients when it comes to switching to a biosimilar product in order to achieve a better acceptance and higher retention rate, minimizing the nocebo effect [5]. However, long-term follow-up data is missing. The aim of our study was to investigate if BI is equivalent to RI to maintain patients with AS in clinical remission compared with continuing RI in a long-term fashion.

2. Materials and Methods

This is a single-center prospective observational cohort study with a total number of 109 consecutive unselected patients with AS who were treated with RI in a tertiary university center. All patients were followed-up at predefined times receiving RI (5 mg/kg/8 weeks) intravenously and were naïve to previous biologic treatments. Patients who were in clinical remission were asked to switch from RI to BI using the same therapeutic dose after shared-decision making. The allocation of the patients was done randomly using an internet-based allocation program in order to minimize any selection bias (Random.org). Patients switched to BI were compared with a matched control group receiving continuous RI. The switching period was from January 2017 until June 2017 and patients were followed-up until December 2018. During follow-up, the demographic, clinical, and laboratory parameters as well as comorbidities were all recorded for at least 18 months. In addition, all adverse events as well as serious adverse events according to the Food and Drug Administration (FDA.gov) were also recorded. Disease activity was measured using the Bath Ankylosing Spondylitis Activity Index (BASDAI) [7] and the Ankylosing Spondylitis Activity Score (ASDAS) [8,9] using the C-reactive protein (CRP). Clinical remission was defined if patients had BASDAI < 4 and ASDAS < 1.3. Statistical analysis was performed using SPSS statistics version 20.0 (IBM Corporation, Armonk, NY, USA) We used the paired samples t-test for variables with normal distribution and Wilcoxon signed ranks test for variables which were not normally distributed. A p-value < 0.05 was considered statistically significant. Written informed consent was obtained from all patients, and the study has been approved by the clinical Research Ethic Committee of the University Hospital of Ioannina, according to the principles in the Declaration of Helsinki (197/2-12-2016).

3. Results

Twenty-one patients were excluded: 9 because they were not in clinical remission and 12 refused to switch from RI to its biosimilar. Thus, the final results comprise 88 patients. From these patients, 45 switched to BI, while 43 continued receiving RI (Figure 1). The demographic and clinical characteristics of our patients are depicted in Table 1. There were no differences between groups regarding the demographic, clinical and laboratory parameters. All patients were in clinical remission with low BASDAI and low ASDAS for approximately 3 years. During the follow-up period, 5 patients from the switched group and 3 from the continuing group discontinued the study (Figure 1). Four patients receiving BI presented nocebo effects after the second infusion while one had recurrent urinary tract infections. The patients with nocebo effects experienced nonspecific, subjective complaints such as headache, somnolence, dizziness, arthralgias, fatigue and pain. The clinical examination of these patients was unremarkable, and the acute phase reactants were within normal limits. These patients were switched to RI. Three responded well, while the fourth did not, and was changed to interleukin-17 (IL-17) inhibitor with good results. On the other hand, from the patients who continued receiving the RI, two patients presented recurrent upper respiratory tract infections while one had a disease flare-up. These patients were treated with an IL-17 inhibitor and responded very well. After 18 months of follow-up, all patients in both groups remained in clinical remission with low BASDAI, low ASDAS as well as low erythrocyte sedimentation rate (ESR) and CRP (Table 2). No significant adverse events, serious adverse events or any comorbidities were noted between the studied groups (Table 3).

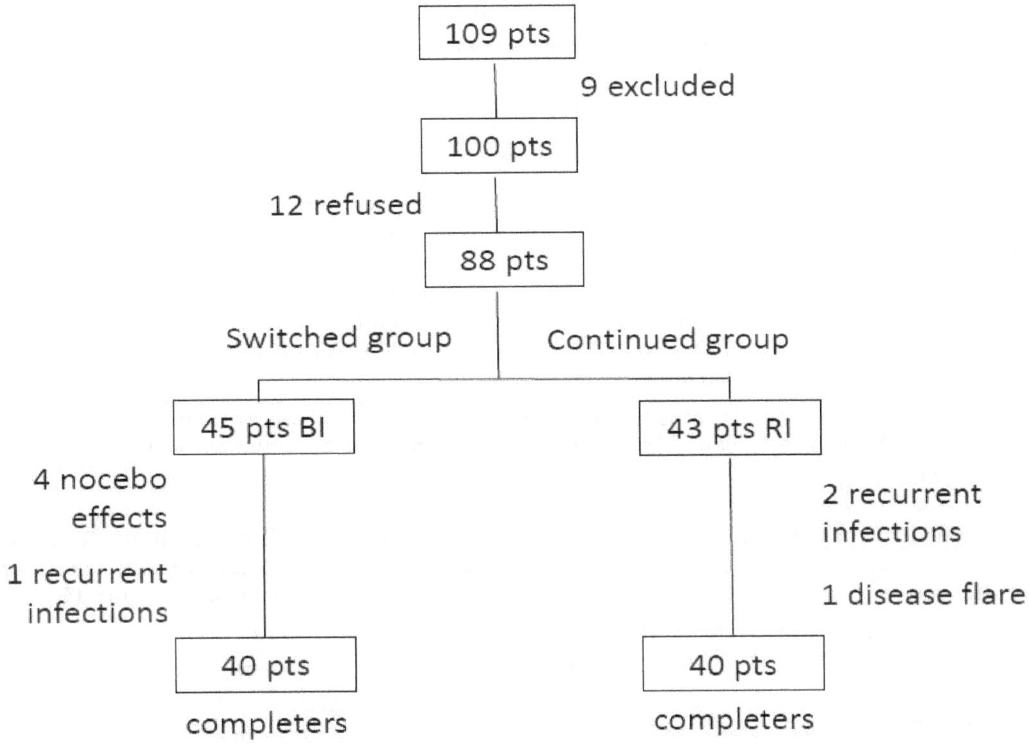

Figure 1. Flow chart of AS patients treated with infliximab.

Table 1. Demographic and clinical characteristic of Ankylosing Spondylitis (AS) patients at switching.

Parameters	Switched Group (BI) *n*:45	Continued Group (RI) *n*:43	*p*-Value
Mean age (years) (SD)	36.1 (4.6)	35.7 (4.3)	NS
Male/female	39/6	40 (3)	NS
Mean disease duration (years) (SD)	7.8 (3.0)	7.6 (2.8)	NS
Mean follow-up (years) (SD)	7.0 (1.1)	6.9 (0.9)	NS
BMI (kgr/m^2) >25	5 (11.1)	4 (9.3)	NS
Current smokers n (%)	10 (22.2)	8 (18.6)	NS
Ex-smokers n (%)	9 (20)	9 (20.9)	NS
Mean treatment with BI/RI	6.4 (0.9)	6.5 (0.8)	NS
Mean treatment with RI and clinical remission (years) (SD)		3.6 (0.8)	NS
Axial disease n (%)	45 (100)	43 (100)	NS
Peripheral disease n (%)	4 (9)	3 (7)	NS
Methotrexate intake n (%)	3 (7)	2 (5)	NS
Mean BASDAI (SD)	3.7 (0.2)	3.6 (0.4)	NS
Mean ASDAS (SD)	1.0 (0.2)	1.1 (0.2)	NS
Mean ESR mm/h (SD)	18.5 (2.2)	19.3 (1.7)	NS
Mean CRP mg/L (SD)	6.0 (0.8)	5.8 (0.6)	NS

BI, biosimilar infliximab; RI, reference infliximab; SD, standard deviation; BMI, body mass index; BASDAI, bath ankylosing spondylitis activity index; ASDAS, ankylosing spondylitis disease activity score; ESR, erythrocyte sedimentation rate; CRP, C-reactive protein; NS, non-statistical.

Table 2. Response to treatment in AS patients switched to BI versus those continuing RI.

Parameters	Switched Group (BI)	Continued Group (RI)	*p*-Value
At switching			
BASDAI (SD)	3.7 (0.2)	3.6 (0.4)	NS
ASDAS (SD)	1.0 (0.2)	1.1 (0.2)	NS
ESR mm/h (SD)	18.5 (2.2)	19.3 (1.7)	NS
CRP mg/l (SD)	6.0 (0.8)	5.8 (0.6)	NS
End of the study			
BASDAI (SD)	3.7 (0.4)	3.8 (0.2)	N5
ASDAS (SD)	1.0 (0.2)	1.1 (0.1)	NS
ESR mm/h (SD)	19.5 (1.5)	20.0 (1.6)	NS
CRP mg/l (SD)	6.0 (1.0)	6.1 (1.1)	NS

BI, biosimilar infliximab; RI, reference infliximab; SD, standard deviation; BASDAI, bath ankylosing spondylitis activity index; ASDAS, ankylosing spondylitis disease activity score; ESR, erythrocyte sedimentation rate; CRP, C-reactive protein; NS, non-statistical.

Table 3. Adverse events during follow-up in AS patients switched to BI versus those continuing RI.

Adverse Events * *n* (%)	Switched Group (BI)	Continued Group (RI)	*p*-Value
Upper respiratory tract infections	3 (6.6)	2 (4.6)	NS
Urinary tract infections	2 (4.4)	2 (4.6)	NS
Skin infections	2 (2.2)	1 (2.3)	NS
Increased liver enzymes	2 (4.4)	2 (4.6)	NS
Diarrhea	1 (2.2)	2 (4.6)	NS
Viral infections	2 (4.4)	1 (2.3)	NS
Headache	1 (2.2)	0 (0)	NS
Hypertension	1 (2.2)	1 (2.3)	NS

*, not requiring discontinuation; BI, Biosimilar Infliximab; RI, Reference Infliximab; n, number of patients; NS, Non-statistical.

4. Discussion

Biosimilars represent an important new generation of drugs in a rheumatologist's armamentarium [10]. Biosimilars have been approved by the European Medical Association (EMA) for rheumatologic indications and those for which the biological originator is no longer patent-protected. CTP-13, under the commercial name Inflectra/Remsima, was the first biosimilar approved by the EMA in 2013 [1]. Approval of BI was based on findings from two pivotal trials in AS [2] and RA [3]. Data from open-label extension studies of the original trials for AS have been reported [5]. Current data supports the proposal that it was possible to switch from RI to BI without any detrimental effects on safety and efficacy [5]. In addition, all available data regarding switching from RI to its biosimilar are reassuring. Switching is also recommended in the European League Against Rheumatism (EULAR) guidelines [11]. Indeed, a 52-week double-blind trial supports the efficacy and safety of the switch from RI to its biosimilar in patients with stable disease [12]. However, long-term follow-up data are required to confirm the efficacy and safety of the switch. The present study tries to cover this gap.

In our study, 88 AS patients receiving RI who were in clinical remission were asked to switch to BI. Half of them received BI, while the rest continued receiving RI. After 18 months of follow-up, no differences of clinical efficacy and safety were found between groups. Both groups remained in clinical remission. Our findings are in line with the PLANETAS study despite the fact that they used different tools in assessing disease activity [2]. Five patients from the BI group and three from the RI group discontinued the treatment. In the switched group, four patients discontinued the treatment due to nocebo effects. Nocebo effects are complex and individualized clinical phenomena that can induce new worsening pain, nonspecific subjective complaints such as malaise, fatigue, headache, weakness and others which are mainly induced by the patients' negative expectations [13]. Thus, physicians should be aware of the potential appearance of nocebo effects which may hinder the transition to biosimilars in some patients [14]. Our patients responded very well to switching from RI to its biosimilar. The reason for this could be the clinical state of the patients that are in clinical remission. Our results are in line with those of other investigators who reported a high retention rate of switching to biosimilars if the patients are stable [5,12]. Another reason could be that the switching was after discussion and decision-making with the patients. Evidence-based recommendations are available for several conditions in order to guide physicians in the switching process with biologics. Data suggests that shared-decision making leads to a better therapeutic response with fewer nocebo effects in contrast to non-medical switching [15,16]. The limitation of our study is that we included a small number of patients. On the other hand, the strength of our study is that it is the longest comparative study regarding switching from the RI to BI in AS.

When biosimilars appeared in the market, they not only had a lower price but also led to the price erosion of the reference products. In our study, there were no differences between the studied groups, and despite the fact that we did not make a cost-effectiveness analysis, we assume that the cost of the BI per patient is lower than that of the RI. Our study offers the promise of substantial savings relative to the RI product, enabling more AS patients to access biological therapy and reducing the cost associated with expensive biological treatment [17].

5. Conclusions

This is the first study in which AS patients in clinical remission receiving RI who were switched to BI remained in clinical remission for at least 18 months. We demonstrated that BI is equivalent to RI in maintaining AS patients in clinical remission.

Author Contributions: E.K., acquisition, analysis and interpretation of the data and manuscript drafting; E.P., acquisition and analysis of the data, editing and manuscript review; P.V.V. acquisition and analysis of the data, editing and manuscript review; and A.A.D. conception and study design and manuscript review. All authors have approved the final manuscript.

References

1. Dörner, T.; Kay, J. Biosimilars in rheumatology: Current perspectives and lessons learnt. *Nat. Rev. Rheumatol.* **2015**, *11*, 713–724. [CrossRef] [PubMed]
2. Park, W.; Yoo, D.H.; Miranda, P.; Brzosko, M.; Wiland, P.; Gutierrez-Ureña, S.; Mikazane, H.; Lee, Y.A.; Smiyan, S.; Lim, M.J.; et al. Efficacy and safety of switching from reference infliximab to CT-P13 compared with maintenance of CT-P13 in ankylosing spondylitis: 102-week data from the PLANETAS extension study. *Ann. Rheum. Dis.* **2017**, *76*, 346–354. [CrossRef] [PubMed]
3. Yoo, D.H.; Prodanovic, N.; Jaworski, J.; Miranda, P.; Ramiterre, E.; Lanzon, A.; Baranauskaite, A.; Wiland, P.; Abud-Mendoza, C.; Oparanov, B.; et al. Efficacy and safety of CT-P13 (biosimilar infliximab) in patients with rheumatoid arthritis: Comparison between switching from reference infliximab to CT-P13 and continuing CT-P13 in the PLANETRA extension study. *Ann. Rheum. Dis.* **2017**, *76*, 355–363. [CrossRef] [PubMed]
4. Tanaka, Y.; Yamanaka, H.; Takeuchi, T.; Inoue, M.; Saito, K.; Saeki, Y.; Lee, S.J.; Nambu, Y. Safety and efficacy of CT-P13 in Japanese patients with rheumatoid arthritis in an extension phase or after switching from infliximab. *Mod. Rheumatol.* **2017**, *27*, 237–245. [CrossRef] [PubMed]
5. Scherlinger, M.; Germain, V.; Labadie, C.; Barnetche, T.; Truchetet, M.E.; Bannwarth, B.; Mehsen-Cetre, N.; Richez, C.; Schaeverbeke, T.; FHU ACRONIM. Switching from originator infliximab to biosimilar CT-P13 in real-life: The weight of patient acceptance. *Joint Bone Spine.* **2018**, *85*, 561–567. [CrossRef] [PubMed]
6. Jones, A.; Ciurtin, C.; Ismajli, M.; Leandro, M.; Sengupta, R.; Machado, P.M. Biologics for treating axial spondyloarthritis. *Expert Opin. Biol. Ther.* **2018**, *18*, 641–652. [CrossRef] [PubMed]
7. Calin, A.; Garrett, S.; Whitelock, H.; Kennedy, L.G.; O'Hea, J.; Mallorie, P.; Jenkinson, T. A new approach to defining functional ability in ankylosing spondylitis: The development of the Bath Ankylosing Spondylitis Functional Index. *J. Rheumatol.* **1994**, *21*, 2281–2285. [PubMed]

8. Lukas, C.; Landewé, R.; Sieper, J.; Dougados, M.; Davis, J.; Braun, J.; van der Linden, S.; van der Heijde, D. Assessment of SpondyloArthritis international Society. Development of an ASAS-endorsed disease activity score (ASDAS) in patients with ankylosing spondylitis. *Ann. Rheum. Dis.* **2009**, *68*, 18–24. [CrossRef] [PubMed]
9. Machado, P.; Landewé, R.; Lie, E.; Kvien, T.K.; Braun, J.; Baker, D.; van der Heijde, D.; Assessment of SpondyloArthritis international Society. Ankylosing Spondylitis Disease Activity Score (ASDAS): Defining cut-off values for disease activity states and improvement scores. *Ann. Rheum. Dis.* **2011**, *70*, 47–53. [CrossRef] [PubMed]
10. Blair, H.A.; Deeks, E.D. Infliximab Biosimilar (CT-P13; Infliximab-dyyb): A Review in Autoimmune Inflammatory Diseases. *Bio Drugs.* **2016**, *30*, 469–480. [CrossRef] [PubMed]
11. Kay, J.; Schoels, M.M.; Dörner, T.; Emery, P.; Kvien, T.K.; Smolen, J.S.; Breedveld, F.C. Task Force on the Use of Biosimilars to Treat Rheumatological Diseases. Consensus-based recommendations for the use of biosimilars to treat rheumatological diseases. *Ann. Rheum. Dis.* **2018**, *77*, 165–174. [CrossRef] [PubMed]
12. Jørgensen, K.K.; Olsen, I.C.; Goll, G.L.; Lorentzen, M.; Bolstad, N.; Haavardsholm, E.A.; Lundin, K.E.A.; Mørk, C.; Jahnsen, J.; Kvien, T.K.; et al. Switching from originator infliximab to biosimilar CT-P13 compared with maintained treatment with originator infliximab (NOR-SWITCH): A 52-week, randomised, double-blind, non-inferiority trial. *Lancet* **2017**, *389*, 2304–2316.
13. Kravvariti, E.; Kitas, G.D.; Mitsikostas, D.D.; Sfikakis, P.P. Nocebos in rheumatology: Emerging concepts and their implications for clinical practice. *Nat. Rev. Rheumatol.* **2018**, *14*, 727–740. [CrossRef] [PubMed]
14. Tweehuysen, L.; van den Bemt, B.J.F.; van Ingen, I.L.; de Jong, A.J.L.; van der Laan, W.H.; van den Hoogen, F.H.J.; den Broeder, A.A. Subjective Complaints as the Main Reason for Biosimilar Discontinuation After Open-Label Transition From Reference Infliximab to Biosimilar Infliximab. *Arthritis Rheumatol.* **2018**, *70*, 60–68. [CrossRef] [PubMed]
15. Scherlinger, M.; Langlois, E.; Germain, V.; Schaeverbeke, T. Acceptance rate and sociological factors involved in the switch from originator to biosimilar etanercept (SB4). *Semin. Arthritis Rheum.* **2019**, *48*, 927–932. [CrossRef] [PubMed]
16. Tweehuysen, L.; Huiskes, V.J.B.; van den Bemt, B.J.F.; Vriezekolk, J.E.; Teerenstra, S.; van den Hoogen, F.H.J.; van den Ende, C.H.; den Broeder, A.A. Open-Label, Non-Mandatory Transitioning From Originator Etanercept to Biosimilar SB4: Six-Month Results From a Controlled Cohort Study. *Arthritis Rheumatol.* **2018**, *70*, 1408–1418. [CrossRef] [PubMed]
17. Lyman, G.H.; Zon, R.; Harvey, R.D.; Schilsky, R.L. Rationale, Opportunities, and Reality of Biosimilar Medications. *N. Engl. J. Med.* **2018**, *378*, 2036–2044. [CrossRef] [PubMed]

16

Golimumab for Rheumatoid Arthritis

Eleftherios Pelechas, Paraskevi V. Voulgari and Alexandros A. Drosos *

Rheumatology Clinic, Department of Internal Medicine, Medical School, University of Ioannina, 45110 Ioannina, Greece; pelechas@doctors.org.uk (E.P.); pvoulgar@cc.uoi.gr (P.V.V.)
* Correspondence: adrosos@cc.uoi.gr

Abstract: Since the advent of infliximab for the treatment of rheumatoid arthritis (RA), new genetically-engineered molecules have appeared. This review aims to present the current data and body of evidence for golimumab (GLM). Safety, efficacy, tolerability and immunogenicity are all being investigated, not only through phase III trials (GO-BEFORE, GO-FORWARD, GO-AFTER, GO-MORE, GO-FURTHER, GO-NICE), but also through studies of real-world data. It seems that GLM in the subcutaneous form is an efficacious molecule with a good safety profile at the standard dosage scheme, but a 100 mg subcutaneous dose is associated with a higher risk of opportunistic infections, lymphoma and demyelination. Furthermore, when compared to other tumor necrosis factor-α molecules, it is non-inferior, and, at some points, such as when it comes to immunogenicity and persistence of the drug, it has a better profile. In summary, GLM is an effective, well-tolerated option for the treatment of RA, for both the clinician and patients who are seeking a convenient dosage scheme.

Keywords: rheumatoid arthritis; TNFα; golimumab; efficacy; tolerability; immunogenicity

---

1. Introduction

Nowadays, rheumatology has been transformed into one of the most impactful specialties in the field of medicine, mainly due to a better understanding of the way our immune system responds to different internal and external stimuli [1]. The idea of neutralizing tumor necrosis factor (TNF)α via a specific antibody emerged in the mid-1980s. The hypothesis was that reducing TNFα levels would restore the balance in the cytokine system. Thus infliximab (INF), a chimeric human-murine monoclonal antibody that binds with high affinity to both soluble and transmembrane forms of TNFα, but not to lymphotoxin α (TNFβ), was developed with the employment of genetic engineering techniques. Since the advent of INF, four more genetically engineered molecules have been marketed: etanercept (ETN), adalimumab (ADA), certolizumab (CTZ) and golimumab (GLM), each employing a slightly different compositional and pharmacodynamic approach. In addition, anti-TNFα biosimilars have come of age and are already on the market [2,3]. Nevertheless, even with the appearance of different molecules targeting rheumatoid arthritis (RA), the unmet needs for the treatment of the disease remain high [4].

2. Golimumab

GLM is a human IgG1κ monoclonal antibody produced by a murine hybridoma cell line with recombinant DNA technology [5], which has been shown to improve the signs and symptoms of RA in adults in large, randomized, placebo-controlled phase III trials [6–10]. It is the latest anti-TNFα approved by the Food and Drug Administration (FDA), in 2009, under the brand name Simponi. In Europe, a once-monthly 50-mg subcutaneous (s.c.) formulation of the TNFα GLM is approved as monotherapy and/or in combination with methotrexate (MTX). Other approved indications of GLM are for the treatment of psoriatic arthritis (PsA) and axial spondyloarthritis (AxSpA)—comprising ankylosing spondylitis (AS) and non-radiographic axial spondyloarthritis (nr-AxSpA) in adults, and polyarticular juvenile idiopathic arthritis (pJIA) in children (50 mg/month if body weight > 40 kg). In patients with body weight greater than 100 kg and for all the above indications who do not achieve an adequate clinical response after 3–4 doses, increasing the dose to 100 mg once a month may be considered, taking into account the increased risk of certain serious adverse drug reactions. Finally, GLM has been also approved for ulcerative colitis. The initial dose should be 200 mg, followed by 100 mg at week two. Patients who have an adequate response should receive 50 mg at week six and every four weeks thereafter, whereas for those with an inadequate response or with body weight greater than 80 kg, 100 mg at week six and every four weeks thereafter.

3. Pharmacological Properties of GLM

GLM acts principally by targeting and neutralizing TNFα with the ultimate goal to prevent inflammation as well as cartilage degradation and bone destruction [11]. In pivotal phase III trials (but also in different sub-studies in patients with RA and other inflammatory arthritides), when administered alone or in combination with MTX, it showed that there is a significant reduction in serum acute phase reactants and other inflammatory biomarkers [12–15].

GLM exhibits dose-proportional pharmacokinetics and this is why patients with different body weights should receive different dosage schemes. The median time to maximum plasma concentration is 2–7 days following a single s.c. injection. Steady-state plasma concentrations can be achieved at 12 weeks of repeated injections and the mean absolute bioavailability is approximately 50% [16]. The mean elimination half-life is estimated to be approximately 12 days. In patients receiving MTX with GLM, the mean steady-state trough concentrations were 30% higher than those receiving GLM alone. The concomitant use of MTX reduces the apparent clearance of GLM by approximately 35% [17].

4. Clinical Efficacy

The clinical efficacy of GLM in inflammatory arthritides has been shown in a series of phase III trials but also in several sub-studies (Table 1) [8–10,18–23]. More specifically, in RA there is sufficient data supporting the therapeutic efficacy of the drug.

In the GO-BEFORE study (NCT00264537), a total of 637 MTX-naïve patients with active RA were randomized (1:1:1:1) to placebo + MTX (group 1), GLM 100 mg + placebo (group 2), GLM 50 mg + MTX (group 3), or GLM 100 mg + MTX (group 4). This study did not detect significant differences in ACR50 response (primary endpoint) between the combination therapy groups (3 and 4) of GLM (50 mg/100 mg) every four weeks plus MTX and MTX as monotherapy. A difference would have been seen if the ACR 20 response had been considered. Thus, the modified intend-to-treat (ITT) analysis of the primary endpoint and other prespecified efficacy measures demonstrated that the efficacy of GLM + MTX is better than, and the efficacy of GLM alone is similar to, the efficacy of MTX alone in reducing RA symptoms in MTX naïve patients, with no unexpected safety concerns [8,18].

In the *GO-FORWARD* study (NCT00264550), a total of 444 patients with active RA despite MTX therapy were randomly assigned (3:3:2:2) to placebo injections + MTX capsules (group 1), GLM 100 mg injections + placebo capsules (group 2) GLM 50 mg injections + MTX capsules (group 3) and GLM 100 mg injections + MTX capsules (group 4). The co-primary endpoints were the proportion of patients with >ACR20% improvement at week 14 and change from baseline in the health assessment questionnaire-disability index (HAQ-DI) score at week 24. In the aforementioned groups ACR20 response at week 14 was achieved by 33.1%/44.4%/55.1%/56.2%, respectively, whereas at week 24, median improvements from baseline in HAQ-DI score (0.13) were: 0.13 ($p = 0.240$); 0.38 ($p < 0.001$); 0.50 ($p < 0.001$), respectively [9,19]. The conclusion of this study was that the addition of GLM to MTX in patients with active RA despite MTX therapy, significantly reduced the signs and symptoms of RA and improvement of physical function.

The *GO-AFTER* study (NCT00299546) evaluated the efficacy and safety of GLM in subjects who have active RA and have been treated previously with >1 dose of a biologic anti-TNFα agent (ETN,

ADA, INF). A total of 461 patients from 10 countries were randomly allocated to receive s.c. injections of placebo (group 1), GLM 50 mg s.c. (group 2) or GLM 100 mg s.c. (group 3) every four weeks. MTX, sulfasalazine (SSZ), hydroxychloroquine (HCQ), oral corticosteroids (CS) and non-steroidal anti-inflammatory drugs (NSAIDs) were carried on at stable doses. As primary endpoint, an ACR20 improvement at week 14 should be achieved by patients who discontinued previous anti-TNFα treatment due to lack of effectiveness or reasons unrelated to effectiveness, such as intolerance and accessibility issues. In groups 1–3, 18%/35%/38% respectively achieved ACR 20 at week 14. The conclusion of this study was that GLM reduces the signs and symptoms of RA in patients with active disease who had previously received >1 anti-TNFα [10,20].

Table 1. Summary of GLM trials.

Trial (Clinical Trial Identifier Number)	Official Title	Study Type (Phase)	Indication	Number of Participants
GO-BEFORE (NCT00264537)	A multicentre, randomized, double-blind, placebo-controlled trial of golimumab, a fully human anti-TNFa monoclonal antibody, administered subcutaneously, in methotrexate-naïve subjects with active rheumatoid arthritis	Clinical Trial (Phase III)	RA	637
GO-FORWARD (NCT00264550)	A multicentre, randomized, double-blind, placebo-controlled trial of golimumab, a fully human anti-TNFa monoclonal antibody, administered subcutaneously, in subjects with active Rheumatoid arthritis despite methotrexate therapy	Clinical trial (Phase III)	RA	444
GO-AFTER (NCT00299546)	A multicentre, randomized, double-blind, placebo-controlled trial of golimumab, a fully human anti-TNFa monoclonal antibody, administered subcutaneously in subjects with active rheumatoid arthritis and previously treated with biologic anti-TNFa Agent(s)	Clinical trial (Phase III)	RA	461
GO-MORE (NCT00975130)	An open-label study assessing the addition of subcutaneous golimumab (GLM) to conventional disease-modifying antirheumatic drug (DMARD therapy in biologic-naïve subjects with rheumatoid arthritis (Part 1), followed by a randomized study assessing the value of combined intravenous and subcutaneous GLM administration aimed at inducing and maintaining remission (Part 2)	Clinical trial (Phase III)	RA	3366
GO-FURTHER (NCT00973479	A multicentre, randomized, double-blind, placebo-controlled trial of golimumab, an anti-TNF alpha monoclonal antibody, administered intravenously, in patients with active rheumatoid arthritis despite methotrexate therapy	Clinical trial (Phase III)	RA	592
GO-NICE (NCT01313858)	Non-interventional study investigating the use of golimumab in patients with rheumatoid arthritis, psoriatic arthritis, and ankylosing spondylitis	Observational	RA, PsA, AS	1613

GLM: golimumab; TNF: tumor necrosis fator; RA: rheumatoid arthritis; PsA: psoriatic arthritis; AS: ankylosing spondylitis; nr-AxSpA: non-radiographic axial spondyloarthritis.

In the *GO-MORE* study (NCT00975130) a total number of 3366 patients were enrolled in order to evaluate the efficacy and safety of s.c. GLM as add-on therapy in patients with active RA in typical clinical practice settings (use of csDMARDs and Cs). A four-weeks add-on of 50 mg s.c. GLM for a period of six months were given in part one of the study whereas in part two, patients not on remission were randomly assigned to receive intravenous (i.v.) + s.c. (group 1) or s.c. GLM to month 12. Neither in part one nor part two of the study a statistically significant difference was observed apart from the efficacy and safety of GLM as an add-on therapy for csDMARD-refractory RA in a typical clinical practice population. This study concluded that there is no additional efficacy of the i.v. + s.c. scheme of GLM over the s.c. regimen [21].

The *GO-FURTHER* study (NCT00973479) evaluated not only the safety and efficacy but also the radiographic progression through two years of treatment with i.v. GLM + MTX in an open-label extension of a phase III trial of patients with active RA despite MTX therapy. A total number of 592 patients with active RA were randomized (2:1) to i.v. GLM 2 mg/kg + MTX (group one), or placebo + MTX (group 2) at weeks 0 and 4, and every eight weeks thereafter. ACR 20/50/70 response criteria were measured as well as the 28-joint count disease activity score using the C-reactive protein (DAS-28-CRP), physical function and quality of life, and changes in the modified Sharp/van der Heijde scores (SHS). The ACR responses at week 100 were 68.1%/43.8%/23.5% respectively. Physical function, quality of life and clinical response were maintained throughout the study period (two years). The SHS score was 0.74 in group 1 and 2.10 in group 2 ($p = 0.005$). As far as it concerns the AE, 79.1% had at least one and 18.2% had a serious AE. This study demonstrated that in patients with active RA, despite MTX, i.v. GLM + MTX showed significant inhibition of structural damage at weeks 24 and 52 and substantial clinical improvement with no safety signs up to one year [22].

The *GO-NICE* study (NCT01313858), aimed to document patient and treatment characteristics as well as clinical effectiveness and safety in adult patients newly treated with the 50 mg s.c. GLM every four weeks under real-life conditions. Of the 1613 patients, 1458 were eligible for final analysis and of those 474 patients were suffering from RA. The mean age of those patients was 54.9 ± 13.4 years, 72.8% were females and 64.7% biologic-naïve. The DAS-28-erythrocyte sedimentation rate (ESR) decreased from 5.0 to 2.9 after 24 months ($p < 0.0001$). As reported, most AE were of mild or moderate nature, and no new safety signals were detected [23].

Finally, there are several other studies regarding the persistence of GLM treatment in patients with RA. Thomas et al. [24] in a retrospective, observational study of all patients treated with GLM in four Academic centers in Greece during a four-year period examined the long-term survival on drug (SOD) of patients not only with RA (166 patients) but also PsA (82 patients) and AS (80 patients). The estimated SOD at two and three years was 68% and 62% respectively (69% and 60% for RA patients) concluding that GLM showed a high three-year SOD with a low rate of discontinuation due to AEs. Furthermore, Rotar et al. [25] analyzed prospectively the collected data of all patients treated with GLM and other TNFs for seven years and were suffering from RA, AS, and PsA. The authors concluded that the persistence of GLM in RA-treated patients is lower compared with the AS and PsA patients but it is higher among those patients treated with other anti-TNFs. Svedbom et al. [26] in a systematic review of real-world evidence in immune-mediated rheumatic diseases including RA, examined the persistence to treatment with s.c. GLM but also to other anti-TNFα molecules. Of 376 available references identified, 12 studies with a total of 4910 patients met the inclusion criteria. In four studies that included comparisons to other biologics, GLM was either statistically noninferior or statistically superior to other treatments. Serrano et al. [27] in a prospective monocentric cohort of RA patients treated with GLM and a total number of 61 patients (mean age 55.1 ± 14.1 years; 85.2% females; RF + 70%; anti-CCP + 78%) showed that GLM survival time was better when used as first or second biological and with concomitant use of csDMARDs. Aaltonen et al., based on Kaplan-Meier survival analysis in a systematic review regarding the anti-TNFα, showed that the probability of discontinuing the treatment within 6, 12, 24, and 36 months was 16%, 27%, 37%, and 43%, respectively in patients with RA. SOD was better among the patients with no prior bDMARD therapy than among those using anti-TNFα as their second or third bDMARD. CTZ (41%) and INF (38%) were associated with higher probability of treatment discontinuation within 12 months compared to ADA (25%), ETN (25%), and GLM (25%) [28].

5. Tolerability and Immunogenicity

Data from the pivotal phase III trials in adults with RA but also the open-label extension studies, support that s.c. GLM is generally a well-tolerated therapeutic option [8–10]. Overall, in these trials, upper-respiratory infections (32.0% vs. 8.8% with placebo), nasopharyngitis (17.4% vs. 6.4%), followed by elevated aminotransferase levels (11.9% vs. 5.2%) and hypertension (9.8% vs. 2.7%) were the most common AE in the 50 mg s.c. dose. Injection-site reactions (ISRs) were reported by 11.0% vs. 2.8% of GLM and placebo recipients, the most common being injection-site erythema (5.8% vs. 1.1%) [29]. Tuberculosis, opportunistic infections, lymphoma, and demyelination incidence appeared to be higher among patients receiving GLM 100 mg s.c. dose.

As far as it concerns the immunogenicity, Thomas et al. documented in a systematic review for the immunogenicity of TNF inhibitors that GLM and ETN were the least immunogenic (3.8% and 1.2% respectively) whereas the most immunogenic were INF (25.3%), followed by ADA (14.1%) and CTZ (6.9%). The clinical significance of the anti-drug antibodies (ADAbs) in the sera of patients with RA is associated with decreased clinical response [30].

6. Conclusions

GLM is one of five anti-TNFα inhibitors approved for the treatment of RA, but also other inflammatory arthritides [31]. It is a newer, second-generation anti-TNFα and for this reason the clinical experience is less in comparison with the older ones such as INF, ETA and ADA (first generation TNFα inhibitors). On the other hand, the growing body of evidence through the open-label extension trials of pivotal studies and those from several medical centers in patients with RA, confirm the efficacy and safety of the drug. Furthermore, with clinical and radiological benefits being sustained and no new safety signals being identified, GLM seems an attractive choice for the treatment of RA. Other, important elements that make this choice attractive, are the low levels of immunogenicity, the low rate of drug discontinuation in comparison with the other anti-TNFs and the dosage scheme (every four weeks) which seems to be a point of major significance when a physician-patient sharing decision occurs. One concern is the tendency of higher incidence of opportunistic infections, lymphoma and demyelination in the 100 mg s.c. injection, and it should be used with caution in patients with higher body weight or poor response to treatment with the 50 mg dosage scheme.

As there are no head-to-head trials comparing it with the other anti-TNFα inhibitors, the indirect comparison of all five agents suggests that possibly GLM is better tolerated than ADA, CTZ and INF in terms of the risks of serious infection and of discontinuing treatment due to AEs. In summary, GLM is an effective, well-tolerated option for the treatment of RA for both the clinician but also for the patients seeking a convenient dosage scheme.

Author Contributions: E.P., P.V.V. and A.A.D. contributed to the design, analysis and writing of the manuscript. All authors have approved the final manuscript.

References

1. McInnes, I.B.; Schett, G. Pathogenetic insights from the treatment of rheumatoid arthritis. *Lancet* **2017**, *389*, 2328–2337. [CrossRef]
2. Pelechas, E.; Voulgari, P.V.; Drosos, A.A. ABP501 for the treatment of rheumatoid arthritis. *Expert Opin. Biol. Ther.* **2018**, *18*, 317–322. [CrossRef] [PubMed]
3. Pelechas, E.; Drosos, A.A. Etanercept biosimilars SB-4. *Expert Opin. Biol. Ther.* **2019**, *19*, 173–179. [CrossRef]
4. Kaltsonoudis, E.; Pelechas, E.; Voulgari, P.V.; Drosos, A.A. Unmet needs in the treatment of rheumatoid arthritis. An observational study and a real-life experience from a single university center. *Semin. Arthritis Rheum.* **2019**, *48*, 597–602. [CrossRef] [PubMed]
5. Summary of Product Characteristics. Available online: https://www.ema.europa.eu/en/documents/product-information/simponi-epar-product-information_en.pdf (accessed on 19 March 2019).
6. Singh, J.A.; Noorbaloochi, S.; Singh, G. Golimumab for rheumatoid arthritis: A systematic review. *J. Rheumatol.* **2010**, *37*, 1096–1104. [CrossRef]
7. Papagoras, C.; Voulgari, P.V.; Drosos, A.A. Golimumab, the newest TNF-α blocker, comes of age. *Clin. Exp. Rheumatol.* **2015**, *33*, 570–577. [PubMed]

8. Emery, P.; Fleischmann, R.M.; Moreland, L.W.; Hsia, E.C.; Strusberg, I.; Durez, P.; Nash, P.; Amante, E.J.; Churchill, M.; Park, W.; et al. Golimumab, a human anti-tumor necrosis factor α monoclonal antibody, injected subcutaneously every four weeks in methotrexate-naïve patients with active rheumatoid arthritis: Twenty-four-week results of a phase III, multicenter, randomized, double-blind, placebo-controlled study of Golimumab before methotrexate as first-line therapy for early-onset rheumatoid arthritis. *Arthritis Rheum.* **2009**, *60*, 2272–2283. [PubMed]
9. Keystone, E.C.; Genovese, M.C.; Klareskog, L.; Hsia, E.C.; Hall, S.T.; Miranda, P.C.; Pazdur, J.; Bae, S.C.; Palmer, W.; Zrubek, J.; et al. Golimumab, a human antibody to tumour necrosis factor α given by monthly subcutaneous injections, in active rheumatoid arthritis despite methotrexate therapy: The GO-FORWARD Study. *Ann. Rheum. Dis.* **2009**, *68*, 789–796. [CrossRef]
10. Smolen, J.S.; Kay, J.; Doyle, M.K.; Landewé, R.; Matteson, E.L.; Wollenhaupt, J.; Gaylis, N.; Murphy, F.T.; Neal, J.S.; Zhou, Y.; et al. Golimumab in patients with active rheumatoid arthritis after treatment with tumour necrosis factor α inhibitors (GO-AFTER study): A multicenter, randomised, double-blind, placebo-controlled, phase III trial. *Lancet* **2009**, *374*, 210–221. [CrossRef]
11. Oldfield, V.; Plosker, G.L. Golimumab: In the treatment of rheumatoid arthritis, psoriatic arthritis, and ankylosing spondylitis. *BioDrugs* **2009**, *23*, 125–135. [CrossRef] [PubMed]
12. Visvanathan, S.; Rahman, M.U.; Keystone, E.; Genovese, M.; Klareskog, L.; Hsia, E.; Mack, M.; Buchanan, J.; Elashoff, M.; Wagner, C. Association of serum markers with improvement in clinical response measures after treatment with Golimumab in patients with active rheumatoid arthritis despite receiving methotrexate: Results from the GO-FORWARD study. *Arthritis Res. Ther.* **2010**, *12*, R211. [CrossRef] [PubMed]
13. Inman, R.D.; Baraliakos, X.; Hermann, K.A.; Braun, J.; Deodhar, A.; van der Heijde, D.; Xu, S.; Hsu, B. Serum biomarkers and changes in clinical/MRI evidence of Golimumab-treated patients with ankylosing spondylitis: Results of the randomized, placebo-controlled GO-RAISE study. *Arthritis Res. Ther.* **2016**, *18*, 304. [CrossRef]
14. Wagner, C.L.; Visvanathan, S.; Elashoff, M.; McInnes, I.B.; Mease, P.J.; Krueger, G.G.; Murphy, F.T.; Papp, K.; Gomez-Reino, J.J.; Mack, M.; et al. Markers of inflammation and bone remodeling associated with improvement in clinical response measures in psoriatic arthritis patients treated with Golimumab. *Ann. Rheum. Dis.* **2013**, *72*, 83–88. [CrossRef] [PubMed]
15. Wagner, C.L.; Visvanathan, S.; Braun, J.; van der Heijde, D.; Deodhar, A.; Hsu, B.; Mack, M.; Elashoff, M.; Inman, R.D. Serum markers associated with clinical improvement in patients with ankylosing spondylitis treated with Golimumab. *Ann. Rheum. Dis.* **2012**, *71*, 674–680. [CrossRef]
16. Zhou, H.; Jang, H.; Fleischmann, R.M.; Bouman-Thio, E.; Xu, Z.; Marini, J.C.; Pendley, C.; Jiao, Q.; Shankar, G.; Marciniak, S.J.; et al. Pharmacokinetics and safety of Golimumab, a fully human anti-TNFα monoclonal antibody, in subjects with rheumatoid arthritis. *J. Clin. Pharmacol.* **2007**, *47*, 383–396. [CrossRef] [PubMed]
17. Xu, Z.; Vu, T.; Lee, H.; Hu, C.; Ling, J.; Yan, H.; Baker, D.; Beutler, A.; Pendley, C.; Wagner, C.; et al. Population pharmacokinetics of Golimumab, an anti-tumor necrosis factor-alpha human monoclonal antibody, in patients with psoriatic arthritis. *J. Clin. Pharmacol.* **2009**, *49*, 1056–1070. [CrossRef] [PubMed]
18. Emery, P.; Fleischmann, R.M.; Strusberg, I.; Durez, P.; Nash, P.; Amante, E.J.; Churchill, M.; Park, W.; Pons-Estel, B.; Han, C.; et al. Efficacy and safety of subcutaneous golimumab in methotrexate-naïve patients with rheumatoid arthritis: Five-year results of a randomized clinical trial. *Arthritis Care Res.* **2016**, *68*, 744–752. [CrossRef]
19. Keystone, E.C.; Genovese, M.C.; Hall, S.; Bae, S.C.; Han, C.; Gathany, T.A.; Xu, S.; Zhou, Y.; Leu, J.H.; Hsia, E.C. Safety and efficacy of subcutaneous golimumab in patients with active rheumatoid arthritis despite methotrexate therapy: Final 5-year results of the GO-FORWARD trial. *J. Rheumatol.* **2016**, *43*, 298–306. [CrossRef] [PubMed]
20. Smolen, J.S.; Kay, J.; Doyle, M.; Landewé, R.; Matteson, E.L.; Gaylis, N.; Wollenhaupt, J.; Murphy, F.T.; Xu, S.; Zhou, Y.; et al. Golimumab in patients with active rheumatoid arthritis after treatment with tumor necrosis factor alpha inhibitors: Findings with up to five years of treatment in the multicenter, randomized, double-blind, placebo-controlled, phase 3 GO-AFTER study. *Arthritis Res. Ther.* **2015**, *17*, 14. [CrossRef]
21. Combe, B.; Dasgupta, B.; Louw, I.; Pal, S.; Wollenhaupt, J.; Zerbini, C.A.; Beaulieu, A.D.; Schulze-Koops, H.; Durez, P.; Yao, R.; et al. GO-MORE investigators. Efficacy and safety of golimumab as add-on therapy to disease-modifying antirheumatic drugs: Results of the GO-MORE study. *Ann. Rheum. Dis.* **2014**, *73*, 1477–1486. [CrossRef]

22. Weinblatt, M.E.; Westhovens, R.; Mendelsohn, A.M.; Kim, L.; Lo, K.H.; Sheng, S.; Noonan, L.; Lu, J.; Xu, Z.; Leu, J.; et al. GO-FURTHER investigators. Radiographic benefit and maintenance of clinical benefit with intravenous golimumab therapy in patients with active rheumatoid arthritis despite methotrexate therapy: Results up to 1 year of the phase 3, randomised, multicenter, double-blind, placebo-controlled GO-FURTHER trial. *Ann. Rheum. Dis.* **2014**, *73*, 2152–2159. [PubMed]
23. Kruger, K.; Burmester, G.R.; Wassenberg, S.; Bohl-Bühler, M.; Thomas, M.H. Effectiveness and safety of golimumab in patients with rheumatoid arthritis, psoriatic arthritis and ankylosing spondylitis under real-life clinical conditions: Non-interventional GO-NICE study in Germany. *BMJ Open* **2018**, *8*, e021082. [PubMed]
24. Thomas, K.; Flouri, I.; Repa, A.; Fragiadaki, K.; Sfikakis, P.P.; Koutsianas, C.; Kaltsonoudis, E.; Voulgari, P.V.; Drosos, A.A.; Petrikkou, E.; et al. High 3-year golimumab survival in patients with rheumatoid arthritis, ankylosing spondylitis and psoriatic arthritis: Real world data from 328 patients. *Clin. Exp. Rheumatol.* **2018**, *36*, 254–262. [PubMed]
25. Rotar, Z.; Tomsic, M.; Praprotnik, S. The persistence of golimumab compared to other tumour necrosis factor-α inhibitors in daily clinical practice for the treatment of rheumatoid arthritis, ankylosing spondylitis and psoriatic arthritis: Observations from the Slovenian nation-wide longitudinal registry of patients treated with biologic disease-modifying antirheumatic drugs. *Clin. Rheumatol.* **2019**, *38*, 297–305. [CrossRef]
26. Svedbom, A.; Storck, C.; Kachroo, S.; Govoni, M.; Khalifa, A. Persistence with golimumab in immune-mediated rheumatic diseases: A systematic review of real-world evidence in rheumatoid arthritis, axial spondyloarthritis, and psoriatic arthritis. *Patient Prefer. Adherence* **2017**, *11*, 719–729. [CrossRef]
27. Serrano, B.; Gonzalez, C.M.; Gonzalez, R.; Martinez-Barrio, J.; Gabriel Ovalles-Bonilla, J.; Carlos Nieto, J.; Janta, I.; Valor, L.; Longo, F.J.L.; Monteagudo, I.; et al. Golimumab retention rate in patients with rheumatoid arthritis. Predictors of long-term retention [abstract]. *Arthritis Rheumatol.* **2017**, *69* (Suppl. 10). Available online: https://acrabstracts.org/abstract/golimumab-retention-rate-in-patients-with-rheumatoid-arthritis-predictors-of-long-term-retention/ (accessed on 27 December 2018).
28. Aaltonen, K.J.; Joensuu, J.T.; Pirila, L.; Kauppi, M.; Uutela, T.; Varjolahti-Lehtinen, T.; Yli-Kerttula, T.; Isomäki, P.; Nordström, D.; Sokka, T. Drug survival on tumour necrosis factor inhibitors in patients with rheumatoid arthritis in Finland. *Scand. J. Rheumatol.* **2017**, *46*, 359–363. [CrossRef]
29. Kay, J.; Fleischmann, R.; Keystone, E.; Hsia, E.C.; Hsu, B.; Zhou, Y.; Goldstein, N.; Braun, J. Five-year safety data from 5 clinical trials of subcutaneous golimumab in patients with rheumatoid arthritis, psoriatic arthritis, and ankylosing spondylitis. *J. Rheumatol.* **2016**, *43*, 2120–2130. [CrossRef]
30. Thomas, S.S.; Borazan, N.; Barroso, N.; Duan, L.; Taroumian, S.; Kretzmann, B.; Bardales, R.; Elashoff, D.; Vangala, S.; Furst, D.E. Comparative immunogenicity of TNF inhibitors: Impact on clinical efficacy and tolerability in the management of autoimmune diseases. A systematic review and Meta-analysis. *BioDrugs* **2015**, *29*, 241–258. [CrossRef]
31. Frampton, J.E. Golimumab: A Review in Inflammatory Arthritis. *BioDrugs* **2017**, *31*, 263–274. [CrossRef]

Effectiveness, Tolerability and Safety of Tofacitinib in Rheumatoid Arthritis: A Retrospective Analysis of Real-World Data from the St. Gallen and Aarau Cohorts

Ruediger B. Mueller [1,2,3,*], Caroline Hasler [2], Florian Popp [1], Frederik Mattow [1], Mirsada Durmisi [2], Alexander Souza [4], Paul Hasler [2], Andrea Rubbert-Roth [1], Hendrik Schulze-Koops [3] and Johannes von Kempis [1]

1 Division of Rheumatology and Immunology, Department of Internal Medicine, Kantonsspital St. Gallen, 9007 St. Gallen, Switzerland; fmpopp@gmail.com (F.P.); fmattow@googlemail.com (F.M.); andrea.rubbert-roth@uk-koeln.de (A.R.-R.); johannes.vonkempis@kssg.ch (J.v.K.)
2 Division of Rheumatology, Medical University Department, Kantonsspital Aarau, 5001 Aarau, Switzerland; carolinehasler4@gmail.com (C.H.); m.durmisi@stud.unibas.ch (M.D.); paul.hasler@ksa.ch (P.H.)
3 Division of Rheumatology and Clinical Immunology, Department of Internal Medicine IV, Ludwig-Maximilians-University Munich, 80336 Munich, Germany; Hendrik.Schulze-Koops@med.uni-muenchen.de
4 Iterata AG, 5722 Gränichen, Switzerland; souza@iterata.ch
* Correspondence: Ruediger.Mueller@ksa.ch

Abstract: Introduction: Tofacitinib is an oral JAK inhibitor indicated for the treatment of rheumatoid arthritis (RA). The efficacy and safety of tofacitinib have been shown in several randomized clinical trials. The study presented here aimed to assess the clinical tolerability and effectiveness of tofacitinib among RA patients in real life. **Methods:** Consecutive patients between January 2015 and April 2017 with RA who fulfilled the American College of Rheumatology (ACR)/European League Against Rheumatism (EULAR) 2010 criteria were included in a prospectively designed analysis of retrospective data. Patients were initiated on tofacitinib 5 mg bid. The primary objective was to analyze the safety of tofacitinib in a real-life cohort. Safety was assessed by the reasons to stop tofacitinib during follow up and changes of liver enzymes, hemoglobin, and creatinine. The secondary outcome was to analyze the frequency of and time to achieve low disease activity (LDA) and remission as defined by 28 joint count disease activity score (DAS28). **Results:** A total of 144 patients were treated with tofacitinib. A total of 84.9% of patients were pre-exposed to at least one biological agent. The average DAS28 at the initiation of tofacitinib was 4.43. A total of 50.0% of patients were positive for rheumatoid factor and 49.0% for ACPA. The mean follow up was 1.22 years (range 10d–3.7a) after initiation of tofacitinib treatment. A total of 94 (64.4%) patients remained on tofacitinib during follow-up. The average time to stop tofacitinib was 190.0 days. Reasons to stop tofacitinib were: insufficient response ($n = 23$), gastrointestinal symptoms ($n = 18$), infection ($n = 5$), myalgia ($n = 2$), remission ($n = 2$), headache ($n = 2$), cough, blue finger syndrome, intolerance, heartburn, psoriasis, and increased liver enzymes (all $n = 1$). Increased alanine amino transferase (ALAT) or aspartate amino transferase (ASAT) > 2× upper limit of normal (ULN) were detected in 3.3% and 4.4% of patients, respectively. Hemoglobin decrease of >10% was detected in 15.1% of the patients and decreased lymphocytes <500/μL in 3.4%. An increase of creatinine >20% was detected in 9.4% of patients. A total of 62.9% and 50.0% of the patients achieved low disease activity (LDA) or remission after a median of 319 and 645 days, respectively. These rates were significantly higher in patients naïve to biologic agents as compared to patients pre-exposed to biologics (LDA: naïve 100% 92 d, pre-exposed 57.0% 434 d, $p \leq 0.001$; remission: naïve 86.7% 132 d, pre-exposed 44.1%, 692 d, $p = 0.001$). **Conclusions:** Tofacitinib is a safe and effective treatment option for patients with RA. Tofacitinib may induce high rates of LDA and remission in patients with active disease, even after the use of one or more biologics, though the rate appeared higher in patients naïve to biologics. Tofacitinib may be a valuable option in a treat-to-target approach. Our data demonstrate that Janus kinase (JAK) inhibitors are safe and efficacious in real life patients.

Keywords: tofacitinib; rheumatoid arthritis; oral

---

1. Introduction

Rheumatoid arthritis (RA) is a chronic autoimmune disease characterized by the inflammation and destruction of joints. It may result in functional impairment, declining health status and reduced quality of life for affected patients [1–3]. The principal goal in the treatment of RA is to achieve and maintain remission, or, if that is not attainable, low disease activity (LDA) [4,5].

Conventional synthetic (cs) disease-modifying anti-rheumatic drugs (DMARDs), especially methotrexate (MTX), have long been the cornerstones of RA treatment. In the last 20 years, biologic agents have broadened the clinical armamentarium [6]. Though biologics have revolutionized the managing of RA [7–24], their effects are limited. Approximately 50% of RA patients treated with biologics meet the criteria for low disease activity (28 joint count disease activity score (DAS28) $\leq$ 3.2) or remission (DAS28 < 2.6), while a significant proportion of patients do not achieve an ACR 20 (American College of Rheumatology) response [14,15]. Furthermore, patients on biologics may experience adverse events (AEs) or loss of effectiveness over time [25], e.g., by developing anti-drug antibodies. To quantify the unmet need for additional therapies, Drosos et al. performed a long-term, real-world observational study of their cases with RA treated according to the European League Against Rheumatism (EULAR) and American College of Rheumatology (ACR) recommendations. Approximately one-fifth of their patients did not respond sufficiently to csDMARDs or bDMARDs (biological disease-modifying anti-rheumatic drugs), substantiating the need for alternative treatments [26].

Tofacitinib is a novel, oral Janus kinase (JAK) inhibitor indicated for the treatment of RA. JAK inhibitors are small-molecule drugs that interfere with the activation of JAKs, a family of enzymes implicated in the signaling of leukocytes. JAK signaling has been shown to play an essential role in immune cell generation, differentiation and responses [27–29]. By inhibiting these signaling mechanisms, JAK inhibitors such as tofacitinib have the potential to successfully interfere with immune activation that is critical for RA [30–32] (Koehler, J. Clin. Med. 2019, 8, 938).

Phase II and III clinical trials have shown that the treatment of RA patients with tofacitinib, either as a monotherapy or in combination with csDMARDs, is capable of significantly reducing disease activity, as measured by ACR response rates, EULAR responses and HAQ-DI scores [33–39]. Studies comparing tofacitinib to other therapeutic strategies in the treatment of RA suggest that the effectiveness of tofacitinib is similar to that of biologic agents [40–43]. The safety profile of tofacitinib does not appear to differ significantly from biologics [34,39–44].

In 2012 and 2014, the FDA and the Swissmedic approved tofacitinib for adult patients with moderate to severe RA who had a prior inadequate response to MTX. Approval from the European Medicines Agency (EMA) was granted in 2017. With JAK inhibitors still representing a relatively novel treatment option in the management of RA, there is a demand to use the experience gained through using tofacitinib in a real-life, clinical setting, to further evaluate its safety and utility. In this study, we aimed to analyze real-life data from routine clinical practice to compare our experience with the results of controlled studies.

2. Methods

2.1. Patient Recruitment

For this retrospective analysis of data, patients were recruited through a chart review of all RA patients at the hospitals of St. Gallen and Aarau, Switzerland. Patients with a clinical diagnosis of RA consistent with the current definition in the 2010 ACR/EULAR criteria were required [45] and initiation of oral tofacitinib 5 mg bid followed. Exclusion criteria were ages younger than 18 years or older than 80 years at disease onset. All patient charts of the cohort from Aarau and St. Gallen were screened sequentially for eligibility. Thus, selected patients were followed until tofacitinib administration was terminated or until the last visit entered in the database. The decision to stop tofacitinib and all other decisions concerning treatment were at the discretion of the treating clinician. Ethical approval for the collection of patient data was given by the regional review board.

2.2. Study Design

This was a longitudinal, retrospective chart review conducted between April 2013 and September 2017 within the St. Gallen and Aarau RA cohorts. The pre-defined primary endpoints were the incidence of adverse events, changes in laboratory values (increase in alanine amino transferase (ALAT) or aspartate amino transferase (ASAT) > 1.2 or 2.0 above the upper limits of normal), decrease in hemoglobin of >10%, lymphocytes <500 or <1000/μL, increase in creatinine >20%, and adverse events leading to the termination of tofacitinib treatment. The pre-defined secondary clinical endpoint was longitudinal disease activity as measured by DAS28 and the achievement of LDA (DAS28 ≤ 3.2) and remission (DAS28 < 2.6). Data were analyzed for the entire cohort of 144 patients, and, as a secondary analysis, separately for patients who had prior exposure to biologic agents and patients who were naïve to biologic agents.

2.3. Statistical Methods

Summary statistics are reported as median (range) or n (%). Kaplan–Meier curves were plotted, and Kaplan–Meier estimates with 95% confidence intervals based on a log–log transformation were computed for the endpoints. Time to LDA and remission was compared between patients with and without prior exposure to biologics with a log-rank test. All analyses were performed in the R programming language (R Foundation, Vienna, Austria, version 3.3.3, R Core Team 2013).

3. Results

3.1. Baseline Demographics

A total of 144 patients from the rheumatology units of the St. Gallen and Aarau rheumatology divisions fulfilled the inclusion criteria and were included in the cohort. The mean age at initiation of tofacitinib was 59.7 years and mean disease duration was 9.1 years. The majority of patients were female (69.4%). A total of 50% were positive for rheumatoid factor (RF), and 48.6% were positive for anti-citrullinated protein antibodies (ACPAs), as described in the records. No additional testing for RF and/or ACPA prior or under tofacitinib treatment was conducted. A total of 56% of the patients were either RF and/or ACPA positive.

Disease activity among the patient cohort was moderate, with a mean DAS28 of 4.43 at the initiation of tofacitinib. A total of 63.3% had a disease classified as erosive. All patients were initiated on a baseline dose of tofacitinib 5 mg bid. Regarding other medications, the mean number of previous csDMARDS was 1.9. A total of 84.7% of patients had been previously exposed to at least one biologic agent; the mean number of previous biologics was 2.2. Mean follow-up was 1.22 years (range 10 days–3.7 years) after initiation of tofacitinib (Table 1).

Table 1. Patient demographics.

	All	Stopped	Remained on	Naïve to	After
	Patients	Tofacitinib		A Biologic Agent	
Number (*n*)	144	57	87	22	122
Gender (%, female)	69.4	64.9	72.4	72.7	68.8
Age at initiation tofacitinib (years, mean)	59.7	59.6	59.8	58.8	59.8
Tofacitinib applied in monotherapy (*n*, %)	65	22	43	14	51
Concomitant medication					
- Methotrexate	36 (25.0)	16 (28.1)	20 (23.0)	5 (22.7)	31 (25.4)
- Sulfasalazine	7 (4.9)	4 (7.0)	3 (3.4)	0 (0)	7 (5.7)
- Leflunomide	25 (17.3)	6 (10.5)	19 (21.8)	3 (13.6)	22 (18.0)
- Hydroxychloroquine	11 (7.6)	5 (8.8)	6 (6.9)	0 (0)	11 (9.0)
- Prednisolone or equivalent	48 (33.3)	16 (28.1)	32 (36.8)	4 (18.2)	44 (36.1)
Disease duration (years, mean)	9.1	9.9	8.7	2.6	10.3
Comorbidities of special interest					
Cardiovascular					
- Coronary heart disease	10	2	8	1	9
- Arterial hypertension	29	13	16	3	26
- Dysipoproteinemia	5	2	3	1	4
- Valvular heart disease	2	1	1	1	1
- Adipositas	12	6	6	0	2
- PAD	3	1	2	0	3
Osteoporosis	39	15	24	4	25
After a biologic agent (%)	84.7	87.2	83.5	0	100
Previous biologic agents (*n*, mean)	2.2	2.3	2.2	0	2.6
Previous csDMARDs (*n*, mean)	1.9	1.9	1.8	1.4	1.9
ACPA pos. (%)	48.6	42.8	52.3	50.0	48.3
Rheumatoid factor pos. (%)	50.0	51.1	48.2	40.9	51.7
Erosive disease (%)	63.3	60.9	66.7	45.5	66.7
DAS28 (mean)	4.4	4.4	4.5	3.7	4.6
ESR (mean)	17.2	18.5	16.6	18.8	16.9
CRP (mean, ULN < 5mg/L)	8.5	8.0	8.8	8.9	8.4

n: number. DAS28: 28 joint count disease activity score. DMARDs: disease modifying drugs. ACPA: anti-citrullinated peptide antibody. ESR: erythrocyte sedimentation rate. CRP: C-reactive protein. pos.: positive. ULN: upper limit of normal. PAD: peripheral artery disease.

3.2. *Disease Activity*

For all patients, the mean DAS28 decreased significantly from 4.4 at baseline to 3.59, 3.22, 3.18, and 3.13 at 90, 180, 270, and 360 days (Figure 1). In total, 53% of patients achieved LDA and 48% DAS28 defined remission. The median time to LDA and remission was 319 days and 645 days, respectively.

The rates of LDA and remission under tofacitinib were higher in patients naïve to biologics compared to patients who had been previously exposed: 100% of naïve patients achieved LDA, and 83.3% achieved remission, as compared to 53.3% and 44.9% of pre-exposed to biologics patients. Also, the duration of tofacitinib treatment until LDA or remission was shorter in patients naïve to biologics. Patients in this cohort achieved LDA after a median 92 days and remission after a median 132 days, while medians for achieving LDA and remission among patients pre-exposed to biologic agents amounted to 434 days and 692 days, respectively. In both cases, the difference between naïve and pre-exposed patients was statistically significant (Figure 2, $p < 0.001$).

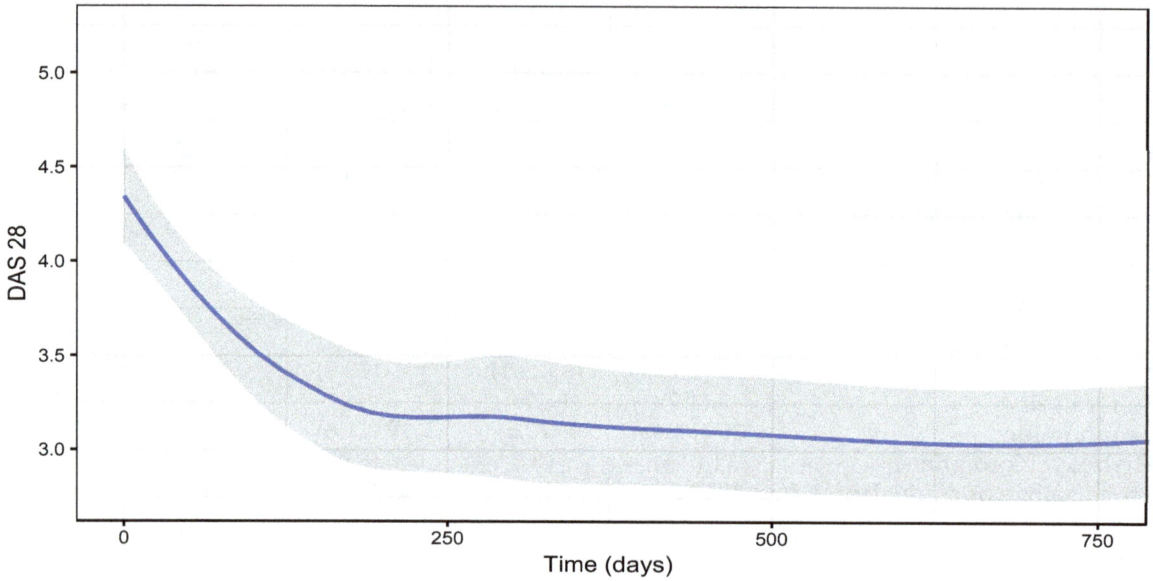

Figure 1. Disease activity: The average disease activity score (DAS28) level is shown for all rheumatoid arthritis (RA) patients treated with tofacitinib with a 95% confidence interval.

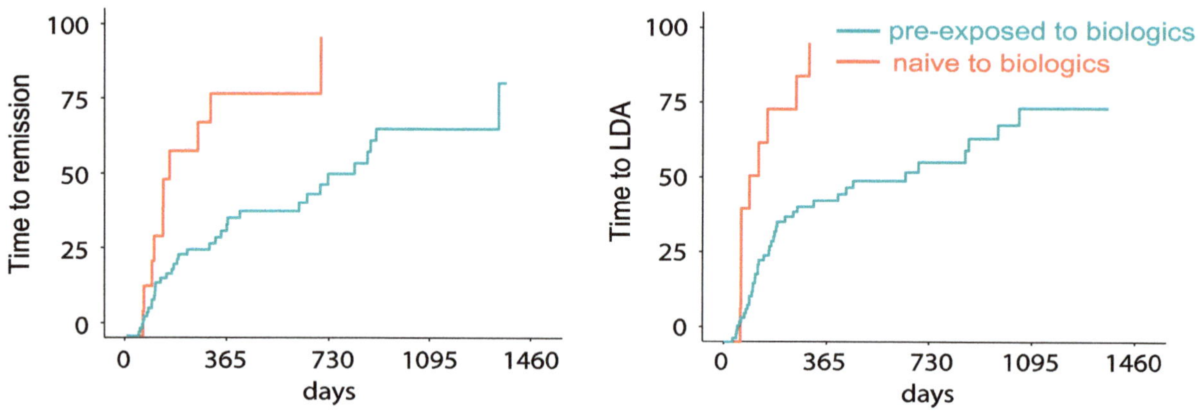

Figure 2. Disease activity: Time to remission (**left panel**) and low disease activity (LDA, **right panel**) is shown for all RA patients treated with tofacitinib. Patients previously exposed to biologic agents are shown in green, and patients naïve to biologics in red.

3.3. Discontinuation

A total of 89 (61.8%) patients remained on tofacitinib during follow-up. The median time to stop tofacitinib was 95 days (range: 4–1106). A total of 21 patients (14.6%) stopped tofacitinib due to insufficient responses and 35 patients (23.6%) stopped due to adverse events (AEs, Table 2). Of these, the most frequent reasons for discontinuing tofacitinib were gastrointestinal symptoms (n = 18), followed by infection (n = 5), myalgia (n = 2), remission (n = 2), headache, cough, blue finger syndrome, intolerance, heartburn, psoriasis, and increased liver enzymes (all n = 1). The median time to stop tofacitinib treatment due to ineffectiveness was 204 days (Figure 3). The median time to stop treatment due to AEs ranged from 10 to 290 days (Figure 3). None of the demographic parameters at baseline was a significant predictor for stopping tofacitinib.

Table 2. Reasons for stopping tofacitinib.

Reason	Number	Time to Stop Tofa
Inefficacy/flare	$n = 22$	median d204, range d21–d1106
Gastrointestinal	$n = 18$	median d28, range d4–d265d
Infection	$n = 5$	median d154, range d85–d877
Myalgia	$n = 2$	range d92–d171
Remission	$n = 2$	range d106–d379
Headache	$n = 2$	d30
Cough	$n = 1$	d22
Blue finger syndrome	$n = 1$	d10
Intolerance	$n = 1$	d42
Heartburn	$n = 1$	d39
Psoriasis	$n = 1$	d287
Increased liver enzymes	$n = 1$	d290

d: day. *n*: number.

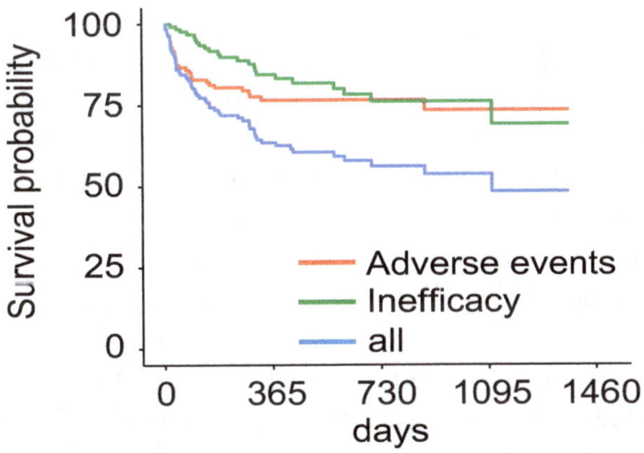

Figure 3. Time to discontinuation of tofacitinib was analyzed for all patients ($n = 57$ out of 144 total patients, blue line). Patients stopping for ineffectiveness ($n = 22$, green line) or adverse events ($n = 35$, red line) are shown separately.

3.4. Laboratory Values

Laboratory values including liver enzymes, creatinine, lymphocyte count, and hemoglobin were followed during tofacitinib treatment. Increased ALAT or ASAT > 2× ULN were detected in 3.3% and 4.4% of patients, respectively. These changes were transient in 50% and 60% of cases, respectively. Hemoglobin decrease of >10% was detected in 15.1% of patients and decreased lymphocytes <500/µL in 3.4%. An increase in creatinine >20% was detected in 9.4% (Figure 4).

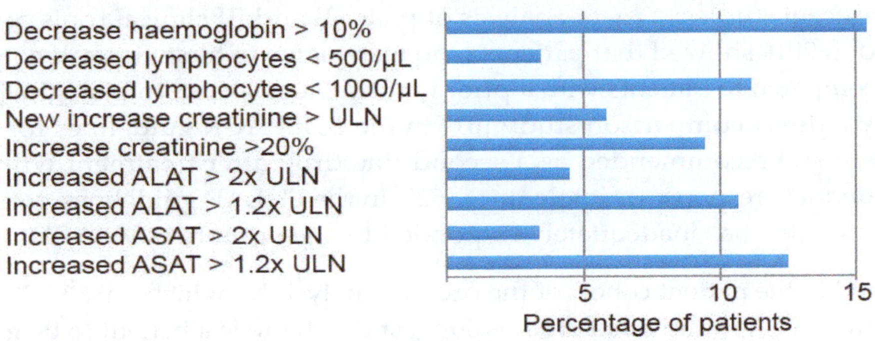

Figure 4. Patients were followed for laboratory changes under treatment with tofacitinib. Data are shown for patients with at least one in- or decrease in one of these parameters during follow-up. Percentages were calculated on patients with available data. ALAT: alanine amino transferase. ASAT: aspartate amino transferase.

4. Discussion

This study retrospectively analyzed real-life data from a cohort of 144 RA patients treated with tofacitinib 5 mg bid, with the aim of assessing the effectiveness and tolerability of tofacitinib in a clinical setting.

4.1. *Effectiveness*

Among the patient cohort, tofacitinib significantly reduced disease activity, with 58.2% of patients achieving LDA and 49.5% achieving remission at follow-up. This is a little higher than in published phase I–III clinical trials. In these clinical trials, the overall proportion of RA patients achieving DAS28 defined as was LDA 5.7%–47.5% [34,37,43,46,47] and remission 7.2%–23.1% [34,36,37,43,46–49], depending on the exposure to and efficacy of previous treatments. Essentially, our findings corroborate those of previous studies that have shown tofacitinib to be effective in the management of RA [33–37,48,50].

A total of 15.9% of our patients stopped tofacitinib due to ineffectiveness. Percentages of inefficacy were not published in the pivotal clinical trials, especially as this is not a defined outcome. Therefore, the best approximation may be missing an ACR 20 response. The ACR 20 response was not reached in 33.9% of the MTX-IR (methotrexate incomplete responders) patients and 48.2% of the TNF-IR (tumor necrosis factor incomplete responders) patients [51] in the phase II and III program for tofacitinib and 28.7% of naïve patients [47]. In a long-term extension study, 20.4% of patients did not achieve ACR 20 after 24 months and 21.5 after 96 months [52]. Importantly, not achieving ACR 20 does not necessarily mean that a patient or a treating physician considers the therapeutic response to, e.g., tofacitinib, ineffective in a clinical setting. Thus, the rate of 15.9% of patients stopping tofacitinib for ineffectiveness appears to be somewhat lower than observed in the clinical studies and long-term extension studies. However, because, as outlined above, missing an ACR 20 response does not necessarily reflect inefficacy, we think that these rates are comparable.

Although tofacitinib demonstrated effectiveness across all patient demographics, a significant difference was observed between patients naïve to biologic agents and patients who had previously been exposed to biologics: naïve patients had a trend of a higher rate of achieving LDA and remission compared to pre-exposed patients. Also, the duration of tofacitinib treatment until LDA and remission was significantly shorter in patients naïve to biologics. However, the small number of patients naïve to biologics have to be taken into account. These patients naïve to biologics had a shorter mean duration of disease at initiation of tofacitinib and lower mean baseline DAS28, which may have influenced the results. Shorter disease duration [53–55] and lower disease activity at initiation of treatment [56–59] have both been shown to correlate with higher rates of LDA and remission in RA patients. However, the indication that previous biologic therapies are associated with a reduced clinical response to tofacitinib is consistent with recent studies: a meta-analysis of phase II and III clinical trials of tofacitinib in RA patients published in 2016 showed that patients who were naïve to biologics had a numerically better clinical response compared to patients with a prior inadequate response to biologics [60]. This finding was confirmed by a direct comparison study [61] In the 2015, ACR guidelines for the treatment of RA tofacitinib were still recommended as a second-line drug after treatment with biologic agents resulted in an inadequate response or intolerance [62]. In the EULAR guidelines, tofacitinib is already recommended for RA that has inadequately responded to one or more csDMARDs [63].

This is reflected in the patient cohort of the present analysis, in which only 15.2% of patients were biologic-naïve. However, this and other studies suggest that there is a benefit to be gained from using tofacitinib early in the treatment of RA, before the initiation of biologics, which may call into question the position of tofacitinib as a second-line drug.

4.2. Adverse Events

Few AEs leading to the discontinuation of tofacitinib treatment were observed in this study. Among the AEs that lead to stopping tofacitinib, the most frequent were gastrointestinal AEs, followed by infections. Patients experienced no severe or life-threatening AEs under tofacitinib. The safety profile was comparable to published data, except for a single case of blue finger syndrome [64]. Following initiation, patients developed an increase in LDL cholesterol, which has been established as a side effect of tofacitinib treatment in previous studies [65,66]; however, a tofacitinib-induced increase in cholesterol does not appear to be associated with a higher incidence of cardiovascular AEs in patients [60,65,67].

It is interesting that AEs are the main reason for stopping tofacitinib in the period directly following initiation of treatment, later superseded by insufficient therapeutic responses. Treatment had to be stopped for AEs, if necessary, usually rather early in the course of treatment, considering that the average time of follow up was 1.22 years and the mean time to stop tofacitinib was 183 days. Most patients (23%) discontinued treatment for AEs as early as within the first month (Figure 3). We found no increase in AEs with longer disease duration. Non-tolerability of the drug seems to become apparent rather early after initiation of treatment.

The rate of 24.3% of patients stopping tofacitinib for adverse events in our study is comparable to the rate of 25% published in the 9.5 year long-term extension study published by Wollenhaupt et al. [52].

4.3. Limitations

A significant limitation of this study is that it deals with real-life data. Follow-ups in real-life practice are not as frequent or consistent as in clinical studies. The size of the patient cohort was also limited, and there was a considerable size difference between the sub-cohorts of patients naïve to biologics and patients with prior exposure. However, the design as a retrospective, whole population real-life analysis also constitutes a strength of this study, as its results reflect the variability of patient populations in medical practice more than data on selected patients in controlled clinical trials.

5. Conclusions

The efficacy and safety of tofacitinib have been established in clinical trials. This retrospective analysis of real-life data shows that tofacitinib is also effective and safe in a real-life setting. Over 50% of the patient cohort achieved LDA or remission on a dose of tofacitinib 5 mg bid, with a higher rate of patients naïve to biologic agents achieving either LDA or remission. The safety profile of tofacitinib was generally consistent with previous studies. In conclusion, our results support the use of tofacitinib in the treatment of RA to achieve a more successful clinical outcome.

Author Contributions: Conceptualization, R.B.M., P.H. and J.v.K.; Data curation, R.B.M. and A.S.; Formal analysis, R.B.M., C.H. and M.D.; Investigation, R.B.M., C.H., F.P., F.M., M.D., A.S., P.H., A.R.-R., H.S.-K. and J.v.K.; Methodology, R.B.M.; Project administration, R.B.M.; Resources, R.B.M.; Software, M.D.; Supervision, R.B.M.; Validation, R.B.M.; Writing—original draft, R.B.M., C.H. and P.H.; Writing—review & editing, R.B.M.

Abbreviations

ACPA	anti-citrullinated protein antibody
ACR	American College of Rheumatology
AE	adverse event
AGREE	Abatacept study to gauge remission and joint damage progression in methotrexate-naïve patients with early erosive rheumatoid arthritis
CAMERA	Computer Assisted Management in Early Rheumatoid Arthritis
COMET	Comparison of methotrexate monotherapy with a combination of methotrexate and etanercept in active, early, moderate to severe rheumatoid arthritis
CRP	C-reactive protein
Cs	Conventional synthetic
DAS	Disease Activity Score
DMARD	disease-modifying antirheumatic drug
ESR	erythrocyte sedimentation rate
EULAR	European League Against Rheumatism
GI	gastrointestinal
LDA	low disease activity
MTX	methotrexate
PREMIER	A multicenter, randomized, double-blind clinical trial of combination therapy with adalimumab plus methotrexate versus methotrexate alone or adalimumab alone in patients with early, aggressive rheumatoid arthritis who had not had previous methotrexate treatment
RA	rheumatoid arthritis
RF	rheumatoid factor
SC	subcutaneous
SWEFOT	Swedish Farmacotherapy Trial
TEAR	Treatment of Early Aggressive Rheumatoid Arthritis
TEMPO	Trial of Etanercept and Methotrexate with Radiographic Patient Outcomes

References

1. Heinimann, K.; Von Kempis, J.; Sauter, R.; Schiff, M.; Sokka-Isler, T.; Schulze-Koops, H.; Müller, R. Long-Term Increase of Radiographic Damage and Disability in Patients with RA in Relation to Disease Duration in the Era of Biologics. Results from the SCQM Cohort. *J. Clin. Med.* **2018**, *7*, 57. [CrossRef] [PubMed]
2. Drossaers-Bakker, K.W.; Zwinderman, A.H.; Vlieland, T.P.M.V.; Van Zeben, D.; Vos, K.; Breedveld, F.C.; Hazes, J.M.W.; Drossaers-Bakker, K.W. Long-term outcome in rheumatoid arthritis: A simple algorithm of baseline parameters can predict radiographic damage, disability, and disease course at 12-year followup. *Arthritis Rheum.* **2002**, *47*, 383–390. [CrossRef] [PubMed]
3. Eberhardt, K.B.; Fex, E. Functional impairment and disability in early rheumatoid arthritis-development over 5 years. *J. Rheumatol.* **1995**, *22*, 1037–1042. [PubMed]
4. Furst, D.E.; Keystone, E.C.; Braun, J.; Breedveld, F.C.; Burmester, G.R.; De Benedetti, F.; Dörner, T.; Emery, P.; Fleischmann, R.; Gibofsky, A.; et al. Updated consensus statement on biological agents for the treatment of rheumatic diseases, 2012. *Ann. Rheum. Dis.* **2013**, *72* (Suppl. 2), ii2–ii34. [CrossRef] [PubMed]
5. Drosos, A.A.; Pelechas, E.; Voulgari, P.V. Rheumatoid Arthritis Treatment. A Back to the Drawing Board Project or High Expectations for Low Unmet Needs? *J. Clin. Med.* **2019**, *8*, 1237. [CrossRef] [PubMed]
6. Upchurch, K.S.; Kay, J. Evolution of treatment for rheumatoid arthritis. *Rheumatology* **2012**, *51* (Suppl. 6), vi28–vi36. [CrossRef] [PubMed]
7. Lipsky, P.E.; Van Der Heijde, D.M.; Clair, E.W.S.; Furst, D.E.; Breedveld, F.C.; Kalden, J.R.; Smolen, J.S.; Weisman, M.; Emery, P.; Feldmann, M.; et al. Infliximab and methotrexate in the treatment of rheumatoid arthritis. Anti-Tumor Necrosis Factor Trial in Rheumatoid Arthritis with Concomitant Therapy Study Group. *N. Engl. J. Med.* **2000**, *343*, 1594–1602. [CrossRef]

8. Breedveld, F.C.; Weisman, M.H.; Kavanaugh, A.F.; Cohen, S.B.; Pavelka, K.; van Vollenhoven, R.; Sharp, J.; Perez, J.L.; Spencer-Green, G.T. The PREMIER study: A multicenter, randomized, double-blind clinical trial of combination therapy with adalimumab plus methotrexate versus methotrexate alone or adalimumab alone in patients with early, aggressive rheumatoid arthritis who had not had previous methotrexate treatment. *Arthritis Rheum.* **2006**, *54*, 26–37.
9. Moreland, L.W.; Schiff, M.H.; Baumgartner, S.W.; Tindall, E.A.; Fleischmann, R.M.; Bulpitt, K.J.; Weaver, A.L.; Keystone, E.C.; Furst, D.E.; Mease, P.J.; et al. Etanercept therapy in rheumatoid arthritis. A randomized, controlled trial. *Ann. Intern. Med.* **1999**, *130*, 478–486. [CrossRef]
10. Clair, E.W.S.; Smolen, J.S.; Maini, R.N.; Bathon, J.M.; Emery, P.; Keystone, E.; Schiff, M.; Kalden, J.R.; Wang, B.; DeWoody, K.; et al. Combination of infliximab and methotrexate therapy for early rheumatoid arthritis: A randomized, controlled trial. *Arthritis Rheum.* **2004**, *50*, 3432–3443. [CrossRef]
11. Weinblatt, M.E.; Keystone, E.C.; Furst, D.E.; Moreland, L.W.; Weisman, M.H.; Birbara, C.A.; Teoh, L.A.; Fischkoff, S.A.; Chartash, E.K. Adalimumab, a fully human anti-tumor necrosis factor alpha monoclonal antibody, for the treatment of rheumatoid arthritis in patients taking concomitant methotrexate: The ARMADA trial. *Arthritis Rheum.* **2003**, *48*, 35–45. [CrossRef] [PubMed]
12. Maini, R.; Clair, E.W.S.; Breedveld, F.; Furst, D.; Kalden, J.; Weisman, M.; Smolen, J.; Emery, P.; Harriman, G.; Feldmann, M.; et al. Infliximab (chimeric anti-tumour necrosis factor alpha monoclonal antibody) versus placebo in rheumatoid arthritis patients receiving concomitant methotrexate: A randomised phase III trial. *Lancet* **1999**, *354*, 1932–1939. [CrossRef]
13. Burmester, G.R.; Mariette, X.; Montecucco, C.; Monteagudo-Saez, I.; Malaise, M.; Tzioufas, A.G.; Bijlsma, J.W.; Unnebrink, K.; Kary, S.; Kupper, H. Adalimumab alone and in combination with disease-modifying antirheumatic drugs for the treatment of rheumatoid arthritis in clinical practice: The Research in Active Rheumatoid Arthritis (ReAct) trial. *Ann. Rheum. Dis.* **2007**, *66*, 732–739. [CrossRef] [PubMed]
14. Klareskog, L.; Van Der Heijde, D.; De Jager, J.P.; Gough, A.; Kalden, J.; Malaise, M.; Mola, E.M.; Pavelka, K.; Sany, J.; Settas, L.; et al. Therapeutic effect of the combination of etanercept and methotrexate compared with each treatment alone in patients with rheumatoid arthritis: Double-blind randomised controlled trial. *Lancet* **2004**, *363*, 675–681.
15. Keystone, E.C.; Kavanaugh, A.F.; Sharp, J.T.; Tannenbaum, H.; Hua, Y.; Teoh, L.S.; Fischkoff, S.A.; Chartash, E.K. Radiographic, clinical, and functional outcomes of treatment with adalimumab (a human anti-tumor necrosis factor monoclonal antibody) in patients with active rheumatoid arthritis receiving concomitant methotrexate therapy: A randomized, placebo-controlled, 52-week trial. *Arthritis Rheum.* **2004**, *50*, 1400–1411. [PubMed]
16. Smolen, J.S.; Kay, J.; Doyle, M.K.; Landewe, R.; Matteson, E.L.; Wollenhaupt, J.; Gaylis, N.; Murphy, F.T.; Neal, J.S.; Zhou, Y.; et al. Golimumab in patients with active rheumatoid arthritis after treatment with tumour necrosis factor alpha inhibitors (GO-AFTER study): A multicentre, randomised, double-blind, placebo-controlled, phase III trial. *Lancet* **2009**, *374*, 210–221. [CrossRef]
17. Fleischmann, R.; Vencovsky, J.; van Vollenhoven, R.F.; Borenstein, D.; Box, J.; Coteur, G.; Goel, N.; Brezinschek, H.P.; Innes, A.; Strand, V. Efficacy and safety of certolizumab pegol monotherapy every 4 weeks in patients with rheumatoid arthritis failing previous disease-modifying antirheumatic therapy: The FAST4WARD study. *Ann. Rheum. Dis.* **2009**, *68*, 805–811. [CrossRef] [PubMed]
18. Smolen, J.; Landewe, R.B.; Mease, P.; Brzezicki, J.; Mason, D.; Luijtens, K.; van Vollenhoven, R.F.; Kavanaugh, A.; Schiff, M.; Burmester, G.R.; et al. Efficacy and safety of certolizumab pegol plus methotrexate in active rheumatoid arthritis: The RAPID 2 study. A randomised controlled trial. *Ann. Rheum. Dis.* **2009**, *68*, 797–804. [CrossRef] [PubMed]
19. Emery, P.; Deodhar, A.; Rigby, W.F.; Isaacs, J.D.; Combe, B.; Racewicz, A.J.; Latinis, K.; Abud-Mendoza, C.; Szczepański, L.J.; Roschmann, R.A.; et al. Efficacy and safety of different doses and retreatment of rituximab: A randomised, placebo-controlled trial in patients who are biological naive with active rheumatoid arthritis and an inadequate response to methotrexate (Study Evaluating Rituximab's Efficacy in MTX iNadequate rEsponders (SERENE)). *Ann. Rheum. Dis.* **2010**, *69*, 1629–1635. [PubMed]
20. Keystone, E.C.; Genovese, M.C.; Klareskog, L.; Hsia, E.C.; Hall, S.T.; Miranda, P.C.; Pazdur, J.; Bae, S.C.; Palmer, W.; Zrubek, J.; et al. Golimumab, a human antibody to tumour necrosis factor {alpha} given by monthly subcutaneous injections, in active rheumatoid arthritis despite methotrexate therapy: The GO-FORWARD Study. *Ann. Rheum. Dis.* **2009**, *68*, 789–796. [PubMed]

21. Schiff, M.; Keiserman, M.; Codding, C.; Songcharoen, S.; Berman, A.; Nayiager, S.; Saldate, C.; Li, T.; Aranda, R.; Becker, J.C.; et al. Efficacy and safety of abatacept or infliximab vs placebo in ATTEST: A phase III, multi-centre, randomised, double-blind, placebo-controlled study in patients with rheumatoid arthritis and an inadequate response to methotrexate. *Ann. Rheum. Dis.* **2008**, *67*, 1096–1103. [CrossRef] [PubMed]
22. Jones, G.; Sebba, A.; Gu, J.; Lowenstein, M.B.; Calvo, A.; Gomez-Reino, J.J.; Siri, D.A.; Tomšič, M.; Alecock, E.; Woodworth, T.; et al. Comparison of tocilizumab monotherapy versus methotrexate monotherapy in patients with moderate to severe rheumatoid arthritis: The AMBITION study. *Ann. Rheum. Dis.* **2010**, *69*, 88–96. [CrossRef] [PubMed]
23. Bykerk, V.P.; Ostor, A.J.K.; Alvaro-Gracia, J.; Pavelka, K.; Ivorra, J.A.R.; Graninger, W.; Bensen, W.; Nurmohamed, M.T.; Krause, A.; Bernasconi, C.; et al. Comparison of tocilizumab as monotherapy or with add-on disease-modifying antirheumatic drugs in patients with rheumatoid arthritis and inadequate responses to previous treatments: An open-label study close to clinical practice. *Clin. Rheumatol.* **2015**, *34*, 563–571. [CrossRef] [PubMed]
24. Nam, J.L.; Ramiro, S.; Gaujoux-Viala, C.; Takase, K.; Leon-Garcia, M.; Emery, P.; Gossec, L.; Landewe, R.; Smolen, J.S.; Buch, M.H. Efficacy of biological disease-modifying antirheumatic drugs: A systematic literature review informing the 2013 update of the EULAR recommendations for the management of rheumatoid arthritis. *Ann. Rheum. Dis.* **2014**, *73*, 516–528. [PubMed]
25. Finckh, A.; Simard, J.F.; Duryea, J.; Liang, M.H.; Huang, J.; Daneel, S.; Forster, A.; Gabay, C.; Guerne, P.A. The effectiveness of anti-tumor necrosis factor therapy in preventing progressive radiographic joint damage in rheumatoid arthritis: A population-based study. *Arthritis Rheum.* **2006**, *54*, 54–59. [CrossRef] [PubMed]
26. Kaltsonoudis, E.; Pelechas, E.; Voulgari, P.V.; Drosos, A.A. Unmet needs in the treatment of rheumatoid arthritis. An observational study and a real-life experience from a single university center. *Semin. Arthritis Rheum.* **2019**, *48*, 597–602. [PubMed]
27. Ghoreschi, K.; Laurence, A.; O'Shea, J.J. Janus kinases in immune cell signaling. *Immunol. Rev.* **2009**, *228*, 273–287. [CrossRef]
28. Meyer, D.M.; Jesson, M.I.; Li, X.; Elrick, M.M.; Funckes-Shippy, C.L.; Warner, J.D.; Gross, C.J.; E Dowty, M.; Ramaiah, S.K.; Hirsch, J.L.; et al. Anti-inflammatory activity and neutrophil reductions mediated by the JAK1/JAK3 inhibitor, CP-690,550, in rat adjuvant-induced arthritis. *J. Inflamm.* **2010**, *7*, 41.
29. Ortmann, R.A.; Cheng, T.; Visconti, R.; Frucht, D.M.; O'Shea, J.J. Janus kinases and signal transducers and activators of transcription: Their roles in cytokine signaling, development and immunoregulation. *Arthritis Res.* **2000**, *2*, 16–32.
30. Ghoreschi, K.; Jesson, M.I.; Li, X.; Lee, J.L.; Ghosh, S.; Alsup, J.W.; Warner, J.D.; Tanaka, M.; Steward-Tharp, S.M.; Gadina, M.; et al. Modulation of innate and adaptive immune responses by tofacitinib (CP-690,550). *J. Immunol.* **2011**, *186*, 4234–4243.
31. O'Shea, J.J.; Laurence, A.; McInnes, I.B. Back to the future: Oral targeted therapy for RA and other autoimmune diseases. *Nat. Rev. Rheumatol.* **2013**, *9*, 173–182. [CrossRef] [PubMed]
32. Maeshima, K.; Yamaoka, K.; Kubo, S.; Nakano, K.; Iwata, S.; Saito, K.; Ohishi, M.; Miyahara, H.; Tanaka, S.; Ishii, K.; et al. The JAK inhibitor tofacitinib regulates synovitis through inhibition of interferon-gamma and interleukin-17 production by human $CD4^+$ T cells. *Arthritis Rheum.* **2012**, *64*, 1790–1798. [CrossRef] [PubMed]
33. Coombs, J.H.; Bloom, B.J.; Breedveld, F.C.; Fletcher, M.P.; Gruben, D.; Kremer, J.M.; Burgos-Vargas, R.; Wilkinson, B.; Zerbini, C.A.; Zwillich, S.H. Improved pain, physical functioning and health status in patients with rheumatoid arthritis treated with CP-690,550, an orally active Janus kinase (JAK) inhibitor: Results from a randomised, double-blind, placebo-controlled trial. *Ann. Rheum. Dis.* **2010**, *69*, 413–416. [CrossRef] [PubMed]
34. Burmester, G.R.; Blanco, R.; Charles-Schoeman, C.; Wollenhaupt, J.; Zerbini, C.; Benda, B.; Gruben, D.; Wallenstein, G.; Krishnaswami, S.; Zwillich, S.H.; et al. Tofacitinib (CP-690,550) in combination with methotrexate in patients with active rheumatoid arthritis with an inadequate response to tumour necrosis factor inhibitors: A randomised phase 3 trial. *Lancet* **2013**, *381*, 451–460. [CrossRef]
35. Fleischmann, R.; Kremer, J.; Cush, J.; Schulze-Koops, H.; Connell, C.A.; Bradley, J.D.; Gruben, D.; Wallenstein, G.V.; Zwillich, S.H.; Kanik, K.S. Placebo-controlled trial of tofacitinib monotherapy in rheumatoid arthritis. *N. Engl. J. Med.* **2012**, *367*, 495–507. [CrossRef] [PubMed]

36. Kremer, J.; Li, Z.-G.; Hall, S.; Fleischmann, R.; Genovese, M.; Martín-Mola, E.; Isaacs, J.D.; Gruben, D.; Wallenstein, G.; Krishnaswami, S.; et al. Tofacitinib in combination with nonbiologic disease-modifying antirheumatic drugs in patients with active rheumatoid arthritis: A randomized trial. *Ann. Intern. Med.* **2013**, *159*, 253–261. [CrossRef] [PubMed]
37. Wollenhaupt, J.; Silverfield, J.; Lee, E.B.; Curtis, J.R.; Wood, S.P.; Soma, K.; Nduaka, C.I.; Benda, B.; Gruben, D.; Nakamura, H.; et al. Safety and efficacy of tofacitinib, an oral janus kinase inhibitor, for the treatment of rheumatoid arthritis in open-label, longterm extension studies. *J. Rheumatol.* **2014**, *41*, 837–852. [CrossRef] [PubMed]
38. Kremer, J.M.; Cohen, S.; Wilkinson, B.E.; Connell, C.A.; French, J.L.; Gómez-Reino, J.; Gruben, D.; Kanik, K.S.; Krishnaswami, S.; Pascual-Ramos, V.; et al. A phase IIb dose-ranging study of the oral JAK inhibitor tofacitinib (CP-690,550) versus placebo in combination with background methotrexate in patients with active rheumatoid arthritis and an inadequate response to methotrexate alone. *Arthritis Rheum.* **2012**, *64*, 970–981. [CrossRef]
39. Tanaka, Y.; Suzuki, M.; Nakamura, H.; Toyoizumi, S.; Zwillich, S.H. Tofacitinib Study I. Phase II study of tofacitinib (CP-690,550) combined with methotrexate in patients with rheumatoid arthritis and an inadequate response to methotrexate. *Arthritis Care Res.* **2011**, *63*, 1150–1158. [CrossRef]
40. Wagner, S.; Forejtova, S.; Zwillich, S.H.; Gruben, D.; Koncz, T.; Wallenstein, G.V.; Krishnaswami, S.; Bradley, J.D.; Van Vollenhoven, R.F.; Fleischmann, R.; et al. Tofacitinib or adalimumab versus placebo in rheumatoid arthritis. *N. Engl. J. Med.* **2012**, *367*, 508–519.
41. Vieira, M.C.; Zwillich, S.H.; Jansen, J.P.; Smiechowski, B.; Spurden, D.; Wallenstein, G.V. Tofacitinib Versus Biologic Treatments in Patients With Active Rheumatoid Arthritis Who Have Had an Inadequate Response to Tumor Necrosis Factor Inhibitors: Results From a Network Meta-analysis. *Clin. Ther.* **2016**, *38*, 2628–2641.e5. [CrossRef] [PubMed]
42. Bergrath, E.; Gerber, R.A.; Gruben, D.; Lukic, T.; Makin, C.; Wallenstein, G. Tofacitinib versus Biologic Treatments in Moderate-to-Severe Rheumatoid Arthritis Patients Who Have Had an Inadequate Response to Nonbiologic DMARDs: Systematic Literature Review and Network Meta-Analysis. *Int. J. Rheumatol.* **2017**, *2017*, 8417249. [CrossRef] [PubMed]
43. Fleischmann, R.; Mysler, E.; Luo, Z.; Demasi, R.; Soma, K.; Zhang, R.; Takiya, L.; Tatulych, S.; Mojcik, C.; Krishnaswami, S.; et al. Efficacy and safety of tofacitinib monotherapy, tofacitinib with methotrexate, and adalimumab with methotrexate in patients with rheumatoid arthritis (ORAL Strategy): A phase 3b/4, double-blind, head-to-head, randomised controlled trial. *Lancet* **2017**, *390*, 457–468. [CrossRef]
44. Fleischmann, R.; Cutolo, M.; Genovese, M.C.; Lee, E.B.; Kanik, K.S.; Sadis, S.; Connell, C.A.; Gruben, D.; Krishnaswami, S.; Wallenstein, G.; et al. Phase IIb dose-ranging study of the oral JAK inhibitor tofacitinib (CP-690,550) or adalimumab monotherapy versus placebo in patients with active rheumatoid arthritis with an inadequate response to disease-modifying antirheumatic drugs. *Arthritis Rheum.* **2012**, *64*, 617–629. [CrossRef] [PubMed]
45. Aletaha, D.; Neogi, T.; Silman, A.J.; Funovits, J.; Felson, D.T.; Bingham, C.O.; Birnbaum, N.S.; Burmester, G.R.; Bykerk, V.P.; Cohen, M.D.; et al. 2010 rheumatoid arthritis classification criteria: An American College of Rheumatology/European League Against Rheumatism collaborative initiative. *Ann. Rheum. Dis.* **2010**, *69*, 1580–1588. [CrossRef] [PubMed]
46. Iwamoto, N.; Tsuji, S.; Takatani, A.; Shimizu, T.; Fukui, S.; Umeda, M.; Nishino, A.; Horai, Y.; Koga, T.; Kawashiri, S.-Y.; et al. Efficacy and safety at 24 weeks of daily clinical use of tofacitinib in patients with rheumatoid arthritis. *PLoS ONE.* **2017**, *12*, e0177057. [CrossRef] [PubMed]
47. Wilkinson, B.; Krishnaswami, S.; Van Vollenhoven, R.F.; Sexton, D.; Yuan, K.; Chen, J.; Xu, A. Tofacitinib versus methotrexate in rheumatoid arthritis. *N. Engl. J. Med.* **2014**, *370*, 2377–2386.
48. Van Der Heijde, D.; Tanaka, Y.; Fleischmann, R.; Keystone, E.; Kremer, J.; Zerbini, C.; Cardiel, M.H.; Cohen, S.; Nash, P.; Song, Y.-W.; et al. Tofacitinib (CP-690,550) in patients with rheumatoid arthritis receiving methotrexate: Twelve-month data from a twenty-four-month phase III randomized radiographic study. *Arthritis Rheum.* **2013**, *65*, 559–570. [CrossRef]
49. Smolen, J.S.; Aletaha, D.; Gruben, D.; Zwillich, S.H.; Krishnaswami, S.; Mebus, C. Brief Report: Remission Rates With Tofacitinib Treatment in Rheumatoid Arthritis: A Comparison of Various Remission Criteria. *Arthritis Rheumatol.* **2017**, *69*, 728–734. [CrossRef]

50. Kremer, J.M.; Bloom, B.J.; Breedveld, F.C.; Coombs, J.H.; Fletcher, M.P.; Gruben, D.; Krishnaswami, S.; Burgos-Vargas, R.; Wilkinson, B.; Zerbini, C.A.F.; et al. The safety and efficacy of a JAK inhibitor in patients with active rheumatoid arthritis: Results of a double-blind, placebo-controlled phase IIa trial of three dosage levels of CP-690,550 versus placebo. *Arthritis Rheum.* **2009**, *60*, 1895–1905. [CrossRef]
51. Charles-Schoeman, C.; Burmester, G.; Nash, P.; Zerbini, C.A.; Soma, K.; Kwok, K.; Hendrikx, T.; Bananis, E.; Fleischmann, R. Efficacy and safety of tofacitinib following inadequate response to conventional synthetic or biological disease-modifying antirheumatic drugs. *Ann. Rheum. Dis.* **2016**, *75*, 1293–1301. [CrossRef] [PubMed]
52. Wollenhaupt, J.; Lee, E.-B.; Curtis, J.R.; Silverfield, J.; Terry, K.; Soma, K.; Mojcik, C.; Demasi, R.; Strengholt, S.; Kwok, K.; et al. Safety and efficacy of tofacitinib for up to 9.5 years in the treatment of rheumatoid arthritis: Final results of a global, open-label, long-term extension study. *Arthritis Res. Ther.* **2019**, *21*, 89. [CrossRef] [PubMed]
53. Anderson, D.R.; Patil, S.; Kamina, A.; Penson, D.F.; Peduzzi, P.; Concato, J. Validation of a staging system for evaluating prognosis in prostate cancer. *Connect. Med.* **2000**, *64*, 459–464.
54. Harrold, L.R.; Litman, H.J.; Connolly, S.E.; Kelly, S.; Hua, W.; Alemao, E.; Rosenblatt, L.; Rebello, S.; Kremer, J.M. A window of opportunity for abatacept in RA: is disease duration an independent predictor of low disease activity/remission in clinical practice? *Clin. Rheumatol.* **2017**, *36*, 1215–1220. [CrossRef] [PubMed]
55. Furst, D.E.; Pangan, A.L.; Harrold, L.R.; Chang, H.; Reed, G.; Kremer, J.M.; Greenberg, J.D. Greater likelihood of remission in rheumatoid arthritis patients treated earlier in the disease course: Results from the Consortium of Rheumatology Researchers of North America registry. *Arthritis Care Res.* **2011**, *63*, 856–864. [CrossRef]
56. Vastesaeger, N.; Kutzbach, A.G.; Amital, H.; Pavelka, K.; Lazaro, M.A.; Moots, R.J.; Wollenhaupt, J.; Zerbini, C.A.F.; Louw, I.; Combe, B.; et al. Prediction of remission and low disease activity in disease-modifying anti-rheumatic drug-refractory patients with rheumatoid arthritis treated with golimumab. *Rheumatology* **2016**, *55*, 1466–1476. [CrossRef]
57. Aletaha, D.; Funovits, J.; Keystone, E.C.; Smolen, J.S. Disease activity early in the course of treatment predicts response to therapy after one year in rheumatoid arthritis patients. *Arthritis Rheum.* **2007**, *56*, 3226–3235. [CrossRef]
58. Smolen, J.S.; Szumski, A.; Koenig, A.S.; Jones, T.V.; Marshall, L. Predictors of remission with etanercept-methotrexate induction therapy and loss of remission with etanercept maintenance, reduction, or withdrawal in moderately active rheumatoid arthritis: Results of the PRESERVE trial. *Arthritis Res. Ther.* **2018**, *20*, 8. [CrossRef]
59. Kavanaugh, A.; Keystone, E.; Greenberg, J.D.; Reed, G.W.; Griffith, J.M.; Friedman, A.W.; Saunders, K.C.; Ganguli, A. Benefit of biologics initiation in moderate versus severe rheumatoid arthritis: Evidence from a United States registry. *Rheumatology* **2017**, *56*, 1095–1101. [CrossRef]
60. Charles-Schoeman, C.; Gonzalez-Gay, M.A.; Kaplan, I.; Boy, M.; Geier, J.; Luo, Z.; Zuckerman, A.; Riese, R. Effects of tofacitinib and other DMARDs on lipid profiles in rheumatoid arthritis: Implications for the rheumatologist. *Semin Arthritis Rheum.* **2016**, *46*, 71–80. [CrossRef]
61. Mori, S.; Yoshitama, T.; Ueki, Y. Tofacitinib Therapy for Rheumatoid Arthritis: A Direct Comparison Study between Biologic-naive and Experienced Patients. *Intern. Med.* **2018**, *57*, 663–670. [CrossRef] [PubMed]
62. Singh, J.A.; Saag, K.G.; Bridges, S.L.; Akl, E.A.; Bannuru, R.R.; Sullivan, M.C.; Vaysbrot, E.; McNaughton, C.; Osani, M.; Shmerling, R.H.; et al. 2015 American College of Rheumatology Guideline for the Treatment of Rheumatoid Arthritis. *Arthritis Rheumatol.* **2016**, *68*, 1–26. [CrossRef] [PubMed]
63. Smolen, J.S.; Breedveld, F.C.; Burmester, G.R.; Bykerk, V.; Dougados, M.; Emery, P.; Kvien, T.K.; Navarro-Compán, M.V.; Oliver, S.; Schoels, M.; et al. Treating rheumatoid arthritis to target: 2014 update of the recommendations of an international task force. *Ann. Rheum. Dis.* **2016**, *75*, 3–15. [CrossRef] [PubMed]
64. Popp, F.; Semela, D.; von Kempis, J.; Mueller, R.B. Improvement of primary biliary cholangitis (PBC) under treatment with sulfasalazine and abatacept. *BMJ Case Rep.* **2018**. [CrossRef] [PubMed]
65. Wu, J.J.; Strober, B.E.; Hansen, P.R.; Ahlehoff, O.; Egeberg, A.; Qureshi, A.A.; Robertson, D.; Valdez, H.; Tan, H.; Wolk, R. Effects of tofacitinib on cardiovascular risk factors and cardiovascular outcomes based on phase III and long-term extension data in patients with plaque psoriasis. *J. Am. Acad. Dermatol.* **2016**, *75*, 897–905. [CrossRef]

66. Wolk, R.; Armstrong, E.J.; Hansen, P.R.; Thiers, B.; Lan, S.; Tallman, A.M.; Kaur, M.; Tatulych, S. Effect of tofacitinib on lipid levels and lipid-related parameters in patients with moderate to severe psoriasis. *J. Clin. Lipidol.* **2017**, *11*, 1243–1256. [CrossRef] [PubMed]
67. Charles-Schoeman, C.; Wicker, P.; Gonzalez-Gay, M.A.; Boy, M.; Zuckerman, A.; Soma, K.; Geier, J.; Kwok, K.; Riese, R. Cardiovascular safety findings in patients with rheumatoid arthritis treated with tofacitinib, an oral Janus kinase inhibitor. *Semin. Arthritis Rheum.* **2016**, *46*, 261–271. [CrossRef] [PubMed]

Permissions

All chapters in this book were first published by MDPI; hereby published with permission under the Creative Commons Attribution License or equivalent. Every chapter published in this book has been scrutinized by our experts. Their significance has been extensively debated. The topics covered herein carry significant findings which will fuel the growth of the discipline. They may even be implemented as practical applications or may be referred to as a beginning point for another development.

The contributors of this book come from diverse backgrounds, making this book a truly international effort. This book will bring forth new frontiers with its revolutionizing research information and detailed analysis of the nascent developments around the world.

We would like to thank all the contributing authors for lending their expertise to make the book truly unique. They have played a crucial role in the development of this book. Without their invaluable contributions this book wouldn't have been possible. They have made vital efforts to compile up to date information on the varied aspects of this subject to make this book a valuable addition to the collection of many professionals and students.

This book was conceptualized with the vision of imparting up-to-date information and advanced data in this field. To ensure the same, a matchless editorial board was set up. Every individual on the board went through rigorous rounds of assessment to prove their worth. After which they invested a large part of their time researching and compiling the most relevant data for our readers.

The editorial board has been involved in producing this book since its inception. They have spent rigorous hours researching and exploring the diverse topics which have resulted in the successful publishing of this book. They have passed on their knowledge of decades through this book. To expedite this challenging task, the publisher supported the team at every step. A small team of assistant editors was also appointed to further simplify the editing procedure and attain best results for the readers.

Apart from the editorial board, the designing team has also invested a significant amount of their time in understanding the subject and creating the most relevant covers. They scrutinized every image to scout for the most suitable representation of the subject and create an appropriate cover for the book.

The publishing team has been an ardent support to the editorial, designing and production team. Their endless efforts to recruit the best for this project, has resulted in the accomplishment of this book. They are a veteran in the field of academics and their pool of knowledge is as vast as their experience in printing. Their expertise and guidance has proved useful at every step. Their uncompromising quality standards have made this book an exceptional effort. Their encouragement from time to time has been an inspiration for everyone.

The publisher and the editorial board hope that this book will prove to be a valuable piece of knowledge for researchers, students, practitioners and scholars across the globe.

List of Contributors

Patrice Fardellone, Vincent Goëb and Laure Le Monnier
Department of Rheumatology, Picardie-Jules Verne University, University hospital of Amiens, 80054 Amiens, France
Department of Rheumatology, Amiens University Hospital, 80000 Amiens, France

Emad Salawati
Assistant Professor, Faculty of Medicine, King Abdulaziz University, 21589 Jeddah, Saudi Arabia

Valentine Deprez, Jean-Marc Sobhy-Danial, Franck Grados, Isabelle Henry-Desailly, Sarah Salomon-Goëb, Thibault Rabin and Sanja Ristic
Department of Rheumatology, Amiens University Hospital, 80000 Amiens, France

Mathurin Fumery
Department of Gastroenterology, Amiens University Hospital, 80000 Amiens, France

Yoon-Jeong Oh and Ki Won Moon
Division of Rheumatology, Department of Internal Medicine, Kangwon National University School of Medicine, Chuncheon 24289, Korea

Igor Grabovac, Sandra Haider and Thomas E. Dorner
Department of Social and Preventive Medicine, Centre for Public Health, Medical University of Vienna, Kinderspitalgasse 15, 1090 Vienna, Austria

Carolin Berner
Department of Rheumatology and Osteology, Kaiser Franz Josef Hospital, Sozialmedizinisches Zentrum Süd, Kundratstrasse 3, 1100 Vienna, Austria

Thomas Lamprecht and Karl-Heinrich Fenzl
Karl Landsteiner Institute for Autoimmune Diseases and Rheumatology, Kundratstrasse 3, 1100 Vienna, Austria

Ludwig Erlacher
Department of Rheumatology and Osteology, Kaiser Franz Josef Hospital, Sozialmedizinisches Zentrum Süd, Kundratstrasse 3, 1100 Vienna, Austria
Karl Landsteiner Institute for Autoimmune Diseases and Rheumatology, Kundratstrasse 3, 1100 Vienna, Austria

Michael Quittan
Karl Landsteiner Institute for Remobilisation and Functional Health, Kundratstrasse 3, 1100 Vienna, Austria
Department of Physical Medicine and Rehabilitation, Kaiser-Franz-Josef-Hospital, Sozialmedizinisches Zentrum Süd, Kundratstrasse 3, 1100 Vienna, Austria

Marialbert Acosta-Herrera, David González-Serna and Javier Martín
Institute of Parasitology and Biomedicine López-Neyra, CSIC, Av. del Conocimiento 17. Armilla, 18016 Granada, Spain

Lena Hirtler and Claus Rath
Division of Anatomy, Center for Anatomy and Cell Biology, Medical University of Vienna, Vienna 1090, Austria

Hannes Platzgummer and Franz Kainberger
Department of Biomedical Imaging and Image-Guided Therapy, Medical University of Vienna, Vienna 1090, Austria

Daniel Aletaha
Division of Rheumatology, Department of Internal Medicine, Medical University of Vienna, Vienna 1090, Austria

Hae-Rim Kim, Hong-Ki Min and Sang-Heon Lee
Division of Rheumatology, Department of Internal Medicine, Research Institute of Medical Science, School of Medicine, Konkuk University, Seoul 05030, Korea

Kyoung-Woon Kim, Bo-Mi Kim and Ji-Yeon Won
Conversant Research Consortium in Immunologic Disease, Seoul St. Mary's Hospital, The Catholic University of Korea, Seoul 06591, Korea

Kyung-Ann Lee
Division of Rheumatology, Department of Internal Medicine, Soonchunhyang University Hospital, Seoul 04401, Korea

Tae-Young Kim
Department of Orthopedic Surgery, School of Medicine, Konkuk University, Seoul 05030, Korea

Mélanie Rinaudo-Gaujous and Stephane Paul
GIMAP EA3064, Laboratory of Immunology and Immunomonitoring, CIC CIE3 Inserm Vaccinology, Hôpital Nord, CHU Saint-Etienne, 42270 Saint-Priest-en-Jarez, France

Vincent Blasco-Baque
Institute of Cardiovascular and Metabolic Diseases, CHU Rangueil, 31400 Toulouse, France

Pierre Miossec
Clinical Immunology Unit, Departments of Immunology and Rheumatology, Hôpital Edouard Herriot, CHU Lyon, 69003 Lyon, France

Philippe Gaudin
Department of Rheumatology, CHU Grenoble, 38130 Échirolles, France

Pierre Farge
Faculty of Odontology, University Lyon I., 69622 Villeurbanne, France

Xavier Roblin
Department of Gastroenterology, Hôpital Nord, CHU Saint-Etienne, 42270 Saint-Priest-en-Jarez, France

Thierry Thomas and Hubert Marotte
Department of Rheumatology, Hôpital Nord, CHU Saint-Etienne, 42055 Saint-Etienne, France
INSERM U1059, Université de Lyon–Université Jean Monnet, 42023 Saint-Etienne, France
SAINBIOSE, INSERM U1059, Université de Lyon, Saint-Etienne, France Service de Rhumatologie, CHU Saint-Etienne, 42055 Saint-Etienne, France

Sang Tae Choi and Ji-Ho Park
Division of Rheumatology, Department of Internal Medicine, Chung-Ang University College of Medicine, Seoul 06973, Korea

Seong-Ryul Kwon
Division of Rheumatology, Department of Internal Medicine, Inha University College of Medicine, Incheon 22332, Korea

Ju-Yang Jung, Hyoun-Ah Kim and Chang-Hee Suh
Department of Rheumatology, Ajou University School of Medicine, Suwon 16499, Korea

Sung-Soo Kim
Division of Rheumatology, Department of Internal Medicine, Ulsan University College of Medicine, Gangneung Asan Hospital, Gangneung 25440, Korea

Sang Hyon Kim and Ji-Min Kim
Division of Rheumatology, Department of Internal Medicine, Keimyung University College of Medicine, Daegu 41931, Korea

Marion Bossennec, Céline Rodriguez, Margaux Hubert, Anthony Di-Roio, Christophe Caux and Christine Ménétrier-Caux
Immunology Department, University of Lyon, Claude Bernard Lyon 1 University, INSERM 1052, CNRS 5286, Cancer Research Center of Lyon (CRCL), Centre Léon Bérard, 69008 Lyon, France
Team "Therapeutic Targeting of the Tumor Cells and Their Immune Stroma", INSERM U1052, CRCL, 69008 Lyon, France

Christelle Machon
Analytical Chemistry Department, ISPB Faculty of Pharmacy, University of Lyon, Claude Bernard Lyon 1 University, 69008 Lyon, France
Biochemistry and Toxicology Laboratory, Lyon Sud Hospital, 69310 Pierre-Bénite, France

Jérôme Guitton
Biochemistry and Toxicology Laboratory, Lyon Sud Hospital, 69310 Pierre-Bénite, France
Toxicology Department, ISPB Faculty of Pharmacy, University of Lyon, Claude Bernard Lyon 1 University, 69008 Lyon, France

Priscilla Battiston-Montagne
Immunology Department, University of Lyon, Claude Bernard Lyon 1 University, INSERM 1052, CNRS 5286, Cancer Research Center of Lyon (CRCL), Centre Léon Bérard, 69008 Lyon, France
Cytometry Platform, CRCL, 69008 Lyon, France

Mathilde Couturier
Rheumatology Department, Lyon Sud Hospital, 69310 Pierre-Bénite, France

Fabienne Coury
Rheumatology Department, Lyon Sud Hospital, 69310 Pierre-Bénite, France
INSERM, UMR 1033, Claude Bernard Lyon 1 University, 69008 Lyon, France

Peter C. Taylor
Botnar Research Centre, University of Oxford, Oxford OX3 7LD, UK

Yvonne C. Lee
Division of Rheumatology, Northwestern University Feinberg School of Medicine, Chicago, IL 60611, USA

Roy Fleischmann
Metroplex Clinical Research Center, University of Texas Southwestern Medical Center, Dallas, TX 75231, USA

Tsutomu Takeuchi
Division of Rheumatology, Department of Internal Medicine, Keio University, Tokyo 162-5882, Japan

Elizabeth L. Perkins
Rheumatology Care Center, Birmingham, AL 35244, USA

Bruno Fautrel
AP-HP, Pitie-Salpetriere Hospital, Dept of Rheumatology, Sorbonne Université, Pierre Louis Institute for Epidemiology and Public Health, 705013 Paris, France
Rheumatology Dept, Institut Pierre Louis d'Epidémiologie et de Santé Publique, Sorbonne Université-Assistance Publique Hôpitaux de Paris, 75013 Paris, France
Department of Rheumatology, Pitié-Salpêtrière Hospital, Assistance Publique-Hôpitaux de Paris, 83 bd de l'hôpital, 75013 Paris, France

Baojin Zhu, Amanda K. Quebe, Carol L. Gaich, Xiang Zhang, Christina L. Dickson, Douglas E. Schlichting, Himanshu Patel, Frederick Durand, Inmaculada de la Torre and Francesco De Leonardis
Eli Lilly and Company, Indianapolis, IN 46285, USA

Paul Emery
Leeds Institute of Rheumatic and Musculoskeletal Medicine University of Leeds, Leeds LS1 3EX, UK

Birgit M. Köhler, Janine Günther, Dorothee Kaudewitz and Hanns-Martin Lorenz
Internal Medicine 5, Division of Rheumatology, University Hospital Heidelberg, 69120 Heidelberg, Germany

Caroline Hasler, Mirsada Durmisi and Paul Hasler
Division of Rheumatology, Medical University Department, Kantonsspital Aarau, 5001 Aarau, Switzerland

Alejandro Balsa Criado
Rheumatology unit, University Hospital La Paz, Institute for Health Research-IdiPAZ, Universidad Autonoma de Madrid, 28046 Madrid, Spain

Anne-Barbara Mongey
St. Vincent's University Hospital, Elm Park, Dublin 4, Ireland

Jerome Avouac
Paris Descartes University, Sorbonne Paris Cité, Rheumatology Department, Cochin Hopital, Assistance Publique-Hôpitaux de Paris, 75014 Paris, France

Rudiger B. Mueller
Division of Rheumatology, Medical University Department, Kantonsspital Aarau, 5001 Aarau, Switzerland

Bruce Kirkham
Department of Rheumatology, Guys and St Thomas' NHS Trust, Great Maze Pond, London SE1 9RT, UK

Janet E. Pope
Department of Medicine, Division of Rheumatology, University of Western Ontario, 1151 Richmond St, London, ON N6A 3K7, Canada

Evripidis Kaltsonoudis, Eleftherios Pelechas, Paraskevi V. Voulgari and Alexandros A. Drosos
Rheumatology Clinic, Department of Internal Medicine, Medical School, University of Ioannina, 45110 Ioannina, Greece

Eleftherios Pelechas, Paraskevi V. Voulgari and Alexandros A. Drosos
Rheumatology Clinic, Department of Internal Medicine, Medical School, University of Ioannina, 45110 Ioannina, Greece

Ruediger B. Mueller
Division of Rheumatology and Immunology, Department of Internal Medicine, Kantonsspital St. Gallen, 9007 St. Gallen, Switzerland
Division of Rheumatology, Medical University Department, Kantonsspital Aarau, 5001 Aarau, Switzerland
Division of Rheumatology and Clinical Immunology, Department of Internal Medicine IV, Ludwig-Maximilians-University Munich, 80336 Munich, Germany

Peter. C. Taylor
Botnar Research Centre, NDORMS, University of Oxford, Windmill Road, Oxford OX3 7LD, UK

Florian Popp, Frederik Mattow, Andrea Rubbert-Roth and Johannes von Kempis
Division of Rheumatology and Immunology, Department of Internal Medicine, Kantonsspital St. Gallen, 9007 St. Gallen, Switzerland

Alexander Souza
Iterata AG, 5722 Gränichen, Switzerland

Hendrik Schulze-Koops
Division of Rheumatology and Clinical Immunology, Department of Internal Medicine IV, Ludwig-Maximilians-University Munich, 80336 Munich, Germany

Index

www.ingramcontent.com/pod-product-compliance
Lightning Source LLC
LaVergne TN
LVHW082201200926
848484LV00008B/2193